Assessment in Health Professions Education

Assessment in Health Professions Education, second edition, provides a comprehensive guide for educators in the health professions—medicine, dentistry, nursing, pharmacy, and allied health fields. This second edition has been extensively revised and updated by leaders in the field. Part I of the book presents an introduction to assessment fundamentals and their theoretical underpinnings from the perspective of the health professions. Part II covers specific assessment methods, with a focus on validity, best practices, challenges, and practical guidelines for the effective implementation of successful assessment programs. Part III addresses special topics and recent innovative approaches, including narrative assessment, situational judgment tests, programmatic assessment, mastery learning settings, and the key features approach. This accessible text addresses the essential concepts for the health professions educator and provides the background needed to understand, interpret, develop, and effectively implement assessment methods.

Rachel Yudkowsky is Professor and Director of Graduate Studies in the Department of Medical Education in the College of Medicine at the University of Illinois at Chicago, USA, and past Director of the UIC Dr. Allan L. and Mary L. Graham Clinical Performance Center.

Yoon Soo Park is Associate Professor and Associate Head of the Department of Medical Education, and Director of Research for Educational Affairs in the College of Medicine at the University of Illinois at Chicago, USA.

Steven M. Downing is Associate Professor, Emeritus, in the Department of Medical Education in the College of Medicine at the University of Illinois at Chicago, USA.

Assessment in Health Professions Education

Second edition

Edited by
**Rachel Yudkowsky, Yoon Soo Park,
and Steven M. Downing**

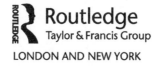

Routledge
Taylor & Francis Group

LONDON AND NEW YORK

First published 2009 by Routledge

Second edition published 2020
by Routledge

Published 2019 by Routledge
2 Park Square, Milton Park, Abingdon, Oxon OX14 4RN
52 Vanderbilt Avenue, New York, NY 10017

Routledge is an imprint of the Taylor & Francis Group, an informa business

Library of Congress Cataloging-in-Publication Data
A catalog record for this book has been requested

ISBN: 978-1-138-05438-7 (hbk)
ISBN: 978-1-315-16690-2 (pbk)
ISBN: 978-1-138-05439-4 (ebk)

Typeset in Minion
by Apex CoVantage, LLC

To my husband Moshe
1.3 billion seconds and counting

To my parents and teachers, Moshe and Mimi Soller
Whose love and values are my bedrock

To our children Eliezer, Channah and Jeff
and our grandchildren Aryeh and Shifra
Who bring us so much pride and joy

And in memory of our son Yehuda Nattan
May his memory be a blessing to all who loved him.

—RY

To my wife Heeyoung
For your love, patience, and encouragement

To my parents Sanghyun Park and Hyeyoung Jin
Whose prayers and love shape my decisions

To my teachers and colleagues
Who inspire me to continue the work we all enjoy.

—YSP

CONTENTS

FIGURES

FOREWORD

Assessment has been a major preoccupation and topic of inquiry in health professions education, as seen by the creation of institutions like national boards or councils of medical and nursing examiners, the presence of highly qualified and respected psychometricians in the field, and the omnipresence of assessment-related articles in scientific journals. This is quite understandable considering the high stakes involved in making sure that examinees have a suitable level of competence to go on to the next level of training or to practice independently. Consequently, attention given to assessment in health professions education has led to great advancements in the development of ever more sophisticated and valid methods of assessments, from multiple-choice items to the use of simulation-based OSCEs, workplace mini-CEXs, and virtual reality mannequins, as well as great advancements in the way assessment is used, from isolated test taking to programs of assessment. These advances, following Shulman's "traveling among the disciplines," have also coincided and influenced measurement and evaluation in general, such as case-content specificity, authentic assessment, rater and scoring models, and programmatic assessment.

The quality of a test hinges on the quality of the items it contains, namely that the items constitute an adequate and representative sample of the domain tested and that each item contributes to discriminating between strong and weak examinees, given the purpose of the test and its position in a program of assessment. Developing, administering, and analyzing results from a single test or sets of tests involve both technical skills, like calculating test score reliability and item difficulty and discrimination indexes, and judgment-related skills, like defining the domain, rating performances, or setting standards, to ensure that threats to validity are kept at a minimum and that inferences and decisions made from the test scores reflect the intended goals, à la Messick and Kane.

During the past half century in health professions education, we have progressively understood and mastered in large part the technical aspects of developing tests that yield valid inferences while seeing at the same time the emergence of new challenges, such as defining competencies that meet the expectations and values of various stakeholders that can be affected by examinee performance—"stakeholders" such as administrators, the diverse cast of professionals in health-care teams and healthcare systems, and faculty and patients, including families and communities; and "expectations" regarding decision-making abilities, communication and collaboration skills, professionalism, and self-improvement. How are the values and beliefs of the stakeholders and raters influencing the definition of competence and their ratings of examinees performance? How can examinee results from classroom promotion tests or national certification exams be used to not only test the adequacy of preparedness but also guide subsequent learning and continuous professional development? How can electronic patient records and health systems databases be used to measure clinical performance in real time and be part of the assessment cycle to promote learning and performance improvement?

Pioneers like George Miller and Christine McGuire in the 1960s proposed new conceptual frameworks to assess health professionals—*Miller's pyramid* (*Does*—*Shows How*—*Knows How*—*Knows*)—and new simulation-based methods to assess clinical problem solving—*Patient Management Problems* (PMPs). Downing, and the new generation of editors in this second edition of *Assessment in Health Professions Education*, called on a cadre of authoritative experts worldwide to share their wisdom and talents. With the rapid expansion of health professions education graduate programs, the first edition of the book proved to be a one-of-a-kind reference for students and alumni, contributing to HPE scholarship and practices of assessment across continents. *Assessment in Health Professions Education* is a standard reference on the bookshelves of colleagues.

This second edition stands to have an even greater impact to train the next generation of HPE educators and uphold the highest standards in the everyday assessment practices and reforms by health professions educators. *Assessment in Health Professions Education* provides the readers with the fundamental principles and basic tools to understand and prepare top-quality tests and programs of assessment but also gives them a footing from which to look into the future and frame new and emerging challenges. Thank you for giving us a solid foundation on which to build our assessment, from admission to training and the workplace, so as to foster learning and, most of all, maximize patient care and healthcare delivery, the ultimate purposes of assessment in the health professions.

Georges Bordage, MD, MSc, PhD
Professor Emeritus, Department of Medical Education
College of Medicine, University of Illinois at Chicago
March 2019

PREFACE

The purpose of this book is to present a basic yet comprehensive treatment of assessment methods for health professions educators. While there are many excellent textbooks in psychometric theory and its application to large-scale standardized testing programs, and many educational measurement and assessment books designed for elementary and secondary teachers and graduate students in education and psychology, none of these books are entirely appropriate for the specialized educational and assessment requirements for health professions. Such books lack essential topics of critical interest to health professions educators and may contain many chapters that are of little or no interest to those engaged in education in the health professions.

Assessment in Health Professions Education presents chapters on the fundamentals of testing and assessment together with some of their theoretical and research underpinnings plus chapters devoted to specific assessment methods used widely in health professions education. Although scholarly, evidence-based, and current, this book is intended to be readable, understandable, and practically useful for the general health professions educator. Validity evidence is an organizing theme and is the conceptual framework used throughout chapters of this book, because the editors and authors think that all assessment data require some amount of scientific evidence to support or refute the intended interpretations of the assessment data and that validity is the single most important attribute of all assessment data.

This second edition of the book has been extensively revised and updated by leaders in the field. It introduces new chapters reflecting developments, innovations, and best-practice guidelines in the assessment of health professionals over the past decade, including chapters on narrative assessment, situational judgment tests, programmatic assessment, assessment in mastery learning settings, and the key features approach. A new chapter on assessment affecting learning provides insightful analysis of a critically important but frequently neglected aspect of assessments in our work. In addition, a new chapter on item response theory introduces modern concepts for scoring and analyzing assessment data. Finally, a new chapter on engaging with your statistician provides useful tips for readers planning to pursue assessment-based research.

PART I: FUNDAMENTALS OF ASSESSMENT

Chapters 1 to 6 present theoretical fundamentals of assessment, from the specialized perspective of the health professions educator. These chapters are basic and fairly non-technical, and they are intended to provide health professions instructors some of the essential background needed to understand, interpret, develop, and successfully apply many of the specialized assessment methods or techniques discussed in Chapters 7 to 19.

In Chapter 1, Yudkowsky, Park, and Downing present a broad overview of assessment in the health professions. This chapter provides the **basic definitions, concepts, and language of assessment** and orients the reader to the conceptual framework for this book. The reader who is unfamiliar with the jargon of assessment or is new to health professions education will find this chapter a solid introduction and orientation to the basics of this specialized discipline.

Lineberry in Chapter 2 discusses **validity** from the perspective of both Kane (framing the validity argument) and Messick (identifying sources of validity evidence) and reviews the classic threats to validity for assessment data. Validity encompasses all other topics in assessment, and thus this chapter is placed early in the book to emphasize its importance. Validity is the organizing principle of this book, so the intention of this chapter is to provide readers with the interpretive tools needed to apply this concept to all other topics and concepts discussed in later chapters.

Chapters 3 and 4 both concern reliability of assessment data. Park discusses the general principles and common applications of **reliability** in Chapter 3. In Chapter 4, Kreiter, Zaidi, and Park present the fundamentals of an important framework for reliability analysis, **generalizability theory**, and apply this methodology to health professions education. The authors present different forms of reliability statistics and their interpretation with examples from the health professions.

In Chapter 5, Downing, Juul, and Park present basic information on the **statistics of testing**, discussing the fundamental score unit, standard scores, item analysis, and some information and examples of practical hand-calculator formulas used to evaluate test and assessment data in typical health professions education settings.

In Chapter 6, Yudkowsky, Downing, and Tekian present **standard setting** or the establishment of passing scores. Defensibility of criterion-based passing scores—as opposed to relative or normative passing score methods—is the focus of this chapter, together with many examples provided for some of the most common methods utilized for standard setting and some of the statistics used to evaluate those standards.

PART II: ASSESSMENT METHODS

The second part of the book—Chapters 7 to 12—covers the basic assessment methods commonly used in health professions education settings, starting with written tests of cognitive knowledge and achievement and proceeding in order of Miller's pyramid (see Chapter 1), through chapters on oral examinations, performance examinations, workplace-based assessment, narrative assessment, and portfolio assessment. Each of these topics represents an important method or technique used to measure knowledge and skills acquisition of students and other learners in the health professions.

In Chapter 7, Paniagua, Swygert, and Downing present an overview of **written tests** of cognitive knowledge. Both constructed-response and selected-response formats are discussed, with practical examples and guidance summarized from the research literature. Written tests of all types are prevalent, especially in classroom assessment settings in health professions education. This chapter aims to provide the basic knowledge and skills needed to effectively assess cognitive learning.

Chapter 8, written by Juul, Yudkowsky, and Tekian, provides basic information on the use of **oral examinations**. Oral exams ranging from vivas to chart-stimulated recall to multiple mini-interviews are used widely in health professions education worldwide. This chapter provides information on the fundamental strengths and limitations of the oral exam and suggestions for improving oral examination processes.

Yudkowsky discusses **performance tests** in Chapter 9. This chapter provides the reader with guidelines for performance assessment leveraging techniques such as human simulation (standardized patients) and objective structured clinical exams (OSCEs) that facilitate direct observation of behavior under controlled conditions. These methods are especially useful in skills testing at all levels of health professions education.

Chapter 10, written by McBride, Adler, and McGaghie, provides an overview of **workplace-based assessment** methods, especially those based on direct observation; these methods are critical for decisions regarding learner autonomy, including decisions regarding entrustable professional activities and developmental milestones (see Chapter 1). The fundamentals of sound workplace-based observational assessment methods are presented, and recommendations are made for ways to improve these methods.

Chapter 11 is a new chapter on **narrative assessment** by Dudek and Cook. Narrative assessment can complement numeric scores by providing rich, qualitative descriptions of performance and identifying specific opportunities for improvement. This chapter lists best practices for obtaining and using narrative assessments, and key considerations for validity.

Chapter 12, written by Schumacher, Tekian, and Yudkowsky, provides guidance on the use of **portfolios** for assessment purposes. Portfolios are enjoying a resurgence in popularity and are widely applied in all levels of health professions education, especially as a component of programmatic assessment in competency-based curricula. This chapter analyzes portfolio design, the role of the mentor, and threats to the validity of portfolios.

PART III: SPECIAL TOPICS

Chapters 13–20 address special topics along with some newer and innovative approaches to assessment in health professions education.

In Chapter 13, Bordage and Page discuss the **key features** approach, which focuses on assessing learners' ability to identify and assess the critical actions or decisions unique to each patient case. They describe the process of developing and scoring KF cases and discuss how the KFs approach can address major threats to assessment validity.

Technology-based **simulations** used in assessment are the focus of Chapter 14 by Devine, McGaghie, and Issenberg. The chapter presents the state of the art of simulation-based assessments and provides the reader with the tools needed to begin to understand and use these methods effectively.

Situational judgment tests (SJTs) are featured in Chapter 15 by Reiter and Roberts. This chapter provides an understanding of design features salient to the use of SJTs to assess personal competencies such as ethics, professionalism, teamwork, and cultural competency, along with caveats for interpreting the results.

Chapter 16 highlights the new emphasis on **programmatic assessment** for competency-based education, in which each assessment "point" is optimized for maximum learning effect, and decisions are based only on aggregated assessment data. Van der Vleuten, Heeneman, and Schut describe what programmatic assessment entails, present guidance on programmatic assessment in practice, and discuss the literature on this topic to date.

The impact of assessment on learning—both positive and negative—has only recently become a focus of attention for assessment designers. In Chapter 17, Lineberry provides an original perspective on **assessment affecting learning** and reviews four mechanisms of action that mediate these effects.

Chapter 18 by Lineberry, Yudkowsky, Park, Cook, Ritter, and Knox provides an overview of noteworthy considerations for **assessments in mastery learning settings**. Repeated testing and the emphasis on well-prepared learners present unique challenges for validity evidence and standard setting; this chapter reviews these challenges and ways to address them.

Park provides a short, non-technical introduction to **item response theory** (IRT) in Chapter 19. IRT links learners and item characteristics to the same measurement scale, thereby generating sample-independent results. Park provides examples of IRT applications in health professions education and compares IRT to classical measurement approaches.

Finally, in Chapter 20, Schwartz and Park provide insightful tips to promote effective **collaboration between assessment researchers and statisticians**. This chapter reviews pitfalls that often ensnare inexperienced assessment researchers and summarizes how to effectively work with a statistician towards the goal of better design, analysis, and reporting of assessment research.

ACKNOWLEDGMENTS

As is often the case in specialized books such as this, the genesis and motivation to edit and produce the book grew out of our teaching and faculty mentoring roles. We continue to learn much from our outstanding students in the Master of Health Professions Education (MHPE) program at the University of Illinois at Chicago (UIC), and we hope that this book provides some useful information to future students in this program and in the many other health professions education graduate and faculty development programs worldwide.

We are most grateful to all of our authors, who dedicated time from their over-busy professional lives to make an outstanding contribution to assessment in health professions education.

We wish to acknowledge and thank all our reviewers. Their special expertise, insight, and helpful comments have made this a stronger publication. We also thank Daniel J. Schwartz and Katie Paton, our editors at Taylor & Francis, for their encouragement and support of this second edition.

Jaime Holden, in the Department of Medical Education at UIC, assisted us greatly in the final preparation of this book, and we are grateful for her help. The value of the mentorship, collaboration, and friendship of our colleagues in the Department of Medical Education cannot be overstated.

Finally, we wish to thank our families, who were most patient with our many distractions over the long timeline required to produce this book.

Rachel Yudkowsky
Yoon Soo Park
Steven M. Downing
Department of Medical Education
University of Illinois at Chicago College of Medicine
March 2019

PART I

FUNDAMENTALS OF ASSESSMENT

1

INTRODUCTION TO ASSESSMENT IN THE HEALTH PROFESSIONS

Rachel Yudkowsky, Yoon Soo Park, and Steven M. Downing

Assessment is defined by the *Standards for Educational and Psychological Testing* (American Educational Research Association, American Psychological Association, & National Council on Measurement in Education, 2014, p. 216) as "a systematic process to measure or evaluate the characteristics or performance of individuals, programs, or other entities, for purposes of drawing inferences." This is a broad definition, but it summarizes the scope of this book, which presents current information about both assessment theory and its practice in health professions education. The focus of this book is on the assessment of learning and skill acquisition in *people*, with a strong emphasis on broadly defined achievement testing, using a variety of methods.

Health professions education is a specialized discipline comprised of many different types of professionals, who provide a wide range of health care services in a wide variety of settings. Examples of health professionals include physicians, nurses, pharmacists, physical therapists, dentists, optometrists, podiatrists, other highly specialized technical professionals such as nuclear and radiological technicians, and many other professionals who provide health care or health related services to patients or clients. The most common thread uniting the health professions may be that all such professionals must complete highly selective educational courses of study, which usually include practical training as well as classroom instruction; those who successfully complete these rigorous courses of study have the serious responsibility of taking care of patients—sometimes in life-and-death situations. Thus, health professionals usually require a specialized license or other type of certificate to practice. It is important to base our health professions education assessment practices and methods on the best research evidence available, with rigorous and accountable standards, since many of the decisions made about our learners ultimately impact health care delivery outcomes for patients and the public more broadly.

The *Standards* (AERA, APA, & NCME, 2014) represent the consensus opinion concerning all major policies, practices, and issues in assessment. This document, revised every decade or so, is sponsored by the three major professional associations concerned with assessment and its application and practice: the American Educational Research Association (AERA), the American Psychological Association (APA), and the National Council on Measurement in Education (NCME). The *Standards* will be referenced frequently in this book because they provide excellent guidance based on the best contemporary research evidence and the consensus view of educational researchers and professionals.

This book devotes chapters to contemporary theory of assessment in the health professions (Part I: Fundamentals of Assessment; Chapters 1 to 6), practical methods typically used to measure learners' knowledge acquisition and their abilities to perform in clinical settings (Part II: Assessment Methods; Chapters 7 to 12), and special topics that address innovative approaches to assessment in health professions education (Part III: Special Topics; Chapters 13 to 20). The theory sections apply to nearly all measurement settings and are essential to master for those who wish to practice sound, defensible, and meaningful assessments of their health professions learners; these principles of validity and sound assessment practices resonate throughout the chapters and form the unifying framework of this book. The methods section deals specifically with common procedures or techniques used in health professions education—written tests, oral examinations, performance tests, workplace-based assessments, narrative assessment, and portfolios—that address the diverse and increasingly complex assessment methods for cognitive achievement, clinical performance, and competence in clinical workplace settings. The special topics section describes cutting-edge innovations and tips for health professions education, introducing advances in methods from the key features approach, technology-based simulations, situational judgment tests, programmatic assessment, assessment affecting learning, assessments in mastery learning settings, item response theory, and guidelines for conducting assessment research with statisticians.

GEORGE MILLER'S PYRAMID

Miller's pyramid (Miller, 1990) is often cited as a useful model or taxonomy of the levels of knowledge and skills assessed in health professions education. In Figure 1.1, Miller's pyramid demonstrates that cognitive knowledge is at the base, as the foundation for all other important aspects or features of learning in the health professions. This is the "knows" level of essential factual knowledge, the knowledge of biological processes and scientific principles on which most of the more complex learnings rest. Knowledge is the essential prerequisite for almost all other types of learning expected of our learners. Miller would likely agree that this "knows" level is best measured by written objective tests, such as selected- and constructed-response tests. The "knows how" level of the Miller pyramid adds a level of complexity to the cognitive scheme, indicating something more than simple recall or recognition of factual knowledge. The "knows how" level indicates a learner's ability to manipulate knowledge in some useful way, to apply this knowledge, and to demonstrate some understanding of the relationships between concepts and principles, and may even indicate the learner's ability to describe the solution to some types of novel problems. This level can also

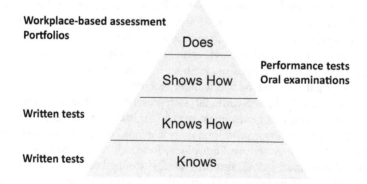

Figure 1.1 Miller's pyramid

Source: Based on Miller (1990)

be assessed quite adequately with carefully crafted written tests, although some health professions educators would tend to use other methods, such as oral exams or other types of more subjective, observational procedures. The "knows how" level deals with cognitive knowledge, but at a somewhat more complex or higher level than the "knows" level. The first two levels of the Miller pyramid are concerned with knowledge that is verbally mediated; the emphasis is on verbal-type knowledge and the learner's ability to describe this knowledge verbally rather than on "doing."

The "shows how" level moves the methods of assessment to performance tests, in which one directly observes learner ability to translate knowledge into practice. All performance exams are somewhat artificial, in that they are contrived situations presented in a standard testing format under more-or-less controlled conditions. Simulation-based assessments, such as a simulated patient encounter to assess communication skills, are good examples of the "shows how" level of assessment. Specific cases or problems are pre-selected for testing and special "standardized patients" are selected and trained to portray the case; performance typically is rated using checklists and/or rating scales. Similarly, standardized oral examinations exams can provide opportunities for learners to demonstrate abilities such as clinical reasoning, decision-making, and presentation skills. These standardization procedures add to the measurement qualities of the assessment but may detract somewhat from the authenticity of it.

Finally, Miller's "does" level is associated with more independent and free-range observations of the learner's performance in actual patient or clinical settings, known as work-based assessment. Some standardization and control of the assessment setting and situation is traded for complete, uncued authenticity of assessment. The learner brings together all the cognitive knowledge, skills, abilities, and experience into their conduct in the real world, which is observed by expert and experienced clinical teachers and raters.

Miller's pyramid can be a useful framework to guide our thinking about teaching and assessment in the health professions. Many other systems or taxonomies of knowledge structure are also discussed in the literature. For example, one of the oldest and most frequently used taxonomies of cognitive knowledge (the "knows" and "knows how" level for Miller) is Bloom's cognitive taxonomy (Bloom, Engelhart, Furst, Hill, & Krathwohl, 1956). It ranks knowledge from very simple recall or recognition of facts to higher levels of synthesizing and evaluating factual knowledge and solving novel problems. Bloom's cognitive taxonomy is often used to guide written testing (Chapter 7). For now, we suggest that for meaningful and successful assessments, there must be some rationale system or plan to connect the content tested to the knowledge, skills, and abilities that we think important for learning.

FOUR MAJOR ASSESSMENT METHODS

In health professions education, almost all of the assessments we construct, select, and administer to our learners can be classified into one (or more) of these four categories: written tests, oral examinations, performance tests, and clinical (workplace-based) observational methods. This section provides an overview of these methods, each of which will be considered in detail in other chapters.

Written Tests

Most formal assessment in health professions education includes some type of written testing. This simply means that the tests consist of written questions or stimuli, to which learners or trainees must respond. There are two major types of written tests: constructed-response (CR) tests and selected-response (SR) tests. Both of these formats can be presented either in the traditional paper-and-pencil format or in computer-based formats, in which the computer presents the test stimuli and records examinee responses or answers. For constructed-response tests, questions or stimuli are presented and examinees respond by writing or typing responses or answers. There are many varieties of constructed-response formats, including "fill-in-the-blanks" type items and short- and long-answer essays. Selected-response tests, on the other hand, present a question or stimulus (referred to as a stem), followed by a number of response options. The multiple-choice (MC) item is the prototype for selected-response formats, but there are many variations on the theme, such as true-false and alternate-choice items, matching items, extended matching items, and many other innovative formats (Sireci & Zenisky, 2006; Lane, Raymond, & Haladyna, 2015) used primarily in computer-based tests (CBTs). While the constructed-response format is probably the most widely used worldwide, the selected-response format is the true "workhorse" of the testing world. This format has many practical advantages and at least 100 years of research to support its validity (Downing, 2002; Welch, 2006). Chapter 7 discusses both constructed- and selected-response written tests. Chapter 13 discusses a specialized form of written test, known as the key features approach, which includes both selected-response and constructed-response formats.

Oral Examinations

Oral examination methods include the formal oral exam, the less formal bedside oral, vivas (the so-called long case and short case assessments), chart-stimulated recall, and other variations (Chapter 8, Oral Examinations). Oral examinations are best deployed to allow demonstration and subsequent probing of the learner's thinking or reasoning, and not for assessment of cognitive knowledge (which is assessed more efficiently and effectively through written tests). Because of the pervasive subjectivity associated with such methods when conducted in the traditional unstandardized format, the threats to validity are strong, particularly for use in high-stakes assessment settings in which serious consequences are possible. Nonetheless, there is a strong tradition supporting their use in many health professions settings. Standardized oral examination formats, including the multiple mini-interview, provide ways to systematically sample content and mitigate some of the threats due to rater subjectivity.

Performance Tests

The term "performance test" is the generic term used to describe many types of formal testing with the primary purpose of measuring "what learners can do," rather than simply "what they know." Systematic, formal performance testing began fairly recently, with the introduction of the objective structured clinical examination (OSCE) by Hart and Harden in the late 1970s (e.g., Harden, Stevenson, Downie, & Wilson, 1975). Medical education in particular has adopted performance testing at all levels of training, from early in the medical school curriculum through graduate or residency training, including its use as one component of the United States Medical Licensure Examination and of post-graduate licensure examinations in Canada.

Simulation-based assessments are a type of performance examination. The term "simulation" refers to a representation of a real-world task. Simulations cover a wide range of methods and modalities, ranging from fairly simple structured oral exams to screen-based simulations (virtual patients), table-top part-task trainers for procedural skills, virtual reality simulators, high-fidelity mannequins, and human simulation (simulated patients). Simulated or standardized patient exams, often used in OSCE stations, are utilized for both teaching and assessment and now comprise a major category of performance testing in many areas of health professions education. Simulated patient examinations date back to the early 1960s, pioneered by Howard Barrows and Stephen Abrahamson (Barrows & Abrahamson, 1964), with the term "standardized patient" credited to Geoff Norman at McMaster University (Wallace, 1997). Some 40 years of research evidence now supports the validity of the standardized patient method and the many different facets of this testing modality (e.g., Swanson & van der Vleuten, 2013).

Chapters 9 (Performance Tests) and 14 (Simulations in Assessment) address the measurement issues and special problems of performance examinations. Human simulation (standardized patients) provides a prototypical example of the performance test methodology in Chapter 9; simulation-based assessment is more broadly addressed in Chapter 14.

Workplace-Based Assessment (Clinical Observational Methods)

Assessment of performance during clinical training is a very common form of assessment in health professions education. These types of assessments range from informal observations of learners in clinical settings to very formal (and sometimes complex) systems of data gathering from multiple raters ("360 evaluations") about the performance of learners in actual clinical settings with real patients over lengthy periods of time. These observational assessment methods rely on checklists, rating forms, and narrative assessments completed by faculty and other instructors and stakeholders in clinical settings.

Many of these observational assessments carry major weight in overall or composite grading schemes, such that the stakes associated with these observations of clinical behavior are high for the learner. Health professions educators rely heavily on these types of observational assessments and value them, but the shortcomings and threats to validity of these methods are well known and difficult to remediate (e.g., William, Klaman, & McGaghie, 2003). Chapter 10 is devoted to a discussion of the issues concerning assessments based on observation of clinical performance in real-life settings (workplace-based assessments) and to best practices that can help mitigate their inherent threats.

NARRATIVE ASSESSMENTS AND PORTFOLIOS

In addition to these four methods, narrative assessments and portfolios are two widely used assessment approaches that cut across assessment methods; they too are described in this section of the book.

Narrative assessments are qualitative descriptions of learners' abilities, usually in the words of the assessor. These can provide a rich source of information in their own right and can supplement and complement quantitative assessment scores derived from any of the four assessment methods (written, oral, performance, and workplace-based assessments). The development and uses of narrative assessments, including their alignment with quantitative assessment scores, are discussed in Chapter 11.

Assessment portfolios similarly cut across methods. A portfolio can be used to prompt a reflective exercise (written test); as a focus for discussion (oral exam); as a demonstration of documentation skills (performance test); or as a procedure log (workplace-based assessment). Assessment portfolios also can be used to organize data across assessment methods to assemble evidence documenting progress and development. Chapter 12 presents assessment portfolios encompassing both reflective and comprehensive components.

SOME BASIC TERMS AND DEFINITIONS

As we begin this journey, some basic terms and definitions may be helpful. The terms and concepts discussed here will be used throughout this book and will be important to many other topics in the book.

Competency-Based Education

Competency-based education in the health professions focuses on ensuring that all of our learners reach a defined level of achievement that will enable them to provide safe and effective care. Competency-based education is often contrasted with the traditional time-based education model, in which promotion decisions are marked by units of time rather than an emphasis on achieving competencies (Park, Hodges, & Tekian, 2016). Well-designed and effectively implemented assessments are a key component of this approach.

Many excellent taxonomies of competencies and roles have been developed by organizations and professions around the world. We will briefly describe here one model, the Accreditation Council for Graduate Medical Education (ACGME) competencies and milestones. These are widely used both in the US and internationally and will be referenced in several chapters of this book.

In the United States, the ACGME and the American Board of Medical Specialties (ABMS) collaborated in a wide-ranging assessment project known as Outcomes Project. The ACGME General Competencies are a product of this collaboration, mandating that residency training programs assess and document their residents' competence in six domains: patient care, medical knowledge, practice-based learning and improvement, interpersonal and communication skills, professionalism, and systems-based practice (Accreditation Council for Graduate Medical Education, 2000). The competencies are sufficiently general to be useful in many different areas of health professions education, and at all levels of training.

In 2012, the ACGME developed and implemented the Next Accreditation System (NAS; Nasca, Philibert, Brigham, & Flynn, 2012). In the NAS, the developmental progress of a learner achieving the competencies is measured using milestones: specialty-specific behavioral descriptors reflecting expected developmental progress in competency subdomains. Examples of milestone subcompetencies for internal medicine residents are listed in Table 1.1, and an example of a milestone scale is shown in Figure 1.2 (Accreditation Council for Graduate Medical Education and the American Board of Internal Medicine, 2015).

Within the competency-based assessment framework, entrustable professional activities (EPAs; ten Cate, 2013) have received increasing attention. EPAs are units of professional work, tasks, or responsibilities that learners are entrusted to perform unsupervised. An example of an EPA for a graduating medical student about to enter residency is "Gather a history and perform a physical exam." EPAs typically require the integration of multiple competencies in a given context; the EPA above might require the application of aspects of patient care, medical knowledge, professionalism, and communication skills. Assessments are used to gather relevant data that can inform entrustment-level decisions for EPAs, including assessments of trustworthiness (e.g., knowing one's own limitations and when to call for help) and required levels of supervision. The *Core Entrustable Professional Activities for Entering Residency* (Association of American Medical Colleges, 2014) are an example of a set of EPAs identified for graduating medical students. EPAs are further discussed in Chapter 10, and an example of a commonly used entrustment scale, the O-SCORE, is shown in Figure 10.2.

Table 1.1 ACGME Competencies and Sample Milestone Subcompetencies for Internal Medicine

ACGME Competency	Example of a Subcompetency
Patient Care	Develops and achieves a comprehensive management plan for each patient
Medical Knowledge	Knowledge of diagnostic testing and procedures
System-based Practice	Works effectively within an interprofessional team
Practice-based Learning and Improvement	Learns and improves via feedback
Professionalism	Accepts responsibility and follows through on tasks
Interpersonal and Communication Skills	Communicates effectively with patients and caregivers

Source: Accreditation Council for Graduate Medical Education and the American Board of Internal Medicine (2015): The Internal Medicine Milestone Project. Accreditation Council for Graduate Medical Education, Chicago, IL. Reprinted with permission of the ACGME and ABIM.

14. Learns and improves via feedback. (PBLI-13)				
Critical Deficiencies			Ready for Unsupervised Practice	Aspirational
Never solicits feedback Actively resists feedback from others	Rarely seeks feedback Responds to unsolicited feedback in a defensive fashion Temporarily or superficially adjusts performance based on feedback	Solicits feedback only from supervisors Is open to unsolicited feedback Inconsistently incorporates feedback	Solicits feedback from all members of the interprofessional team and patients Welcomes unsolicited feedback Consistently incorporates feedback	Performance continuously reflects incorporation of solicited and unsolicited feedback Able to reconcile disparate or conflicting feedback
☐ ☐ ☐ ☐ ☐ ☐ ☐ ☐ ☐				
Comments:				

Figure 1.2 Sample milestone for internal medicine residents

Source: From the Accreditation Council for Graduate Medical Education and the American Board of Internal Medicine (2015): The Internal Medicine Milestone Project. Accreditation Council for Graduate Medical Education, Chicago, IL. Reprinted with permission from the Accreditation Council for Graduate Medical Education and the American Board of Internal Medicine. Available from www.acgme.org/Portals/0/PDFs/Milestones/InternalMedicine Milestones.pdf

Competencies, milestones, and entrustable professional activities address the "what" of assessment rather than the "how." These frameworks provide a basis for systematically blueprinting or sampling the knowledge, skills, attitudes, and other characteristics of our learners, which are the objects of our assessments.

Instruction and Assessment

While the major focus of this book is on assessment, it is important to remember that assessment and instruction are intimately related. Chapters 16 through 18 address strategies to promote the positive impact of assessment on learning and avoid unintended negative effects.

Teaching, learning, and assessment form a closed circle, with each entity tightly bound to the other. Assessments developed locally (as opposed to large-scale standardized testing) must be closely aligned with instruction, with adequate, timely, and meaningful feedback provided to learners wherever possible. Just as we provide learners with many different types of learning experiences from classroom to clinic, we must also utilize multiple methods to assess their learning across competencies, from "knows" to "does." An exclusive reliance on a single method such as written tests, or reliance on a single, high-stakes summative assessment will provide a skewed view of the learner. In programmatic assessment (Chapter 16), multiple low-stakes assessments utilizing a variety of assessment methods are leveraged to provide a holistic and longitudinal view of the learner. Since assessment ultimately drives learning, judicious use of assessment methods at different levels of the Miller pyramid can help ensure that learners focus their learning in ways that are most valuable for their future practice. Specific assessment practices affect different phases of learning, from suggesting strategies for preparing for the exam to facilitating learners' and instructors' use of post-examination feedback. Chapter 17 includes an extended analysis of these effects and their underlying mechanisms of action.

Assessment, Measurement, and Tests

The *Standards* (AERA, APA, & NCME, 2014) define "assessment" very broadly to include just about any method, process, or procedure used to collect any type of information or data with which to make inferences about people, objects, or programs. The focus of this book is on the assessment of learners and not on the evaluation of educational programs or educational products. We use the term *assessment* to cover almost everything we do to measure the educational learning or progress of our students or other trainees. Embedded within this definition are three important characteristics—assessment is a systematic process for obtaining a *sample* of behaviors or characteristics under *structured* conditions to make *inferences* about individuals in non-assessment settings (Thissen & Wainer, 2001). In other words, regardless of the type of assessment administered, the questions, cases, or encounters observed are samples of knowledge, skills, and attitudes of learners that are systematically captured—as such, careful sampling is an important property of sound assessments. Assessments also have a range of structure—from more standardized settings, as reflected in multiple-choice tests that have fixed format and administration regulations, to less structured settings in workplace-based assessments. Finally, assessments generally have the goal of making inferences about learners: using assessment data gathered under "testing situations" to make inferences about "non-testing situations"; for example, performance on licensure or certification examinations is used to make inferences about the future performance of health professionals in their daily activities in the workplace. Consistent with the revised *Standards*, assessment is also used synonymously with the term "test."

The term "measurement" refers to some type of quantification used as an assessment. *Measurement* implies the assignment of numbers, based on some systematic rules and specific assessment process. While the measurement process may include some types of qualitative assessment (see Chapter 11 regarding narrative assessment), the major emphasis in this book is on quantitative measurement. Unlike objects that can be directly counted (e.g., counting the number of cars in the parking area), also referred to as *manifest* variables, educational and psychological constructs are *latent* variables that cannot be directly measured. We discuss measurement issues associated with assessment of latent variables in greater detail in Chapters 2 (Validity and Quality) and 3 (Reliability).

Types of Numbers

Since a book on assessment in the health professions must deal with quantitative matters and numbers, it seems appropriate to begin with a brief overview of the types of number scales commonly used. There are four basic types of number scales that will be familiar to many readers (e.g., Howell, 2002). The most basic number scale is the *nominal scale*, which uses numbers only as arbitrary symbols. Coding a questionnaire demographic question about gender as a nominal response such as 1 = Female and 2 = Male is an example of a nominal number scale. The numbers have no inherent meaning, only the arbitrary meaning assigned by the researcher. The key point is that we can do only very limited mathematical procedures, such as counting, on nominal numbers. We cannot legitimately compute averages for nominal numbers, since the average "score" has no meaning or interpretation.

An *ordinal* number has some inherent meaning, although at a very basic level. Ordinal numbers designate the order or the rank order of the referent. For example, we can rank the height in meters of all students in an entering pharmacy class, designating the rank of 1 as the tallest student and the last number rank as the shortest student. The distance or interval between rank 4 and rank 5 is not necessarily the same as the distance between ranks 6 and 7, however. With ordinal numbers, we can compute averages or mean ranks, take the standard deviation of the distribution of ranks, and so on. In other words, ordinal numbers have some inherent meaning or interpretation and, therefore, summary statistics are useful and interpretable.

Interval numbers are a bit more sophisticated than ordinal numbers in that the distance between numbers is meaningful and is considered equal. This means that the meaning or interpretation associated with the score interval 50 to 60 (10 points) is the same as the interval or distance between scores 30 and 40. This is an important characteristic, since the interval nature of these numbers permits all types of statistical analyses, the full range of which are called parametric statistics.

A *ratio* scale of numbers is the most sophisticated number scale, but it is rarely if ever possible to obtain in educational measurement or the social sciences. A true ratio scale has a meaningful zero point, so that zero means "nothingness." This means that if we could devise a legitimate ratio testing instrument for measuring the achievement of nursing students in biochemistry, students scoring 0 would have absolutely no knowledge of the biochemistry objectives tested. This is not possible in educational measurement, obviously, since even the least capable student will have some minimal knowledge. (True ratio scales are often found in the physical sciences, but not in the social sciences.)

The main point of this discussion of number types is that most of the assessment data we obtain in health professions education are considered or assumed to be interval data, so that we can perform nearly all types of statistical analyses on the results. For instance, data from a multiple-choice achievement test in pharmacology is always assumed to be interval data, so that we can compute summary statistics for the distribution of scores (means, standard deviations), correlations between scores on this test and other similar tests or subtests, and may even perform a paired *t*-test of mean pre-post differences in scores. If these data were ordinal, we would have some limitations on the statistical analyses available, such as using only the Spearman rank-order correlation coefficient. All psychometric models of data used in assessment, such as the various methods used to estimate the reproducibility or reliability of scores or ratings, are derived with the underlying assumption that the data are interval in nature.

Fidelity to the Criterion

Another familiar concept in assessment for the health professions is that of "fidelity." The full term, as used by most educational measurement professionals, is "fidelity to the criterion," implying some validity-type relationship between scores or ratings on the assessment and the ultimate "criterion" variable in real life. "Fidelity to the criterion" is often shortened to "fidelity." What does this actually mean? Think of a dichotomy between a high-fidelity and a low-fidelity assessment. A simulation of an actual clinical problem, presented to pharmacy students by highly trained actors, is thought to be "high fidelity," because the test appears to be much like an authentic, real-life situation that the future pharmacists may encounter with a real patient. On the other hand, a multiple-choice test of basic knowledge in chemistry might be considered a very low-fidelity simulation of a real-life situation for the same learners. High-fidelity assessments are said to be "more proximate to the criterion," meaning that the assessment itself appears to be fairly lifelike and authentic, while low-fidelity assessments appear to be far removed from the criterion or are less proximate to the criterion (Haladyna, 1999). Most highly structured performance exams, complex simulations, and less well-structured observational methods of assessment are of higher fidelity than written exams and are intended to measure different facets of learning.

The concept of fidelity is important only as a superficial trait or characteristic of assessments. Fidelity may have little or nothing to do with true validity evidence and may, in fact, actually interfere with objectivity of measurement, which tends to decrease validity evidence (Downing, 2003). Learners and their faculty, however, often prefer (or think they prefer) more high-fidelity assessments, simply because they look more like real-life situations. One fact is certain: the higher the fidelity of the assessment, the higher the cost and the more complex are the measurement issues of the assessment.

Formative and Summative Assessment

The concepts of formative and summative assessment are pervasive in the assessment literature and date to the middle of the last century; these concepts originated in the program evaluation literature and have come to be used in all areas of assessment (Scriven, 1967). These useful concepts are straightforward in meaning. The primary purpose of formative testing is to provide useful feedback on learner strengths and weaknesses with respect to the learning objectives. Classic formative assessment takes place *during* the course of study, such that student learners have the opportunity to understand what content they have already mastered and what content needs more study (or for the instructor, needs more teaching). Examples of formative assessments include weekly short quizzes during a microbiology course and short written tests given at frequent intervals during a two-semester-long course in pharmacology.

Summative assessment "sums up" the achievement in a course of study and typically takes place at or near the end of a formal course of study, such as an end-of-semester examination in anatomy that covers the entire cumulative course. Summative assessments emphasize the final measurement of achievement and usually count heavily in the grading scheme. Feedback to learners may be one aspect of the summative assessment, but the primary purpose of the summative assessment is to measure what learners have achieved during the course of instruction. The ultimate example of a summative assessment is a test given at the conclusion of long, complex courses of study, such as a licensure test in nursing, which must be taken and passed at the very end of the educational sequence and before the newly graduated nurse can begin professional work.

Norm- and Criterion-Referenced Measurement

The basic concept of norm- and criterion-referenced measurement or assessment is also fairly simple and straightforward. Norm-referenced test scores are interpreted relative to some well-defined normative group, such as all learners who took the test. The key word is *relative*; norm-referenced scores or ratings tell us a lot about how well learners score or are rated relative to some group of other learners, but may tell us less about what exact content they actually know or can do. Criterion-referenced scores or ratings, on the other hand, tell us how much of some specific content learners actually know or can do. Criterion-referenced testing has been popular in North America since the 1970s (Popham & Husek, 1969). This type of assessment is most closely associated with competency- or content-based teaching and testing. Other terms used somewhat interchangeably with criterion-referenced testing are *domain-referenced, objectives-referenced, content-referenced,* and *construct-referenced.* There are some subtle differences in the usage of these terms by various authors and researchers, but all have in common a strong interest in the content actually learned or mastered by the learners and a lack of interest in rank ordering learners by test scores.

Mastery testing is a special type of criterion-referenced testing, in that the assessments are constructed to identify *well-prepared* rather than *minimally competent* learners. Mastery learning strategies and testing methods posit that virtually all learners can achieve the criterion of "mastery," although learners will differ in the time needed to achieve that criterion. Mastery tests are often attempted multiple times before the criterion is met. In general, norm-referenced testing statistics are inappropriate for tests in true mastery settings. Chapter 18 provides an extended discussion of validity and standard-setting challenges in mastery learning assessments.

A final note on this important topic. Any assessment score or rating can be interpreted in either a norm-referenced or a criterion-referenced manner. The test itself, the methods used to construct the test, the overarching philosophy of assessment and learning, and the intended inferences or decisions to be made based on the test determine the basic classification of the test as either norm- or criterion-referenced. It is perfectly possible, for example, to interpret an inherently normative score, like a percentile or a z-score, in some absolute or criterion-referenced manner. Conversely, some criterion-referenced tests may report only percent-correct scores or raw scores but interpret these scores relative to the distribution of scores (i.e., in a normative or relative fashion).

The concepts of norm- and criterion-referenced testing will be revisited often in this book, especially in our treatment of standard setting or establishing effective and defensible passing scores (Chapter 6). For the most part, the orientation of this book is criterion-referenced. We are most interested in assessing what our learners have learned and achieved and about their competency in our health professions disciplines rather than ranking them in a normative distribution.

High-Stakes and Low-Stakes Assessments

Other terms often used to describe assessments are high- and low-stakes assessments. These terms are descriptive of the consequences of testing. If the results of a test can have a serious impact on an examinee, such as gaining or losing a professional job, the stakes associated with the test are clearly high. High-stakes tests require a much higher burden, in that every facet of such tests must be of extremely high quality, with solid research-based evidence to support validity of interpretations. There may even be a need to defend such high-stakes tests legally, if the test is perceived to cause some individuals or groups harm. Examinations used to admit learners to professional schools and tests used to certify or license graduates in the health professions are good examples of very high-stakes tests. Assessments used to determine final grades in important classes required for graduation or final summative exams that must be passed in order to graduate are also high stakes for our learners.

A low- to moderate-stakes test carries somewhat lower consequences. Many of the formative-type assessments typically used in health professions education are low to moderate stakes. If the consequences of failing the test are minor, or if the remediation (test retake) is not too difficult or costly, the exam stakes might be thought of as low or moderate.

Very high-stakes tests are usually professionally produced by testing experts and large testing agencies using major resources to ensure the defensibility of the resulting test scores and pass-fail decisions. Lower stakes tests and assessments, such as those used by many health professions educators in their local school settings, require fewer resources and less validity evidence, since legal challenges to the test outcomes are rare. Since this book focuses on assessments developed at the local (or classroom) level by highly specialized content experts, the assessments of interest are low to moderate stakes. Nevertheless, even lower-stakes assessments should meet the basic minimum standards of quality, since important decisions are ultimately being made about our learners from our cumulative assessments over time.

Large-Scale and Local or Small-Scale Assessments

Another reference point for this book and its orientation toward assessment in the health professions is the distinction between large- and small-scale assessments. Large-scale assessments refer to standardized testing programs, often national or international in scope, which are generally designed by testing professionals and administered to large numbers of examinees. Large-scale tests such as the Pharmacy College Admissions Test (PCAT) and the Medical College Admissions Test (MCAT) are utilized to help select among applicants for pharmacy and medical schools. The National Council Licensure Examination for Registered Nurses (NCLEX-RN®) is another example of a large-scale test, which is used for licensure of registered nurses by jurisdictions in the United States.

Small-scale or locally developed assessments—the main focus of this book—are developed, administered, and scored by "classroom" instructors, clinical teaching faculty, or other educators at the local school, college, or university level. Too frequently, health professions educators "go it alone" when assessing their learners, with little or no formal educational background in assessment and with little or no support from their institutions for the critically important work of assessment. This book aims to provide local instructors and other health professions educators with sound principles, effective tools, and defensible methods to assist in the important work of learner assessment.

TRANSLATIONAL SCIENCE IN EDUCATION

To conclude this chapter, we look to the translational model of science in education, which provides an overarching view of the important role that education plays in improving the skills and abilities of learners, patients, and the healthcare system more broadly. Traditionally, the translational model of science is used to examine the bench-to-bedside transition of discoveries in basic biomedical science and clinical research. The focus is on the *translation* of knowledge from biomedical science to practice, resulting in new treatments for patients. This paradigm of translating discovery from basic laboratory and biomedical science to clinical research (T1), to identifying evidence of clinical effectiveness and treatment policies (T2), and finally to healthcare delivery systems, community, and preventive services (T3), is commonly referred to as the model of translational science or translational research (Woolf, 2008; see Figure 1.3).

This approach to translational science has been adapted for general education in the K–12 education setting as well as to health professions education. Similar to the general translational science model, the K–12 model for education translates the impact of teacher and teaching education to enhance the knowledge and skills of teachers, which leads to improvements in classroom teaching and ultimately to student achievement (Allen, Pianta, Gregory, Mikami, & Lun, 2011; Yoon, Duncan, Lee, Scarloss, & Shapley, 2007).

As applied to health professions education (McGaghie, 2010), education directed toward learners in the health professions can improve their clinical skills and knowledge in the learning environment (T1), which translates to improved performance in the clinical environment (T2), and results in better patient or public health outcomes for the public and community (T3). Barsuk and Szmuilowicz (2015) recently extended this model to include "T4," representing impact on unplanned populations or targets in the clinic, at the bedside, and in the community—for example, the impact of a mastery learning and testing program on non-participating trainees and

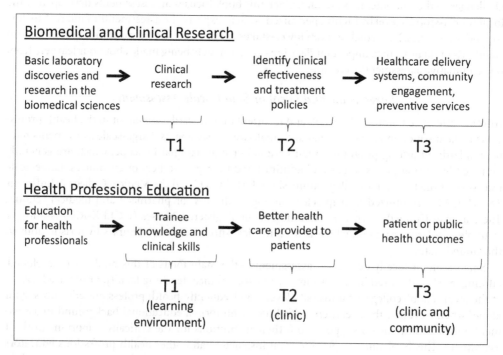

Figure 1.3 Translational science in health professions education

the learning culture. Consideration of the intended and unintended impact or consequences of assessment programs is discussed in detail in Chapters 2 and 17.

The translational science model reminds us that the ultimate goal of educating health professionals through robust assessments and instructional approaches is to improve our learners' performance in clinical settings, and ultimately, to improve patient outcomes and the health of the community.

SUMMARY

This introduction provided the general context and overview for this book. Most of the concepts introduced in this chapter are expanded on and detailed in later chapters. We hope that this introductory chapter provides the basic vocabulary and most essential concepts and principles needed to comprehend some of the more technical aspects of following chapters.

Christine McGuire, a major contributor to assessment theory and practice in medical education, once said: "Evaluation is probably the most logical field in the world and if you use a little bit of logic, it just fits together and jumps at you. . . . It's very common sense" (Harris & Simpson, 2005, p. 68). We agree with McGuire's statement. While there is much technical nuance and much statistical elaboration to assessment topics in health professions education, we should never lose sight of the mostly commonsense nature of the enterprise. On the other hand, as Voltaire noted, "Common sense is very rare" (1962, p. 467)! The goal of this book is to bring state-of-the-art assessment theory and practice to health professions educators, so that their learners will benefit from quality assessments that become "common" in their curricula.

Note: Additional material and resources may be available at the UIC AHPE website: https://go.uic.edu/AHPE

REFERENCES

Accreditation Council for Graduate Medical Education. (2000). *ACGME outcome project*. Chicago, IL: ACGME.

Accreditation Council for Graduate Medical Education and the American Board of Internal Medicine. (2015). *The internal medicine milestone project*. Chicago, IL: Accreditation Council for Graduate Medical Education. Retrieved from www.acgme.org/Portals/0/PDFs/Milestones/InternalMedicineMilestones.pdf. Accessed March 11, 2019.

Allen, J.P., Pianta, R.C., Gregory, A., Mikami, A.Y., & Lun, J. (2011). An interaction-based approach to enhancing secondary school instruction and student achievement. *Science, 333*, 1034–1036.

American Educational Research Association, American Psychological Association, & National Council on Measurement in Education. (2014). *Standards for educational and psychological testing*. Washington, DC: American Educational Research Association.

Association of American Medical Colleges. (2014). *Core entrustable professional activities for entering residency*. Washington, DC: AAMC.

Barrows, H.S., & Abrahamson, S. (1964). The programmed patient: A technique for appraising student performance in clinical neurology. *Journal of Medical Education, 39*, 802–805.

Barsuk, J.H., & Szmuilowicz, E. (2015). Chapter 10: Evaluating medical procedures: Evaluation and transfer to the bedside. In L.N. Pangaro & W.C. McGaghie (Eds.), *Handbook on medical student evaluation and assessment*. North Syracuse, NY: Gegensatz Press.

Bloom, B.S., Engelhart, M.D., Furst, E.J., Hill, W.H., & Krathwohl, D.R. (1956). *Taxonomy of educational objectives*. New York: Longmans Green.

Downing, S.M. (2002). Assessment of knowledge with written test forms. In G.R. Norman, C.P.M. van der Vleuten, & D.I. Newble (Eds.), *International handbook for research in medical education* (pp. 647–672). Dordrecht, The Netherlands: Kluwer Academic Publishers.

Downing, S.M. (2003). Validity: On the meaningful interpretation of assessment data. *Medical Education, 37*, 830–837.

Haladyna, T.M. (1999). When should we use a multiple-choice format? A paper presented at the annual meeting of the American Educational Research Association, Montreal, CA, April.

Harden, R., Stevenson, M., Downie, W., & Wilson, M. (1975). Assessment of clinical competence using objective structured examinations. *British Medical Journal, 1,* 447–451.

Harris, I.B., & Simpson, D. (2005). Christine McGuire: At the heart of the maverick measurement maven. *Advances in Health Sciences Education, 10,* 65–80.

Howell, D.C. (2002). *Statistical methods for psychology* (5th ed.) Pacific Grove, CA: Duxbury-Wadsworth Group.

Lane, S., Raymond, M.R., & Haladyna, T.M. (2015). *Handbook of test development* (2nd ed.). New York: Routledge.

McGaghie, W.C. (2010). Medical education research as translational science. *Science Translational Medicine, 2*(19), 1–3.

Miller, G. (1990). The assessment of clinical skills/competence/performance. *Academic Medicine, 65,* s63–67.

Nasca, T.J., Philibert, I., Brigham, T., & Flynn, T.C. (2012). The next GME accreditation system—rationale and benefits. *The New England Journal of Medicine, 366*(11), 1051–1056.

Park, Y.S., Hodges, B., & Tekian, A. (2016). Evaluating the paradigm shift from time-based toward competency-based medical education: Implications for curriculum and assessment. In P.F. Wimmers & M. Mentkowski (Eds.), *Assessing competence in professional performance across disciplines and professions* (pp. 411–425). New York: Springer.

Popham, W.J., & Husek, T.R. (1969). Implications of criterion-referenced measurement. *Journal of Educational Measurement, 7,* 367–375.

Scriven, M. (1967). The methodology of evaluation. In R. Tyler, R. Gagne, & M. Scriven (Eds.), *Perspectives of curriculum evaluation* (pp. 39–83). Chicago, IL: Rand McNally.

Sireci, S.G., & Zenisky, A.L. (2006). Innovative item formats in computer-based testing: In pursuit of improved construct representation. In S.M. Downing & T.M. Haladyna (Eds.), *Handbook of test development* (pp. 329–348). Mahwah, NJ: Lawrence Erlbaum Associates.

Swanson, D.B., & van der Vleuten, C.P.M. (2013). Assessment of clinical skills with standardized patients: State of the art revisited. *Teaching and Learning in Medicine, 25*(sup1), S17–S25.

ten Cate, O. (2013). Nuts and bolts of entrustable professional activities. *Journal of Graduate Medical Education, 5*(1), 157–158.

Thissen, D., & Wainer, H. (2001). *Test scoring.* Mahwah, NJ: Lawrence Erlbaum Associates.

Voltaire. (1962). *Philosophical dictionary* (Gay, P., trans.). New York: Basic Books, Inc.

Wallace, P. (1997). Following the threads of an innovation: The history of standardized patients in medical education. *CADUCEUS, 13*(2), 5–28.

Welch, C. (2006). Item and prompt development in performance testing. In S.M. Downing & T.M. Haladyna (Eds.), *Handbook of test development* (pp. 303–328). Mahwah, NJ: Lawrence Erlbaum Associates.

William, R.G., Klaman, D.A., & McGaghie, W.C. (2003). Cognitive, social, and environmental sources of bias in clinical performance ratings. *Teaching and Learning in Medicine, 15*(4), 270–292.

Woolf, S.H. (2008). The meaning of translational research and why it matters. *JAMA, 299*(2), 211–213.

Yoon, K.S., Duncan, T., Lee, S., W.Y., Scarloss, B., & Shapley, K. (2007). *Reviewing the evidence on how teacher professional development affects student achievement.* [Issues & Answers Report, REL 2007-No. 033]. Washington, DC: U.S. Department of Education, Institute of Educational Sciences, National Center for Education Evaluation and Regional Assistance, Regional Educational Laboratory Southwest.

2

VALIDITY AND QUALITY
Matthew Lineberry

The reasons for educational testing or assessment can seem straightforward—for instance, "to measure learners' ability to conduct a basic physical examination." However, there are always many questions underlying such seemingly simple purposes. For instance, how do we define this knowledge, skill, or ability we are interested in—what is it, and what is it not? How might we best measure it, and how will we know we are measuring it accurately? What do we hope to achieve by measuring it? How might our measurement activities lead to expenses, logistical hurdles, or even unexpected negative outcomes?

Done well, assessments can be powerful tools to inform decision-making and foster learning and growth in health professions education. However, it can be difficult to know what the criteria should be for a "good" and "valid" assessment for some given purpose and to determine whether a certain assessment meets those criteria. Leading assessment theorists still disagree even on what the term "validity" should mean (Messick, 1995; Borsboom, Mellenbergh, & van Heerden, 2004; Cizek, 2012; Kane, 2013; St-Onge, Young, Eva, & Hodges, 2017)! This chapter is meant to clarify important concepts and frameworks, so practitioners and scholars can apply more effective critical thinking in the design, practice, and evaluation of assessments.

THE PRINCIPLE OF PURPOSE-DRIVEN ASSESSMENT

I suspect many people hold a value that assessments, and measurements generally, should be *objective*, measuring some attribute without our biases contaminating the scores. For instance, we might suppose we should be able to measure the length of a rock without regard for *why* the measurement is taking place. Length is a real attribute of objects, after all, and rulers cannot be affected by our inner assumptions and motives. Can they?

Actually, the "why" behind measurement does matter, even for attributes as basic as length. After all, that measurement system is comprised of not just a ruler, but also a human who decides which ruler to use, what to treat as the longitudinal aspect of the rock, and how precise to be. They also perceive the score along the ruler with whatever visual acuity they possess, and record the value in some way, given their abilities and motivations, then share that score with others as information in some fashion. The length a high school student might desultorily scratch down to satisfy a science class requirement could be quite different than that measured by, say, a geologist for whom slight differences could suggest different interpretations about geological history among their scholarly community.

The appropriate way forward is not just to "be more objective" in the abstract, as if we could or should eliminate all our values and goals for conducting assessments. Rather, we should be reflective about our values and goals. Assessment in health professions education is always first and foremost *instrumental*: it is a deliberate intervention we take in the world, meant to accomplish some goals (Cook & Lineberry, 2016). Our final purpose in an assessment is almost never really "to measure [*x* attribute] as accurately as possible," for instance. Our *real* goals are often more like, "to provide learners with prompt feedback, which we hope that they use to improve their self-directed learning later that month during clerkships; also, to identify and remediate learners who might not be ready for the next educational experience otherwise; all within our resources, and hopefully without any negative consequences." If an assessment vendor told you they could improve how accurately you measure [*x*], but it would delay feedback to learners by a month and break your budget, you would probably decline their services—because "accuracy" only matters to the extent it serves your true goals.

So, we might say that a "good" assessment indeed measures what it is meant to measure, but most importantly, that it helps us achieve our specific goals with reasonable expense and minimal negative outcomes. For this chapter, I will define assessment "validity" as the extent to which an assessment system supports valid inferences about the attribute meant to be measured. More broadly, assessment "quality" is the extent to which a given application of an assessment and use of its scores leads to outcomes that are positive, on the balance, given one's values and goals.

UNDERSTANDING YOUR PURPOSES

A first step in any assessment endeavor is to thoroughly describe your **target attribute**: what you hope your assessment scores will mean. Think for now not of a certain *format* of assessment, only about the actual underlying attribute of interest.

Suppose you want to measure learners' "unprofessionalism," for instance. Well, what is and is not included in "unprofessionalism": knowledge, attitudes, beliefs, behaviors, or some combination? What are the prototypical features of an "unprofessional" behavior: is it that the behavior is against prevailing norms, and if so, whose norms, and which ones, for what era? Are *potentially* harmful behaviors unprofessional, or must an actual harm have occurred? Is ill intent required, or can mistakes also be unprofessional? Are certain behaviors universally unprofessional, or does it depend on the context in which it happens, and if so, how? How is "unprofessionalism" similar to and different from related ideas, like "counterproductive work behaviors" and "workplace deviance"? Are you interested in "unprofessionalism" as some fixed trait each person possesses, or do you suppose it might vary for each person across different contexts? These questions help define your target attribute, aka your "construct." Any lack of clarity here will only cause confusion later.

Next, consider your **planned uses** of scores. For instance, are you mostly interested in identifying learners with especially unprofessional behaviors so you can try a remediation program for them, or are you hoping to select the "Most Professional Student of the Year" for an award, or something in between? Will you be giving feedback to those assessed, and if so, how do you hope they will apply that feedback? Will you share the results with other educators or administrators? Might the results be used to select those assessed for sanctions or dismissal? Will aggregated scores be used to compare your institution to other institutions? Different answers to these questions call for quite different assessment approaches and have different implications for validity and quality.

Finally, broadly consider your **goals** and **anti-goals** for pursuing an assessment endeavor—that is, what you hope will and will not happen. Do you care if those assessed consider the process fair, useful, or enjoyable? Is it important that certain stakeholders support and promote the assessment endeavor? What costs are acceptable? Are there any ways people might react negatively to the assessment, and do you want to detect or avoid those? Do you hope that other institutions will consider your assessment so good that they want to use it?

With all these considerations in mind, we can almost talk of validity and quality, but we need one more element.

TYING METHODS TO YOUR PURPOSES

You get to imagine "perfection" in defining your intentions above, but of course you then must *operationalize* that into an actual system of assessment—the specific methods by which you will collect observations that hopefully reflect your target attribute, the rules you'll use for assigning scores to those observations, the format in which you will give feedback, any informational or public relations efforts you will pursue, and so on. Making good choices about those methods is of course complex and comprises much of the guidance for the rest of this book. Whatever methods you select, though, you ought to have a reasonable—and preferably explicit—**logical argument** for why those methods are suitable to the interpretations, uses, and goals you outlined earlier. Formal logic is an entire subdiscipline within philosophy, so it is not possible to guide every aspect of building an argument here. Thankfully, in many cases, relatively simple chains of logic likely suffice, and even just lists of assumptions are very useful.

For example, suppose you decided to assess the attribute "conflict management skill" among third-year medical students by having examinees converse with simulated colleagues or patients (SPs for short). One encounter might feature an SP portraying a colleague that just verbally mistreated a patient, for instance. The examinee's goal in that encounter might be to de-escalate the situation and prompt the colleague to reflect on their behavior, then apologize and make amends with the patient. At the end of each encounter, suppose you decide the SPs will complete a score sheet and immediately give examinees feedback. You mostly hope that as a result, through the rest of their clerkships, all examinees will better take advantage of opportunities to practice and improve their conflict management. Finally, whenever learners' scores are especially low, you will have them return for one or more extra encounters until they can demonstrate acceptable performance.

A thorough chain of logical assumptions for why those methods should lead to valid and useful scores, and an overall effective assessment endeavor, might include:

1. The rubric of behaviors to observe and the scoring rules for each possible behavior assign credit properly, weighted according to how effective vs. ineffective behaviors are in the actual work environment.
2. The number of encounters each examinee completes and the variety of behaviors displayed across encounters suitably sample what they are likely to encounter in the actual work environment.
3. All examinees *know* what ineffective and effective management behaviors are, so if they do not show them in the assessment, it is correct to call that a lack of "skill" (rather than an undiagnosed knowledge deficit).
4. All examinees understand the purpose of the assessment, e.g., no one believes these are "physical self-defense"-focused encounters.
5. All SPs portray behaviors that prompt skilled examinees to act appropriately—so for instance, no SPs are acting so agitated that examinees might reasonably think, "this person is dangerous; I should be trying to isolate them and call police."
6. SPs respond realistically to effective vs. ineffective examinee behaviors, e.g., they do not de-escalate irrespective of examinee mistakes, nor do they overreact to early mistakes in a way that makes the rest of the encounter unrealistically difficult or unfair.

7. SPs behave similarly across different examination days, and examinees perform similarly well across days, such that the certain day to which an examinee is assigned for the assessment makes no difference.
8. Even while portraying their role, SPs can . . .

    a. thoroughly notice relevant examinee behaviors;
    b. remember examinee behaviors after the encounter;
    c. score behaviors accurately and consistently; and
    d. give feedback that is comprehensible, memorable, and which prompts examinees' reflection and improvement.

9. Examinees are able and motivated to . . .

    a. attend to feedback;
    b. remember feedback; and
    c. formulate effective plans for how to improve their performance.

10. Soon enough after the assessment to reinforce their learning, examinees . . .

    a. have opportunities to practice conflict management;
    b. notice those opportunities;
    c. are able and motivated to experiment with new behaviors in those opportunities; and
    d. receive feedback on their performance that supports further learning (e.g., no peers or supervisors of theirs will give feedback that contradicts the intended learning objectives).

11. Examinees are suitably identified for remediation, according to either especially subpar performance in one encounter or modestly subpar performance across several encounters.
12. The threshold for picking examinees to remediate discriminates well between those prepared vs. not prepared to acceptably practice and learn conflict management independently going forward.
13. Examinees who are selected for remediation value the opportunity for additional practice and do not have any serious negative sequelae (e.g., hopelessness; judgment or isolation from other students; adversarial attitude toward educators).
14. The entire assessment system is feasible within acceptable expenditures of resources.

This is admittedly a long list, but its power is in its thoroughness. If all these assumptions hold true, you probably have a very valid and effective assessment system! But, if any *one* assumption is severely broken, later assumptions might be difficult or impossible to meet, and the endeavor may not meet your goals. If, for instance, your SPs are very capricious in the examinee behaviors that they notice, remember, score, and give feedback on, your assessment might have lots of false positives and false negatives for the remediation decision, and examinees may not learn much from the experience. They might even lose trust in the educational environment. So, it is worth defining these assumptions, then being attentive to whether they hold true—that is, conducting some degree of both "validity investigation" and "quality evaluation."

INVESTIGATING VALIDITY, EVALUATING QUALITY

For any assessment endeavor, we should ask, "Am I measuring the attribute that I meant to, given how I am interpreting and using scores?" When you systematically ask that and seek discriminating data, I suggest calling that a **validity investigation**. (Many people currently call that "validation," but that term implies a problematic bias toward confirmatory results. If a friend calls me and asks me to "validate" their emotions about a personal crisis, I do not think they mean that they want me to rigorously test whether they should be having those emotions!) We should also be asking, "Is pursuing this assessment endeavor accomplishing what I hoped it would, without too many negative consequences?" This is a somewhat separate question from the earlier one, and so I propose calling that a **quality evaluation**. Hopefully that term better conveys what is really being questioned, which is "quality" (or if you prefer, "suitability"). After all, a test might be "valid" in the above sense, but lead to unacceptable negative effects and therefore be of low quality or suitability for one's ultimate purposes. "Evaluation" also reminds us to take a broad view of this question, in the spirit of the relevant field of *program evaluation*, since we are questioning how the assessment exerts positive and negative influences in the big, messy education and healthcare systems within which it is being used.

Up to this point, I avoided referring to formal theories or frameworks from the science and practice of assessment, hoping that two things are apparent without reference to such formal approaches: (1) there are many critical-thinking questions to ask oneself when conducting an assessment, and (2) those questions are not especially technical, but rather flow logically from a consideration of what you are trying to accomplish and its underlying assumptions. I believe there is a risk of seeing assessment development and evaluation as *formulaic* and *technical*, when it really should seem *logical*, specific to your context. There is no one gold standard assessment design, nor is there a universal best possible design of a validity investigation or quality evaluation; it all depends on your goals and context.

That said, with a clear view of what you are trying to accomplish, technical standards and theoretical guidance become very useful to help shape your critical thinking, as well as to communicate with other education professionals and scholars in commonly accepted terms. In my personal practice of assessment leadership and management, I prefer to "think for myself" first and then check my thinking against several frameworks. Below, I will review several of the more influential contemporary concepts and frameworks.

KANE'S VALIDITY FRAMEWORK: THE VALIDITY ARGUMENT

One recent and influential validity framework comes from Kane (2013), a scholar from the Educational Testing Service (ETS), which administers several large-scale standardized assessments primarily in the United States. A health-professions-specific guide to Kane's framework is also available (Cook, Brydges, Ginsburg, & Hatala, 2015). Perhaps the most significant new contribution the framework makes to prior assessment validity thinking is its focus on your *purposes* and closely accompanying *argument* for an assessment. Kane refers to your assessment purpose statement and underlying assumptions as your "interpretation/use argument" (IUA), akin to the list of assumptions we outlined earlier. Once you rigorously evaluate that IUA with logic and data, that results in what Kane calls your "validity argument."

Kane suggests there are four broad categories of assumptions (or "inferences") that should at least be considered in all cases, organized from narrow to broad:

1. **Scoring**: that the observed scores accurately reflect how well examinees performed on the assessment they experienced;
2. **Generalization**: that the observed scores are an unbiased, reliable reflection of examinees' "universe" scores—the imaginary scores produced if we could observe performance across all possible ostensibly irrelevant or trivial differences in assessment conditions (e.g., different but similar items, raters, days of the week, response formats, etc.);
3. **Extrapolation**: that the observed scores are suitably predictive of performance that we really care about (e.g., clinical reasoning with real patients, rather than the simulated patients in the assessment environment); and
4. **Decisions**: that the observed scores inform decisions suitably (e.g., without introducing biases) and lead to suitable consequences for anyone affected by the assessment.

Many of our assumptions in the previous example can be mapped to Kane's inferences. For instance:

- If examinees display effective conflict-management behaviors, but SPs fail to notice, remember, and score those (Assumptions 8a–c), the "Scoring" inference is compromised. In a nutshell: *Performance happened in the assessment, but it didn't make it into the score.*
- If the day of the week on which assessments take place relates to scores—e.g., if examinees on Fridays are stressed by additional exams that take place then, or early examinees give performance hints to subsequent examinees—that would violate Assumption 7 above and compromise the "Generalization" inference.
  Trivial particulars about the assessment procedures mattered in a way they should not have.
- If the cues and challenges in the assessment experience don't really correspond to important cues and challenges in real-world conflict management (Assumption 2), the "Extrapolation" inference is compromised.
  Assessment performance did not correspond to our real-world attribute of interest.
- If the remediation decision rule yields lots of false positives and negatives—or if there is not any benefit to discriminating between examinees that way, and everyone would benefit equally from remediation (Assumptions 11–13)—then the "Decision" inference is compromised.
  Scores did not help make better decisions and/or support better consequences.

Besides Kane's organizing framework, there are many other important insights from his writing. One comforting point is that Kane does not encourage boundaryless validity investigation. Rather, one should always clearly spell out their IUA, then ask: (a) which assumptions are the weakest (i.e., their *prior uncertainty*), (b) for which assumptions can a study give discriminating answers (*information yield*), (c) how *affordable* would a study be, and (d) how much will resolution of this uncertainty affect decision makers' considerations for or against implementing the assessment (*leverage*, or perhaps "political yield")? If you multiply those answers together, you will have a sense of how suitable a certain assumption is for empirical testing. That is, if the answer to any of these questions is effectively zero for some assumption, then that assumption should probably not be tested empirically—at least not yet. Table 2.1 shares an interpretation and use statement, and

Table 2.1 Example Interpretation and Use Statement, and Selected Interpretation and Use Argument Considerations, for an Objective Structured Clinical Examination

---

Interpretation and use statement:

"Our goals are to ensure all students are prepared to pass the USMLE Step 2 Clinical Skills Examination, and to apply basic history and physical examination abilities during their clerkships for common patient conditions.

"As part of meeting these goals, we intend to measure our third-year medical students' abilities to perform a suitable history and physical examination for patients presenting with any of 40 common underlying conditions. (We will use a separate assessment to support their learning regarding the creation of suitable patient notes with diagnoses and initial plans for follow-up.)

"We will assess this by having students perform history and physical examinations in eight different encounters with standardized patients. For each encounter, there will be a case-specific checklist of history questions and physical examination maneuvers that should be performed during the encounter. After each encounter, the standardized patients will complete that checklist. At the end of the eight-encounter circuit, scores will be combined for each learner and e-mailed to them. Learners who score below an established cut score on an encounter will be required to retake that encounter; if they score below the cut score for three or more encounters, they will be required to retake the entire circuit. However, only a few days and a limited number of remediation encounters are available; priority will be given to scheduling retakes for students scoring below the cut score on the most encounters."

Inference	Example assumptions (not comprehensive)	Example considerations for each assumption (including *prior uncertainty, information yield, affordability to study, and/or political yield*)
Scoring	Each case's checklist of history and physical examination maneuvers contains all items essential for safe and effective care, and no nonessential items.	"We belong to a consortium that develops these checklists and has them reviewed by many clinicians, so I am pretty certain this assumption is met. Then again, there has been some recent research suggesting even well-designed checklists often miss important items. All the same, I think we can accept some risk here without collecting new data."
Generalization	SPs are consistently displaying the cues that should trigger learners' recognition of suitable history questions and physical examination maneuvers.	"We have thorough training for SPs, but I have heard concerns about their performance consistency. Student workers could watch a small sample of encounters and see whether cues were being displayed consistently. That would be affordable and informative, and we could address issues if we see any; for instance, we might bolster SP refresher training. So, let's collect that data."
Extrapolation	Performance challenges in the SP encounters closely correspond to challenges with actual patients.	"For several of our physical examination maneuvers, we aren't really simulating findings—for instance, SPs can't manipulate their cardiac rhythm, so we just tell the learner what they would hear. I'm also not sure our SP portrayals are consistent with the styles of communication our patients use. We could do a structured investigation about the fidelity of our cases in relation to what learners are seeing on their clerkships . . . perhaps using structured interviews? That sounds like it will require time to develop, to determine the right questions. That might become affordable if we can make that part of an education master's degree student's thesis project. It could provide useful information, and we have the ability to act on that information."
Decisions (or "Consequences")	Learners recall their areas for improvement into the future, to watch for opportunities to practice those areas.	"I saw an article suggesting that learners often don't recall much feedback from an OSCE, so I am concerned about this assumption. All our learners complete a survey during a different simulation a month after this OSCE; we could ask them what top two learning points they recall from the OSCE and cross-reference that with the feedback we e-mailed them initially. Collecting that data is easy, but the cross-referencing could be difficult, since learners might recall a feedback point but phrase it in a unique way. Here again, this might be a good candidate for a small formal study as part of a capstone project or thesis, so perhaps we can find someone with time and motivation to code those survey responses. If we found that learners rarely recall their feedback points, we could do something about that—maybe create a more memorable environment for sharing the feedback, like a formal review with a faculty member."

several considerations for key inferences, for an SP-based objective structured clinical examination (OSCE) of history taking and physical examination ability.

It will be impossible to collect data about all assumptions, and that is fine, just as lawyers craft legal arguments, trusting that jurors will believe very logical assumptions but need evidence for the least obvious assumptions. So, validity arguments should include explicit acknowledgements when assumptions are not yet tested and why, with no guilt over making wise decisions *not* to test certain assumptions. For instance, in a recent paper on assessment of examinees' learning curves in developing electrocardiogram interpretation skill, Hatala, Gutman, Lineberry, Triola, and Pusic (2018) stated clearly that they were unable to test the Generalization inference, due to limitations in the data available and complexities inherent in the IUA (since analyzing "learning curves" rather than discrete "points in time" made for novel, yet-unresolved conceptual issues). Reviewers and consumers of assessment work should not expect impossibly or unnecessarily comprehensive validity investigations, and instead should value clear statements of one's IUA accompanied with judicious data collection. Similarly, we hope that when users make arguably very minor changes to assessment systems, they do not feel compelled to "start from scratch" with validity investigation efforts, or even necessarily to collect any new data at all.

MESSICK'S VALIDITY FRAMEWORK: SOURCES OF EVIDENCE

A predecessor of Kane, Samuel Messick, is credited with a validity framework that is dominant within the joint *Standards for Educational and Psychological Testing* of the American Educational Research Association (AERA), American Psychological Association (APA), and the National Council on Measurement in Education (NCME) (2014). When cited, Messick's validity thinking (1995) is most often characterized in reference to defining five sources of "validity evidence":

1. **Content evidence**: that assessment tasks, phrasing of items or formatting of performance challenges, and scoring are all suitably aligned with the target attribute;
2. **Response process evidence**: that examinees' cognitions and behaviors when responding to assessments tasks are consistent with the intended interpretation and uses of scores—and so too are the cognitions and behaviors of any observers or raters who generate scores;
3. **Internal structure evidence**: that scores on items within an assessment relate to one another in the way predicted by one's intended interpretation and uses—e.g., that several items all meant to measure the same attribute indeed correlate to one another accordingly;
4. **Relations to other variables evidence**: that scores relate to other attributes the test is meant to predict and to measures of similar constructs, and that they do *not* relate to conceptually distinct or irrelevant variables (e.g., that scores do not vary by examinee gender or race); and
5. **Consequences evidence**: that score interpretation and use leads to suitable positive consequences and minimal negative consequences.

Messick's later work (1995) referred to a sixth source of evidence, **generalizability**, which he indicated was synonymous with the term **reliability** and deemed an "aspect of construct validity." However, the joint *Standards* (AERA, APA, & NCME, 2014) cast reliability as "an independent characteristic of test scores," though one with "implications for validity," and relegate it to a separate chapter. All that to say, there is some confusion here, and it manifests in continuing variability in how people categorize reliability-related evidence. For instance, some HPE articles fold reliability in with "internal structure" validity evidence (Cook, Zendejas, Hamstra, Hatala, & Brydges, 2014; Downing, 2003), though reliability is distinct conceptually from internal structure concerns. For instance, you can have an assessment where the items' relationships to each other are consistent with your theory about the internal structure of the underlying construct(s), but the reliability of scoring can still be unacceptably low, and vice versa (Cortina, 1993; Schmitt, 1996).

Table 2.2 lists common types of evidence under each category of the Messick framework, and for clarity, I separate "Generalizability/Reliability" into a sixth category. These can be thought of as a "menu" of specific types of evidence you can select from when your IUA reveals controversial or uncertain assumptions. Depending on which of Kane's inferences you are considering, certain "menu options" in Messick's framework are more relevant. Sometimes this is very straightforward:

Table 2.2 Examples of Evidence for Written Examinations and Performance Tests Within Each of Messick's Sources of Validity Evidence

Source of Validity Evidence	Example Evidence for Written Examinations	Example Evidence for Performance Examinations
Content	• Degree of agreement between the assessment "blueprint" for proportions of items covering each content area and the relative importance of those content areas • Quality of item development specifications and processes • Actual adherence to item development specifications and processes • Expertise, relevant experience, and/or training of item writers • Correspondence between intended construct and item format (e.g., proper formatting for items meant to assess "memory" vs. "application" of knowledge) • Suitability of observed item difficulties, given expectations for learner population performance	• Degree of agreement between the assessment "blueprint" for underlying disease states, challenges, etc., and the relative importance or prevalence of those • If simulation-based: Quality of case development specifications and simulation processes • If simulation-based: Actual adherence to case development specifications and simulation processes • Expertise, relevant experience, and/or training of item writers • Correspondence between intended construct and performance format (e.g., requiring actual performance of psychomotor tasks, rather than saying "I would cannulate the vein now") • Suitability of observed case and/or difficulties, given expectations for learner population performance
Response Process	• "Think aloud" with examinees and/or direct observation, to ensure the intended construct is determining their responses (not, for instance, confusion over item wording, construct-irrelevant clues to correct answers, or use of "cheat sheets") • "Think aloud" with item raters for manually scored responses (e.g., essays) to ensure the intended construct is determining their ratings (not, for instance, construct-irrelevant cues such as "length of text") • Quality control checks on any score processing (e.g., use of scanning to convert written responses into digital data)	• "Think aloud" with examinees to ensure the intended construct is determining their responses (not, for instance, confusion over poorly simulated aspects of the encounter or construct-irrelevant clues to correct performance) • "Think aloud" with performance raters to ensure the intended construct is determining their ratings (not, for instance, construct-irrelevant cues such as "learners' apparent confidence") • Quality control checks on any score processing (e.g., computer-based computation of composite scores)
Internal Structure	• Internal consistency estimates across items (e.g., coefficient alpha) • Exploratory and/or confirmatory factor analyses consistent with any use of total scores and/or subscores	• Internal consistency estimates across cases and/or observation items (e.g., coefficient alpha) • Exploratory and/or confirmatory factor analyses consistent with any use of total scores and/or subscores
Relations to Other Variables	• Suitable correspondence (or not) with scores from similar (or unrelated) variables, e.g., differential test functioning studies showing no bias according to gender, ethnicity, etc.	• Suitable correspondence (or not) with scores from similar (or unrelated) variables (e.g., positive correlation between assessment scores and performance in the clinical environment)

(Continued)

Table 2.2 (continued)

Source of Validity Evidence	Example Evidence for Written Examinations	Example Evidence for Performance Examinations
Conse-quences	• Suitability of pass/fail processes and decisions • Effects on examinees, e.g., change in knowledge or skill, attitude, motivation, or well-being • Effects on educators, e.g., change in content focus during instruction, individualization for learners based on assessment results, etc. • Broader effects, e.g., improvement in diagnostic accuracy for patients • Detection of unintended consequences (either positive or negative)	• Suitability of pass/fail processes and decisions • Effects on examinees, e.g., change in knowledge or skill, attitude, motivation, or well-being • Effects on educators, e.g., change in content focus during instruction, individualization for learners based on assessment results, etc. • Broader effects, e.g., improvement in sterility during patient procedures • Detection of unintended consequences (either positive or negative)
Generaliza-bility/ Reliability*	• Adequate number of items to sample targeted content areas • Adequate number of assessment occasions to sample across any construct-irrelevant variations over time • Adequate number of raters (for manually scored assessments) to sample across construct-irrelevant rater variance	• Adequate number of cases and/or items to sample targeted content areas • Adequate number of assessment occasions to sample across any construct-irrelevant variations over time • Adequate number of raters to sample across construct-irrelevant rater variance

* Despite inconsistency in the assessment literature as to whether Generalizability/Reliability should be considered an aspect of validity, most health professions education validity studies using the Messick framework consider generalizability/reliability within internal structure validity evidence (Downing, 2003).

Kane "Generalization" inferences usually call for elements in the "Generalizability/Reliability" evidence source, for instance. Similarly, Kane "Decision" inferences seem to exclusively call for "Consequences" evidence sources. In other cases, there is not a simple mapping between Kane inferences and Messick evidence sources, so it may be safest to thoroughly consider many or all Messick evidence sources as being potentially relevant to each Kane inference (Cook & Hatala, 2016). For instance, there are several types of Messick evidence sources that are relevant to Kane's "Scoring" inference: setting an appropriate scoring key falls under Messick's "Content" source, making observations accurately falls under "Response process," and the justification for items to be combined into a total score falls under "Internal structure". To test Kane's "Extrapolation" evidence, it can be suitable to see whether test scores relate to scores on some important real-world criterion like patient outcomes, which is Messick's "Relations to other variables"; making sure that your blueprint for items corresponds well to the domains that are important in the real world falls under Messick's "Content" source.

Messick's framework may be most familiar to HPE scholars and practitioners currently. However, even it is rarely cited in HPE research, being applied in only 3% of reports in one review of simulation-based assessment studies (Cook et al., 2014). A key weakness of the Messick framework is the relative inattention to how sources of validity evidence should be prioritized and connected to one's purposes (Cook & Hatala, 2016), or how sources of evidence should support one another in a logical chain. Understandably but unfortunately, this can encourage scholars to conduct assessment validity investigations aimed at collecting at least one bit of evidence from each of the five Messick sources, without consideration for whether they were collecting *discriminating* evidence about *controversial* assumptions. Using Kane to guide logic, and Messick to think broadly about potential sources of evidence, makes for a powerful combination.

EVALUATION FRAMEWORKS

The evaluation of broad consequences of assessment has been somewhat of an afterthought in assessment scholarship and practice, and it is rarely reported (Cook et al., 2014). Part of this may be due to the conceptual confusion from past attempts to combine consequences with other validity considerations. After all, if validity reflects "measuring what one meant to," then it seems strange to say a test is "invalid" just because it is too expensive, for instance. Borsboom et al. (2004), Cizek (2012), Shadish, Cook, and Campbell (2002), and van der Vleuten (1996) suggest using other terms such as "justification," "overall quality," or "utility" when referring to the consequences of assessment interpretation and use.

Cook and Lineberry (2016) proposed a framework for identifying potential consequences of assessment interpretation and use, meant to help scholars envision the diverse ways that consequences might arise. Slightly adapted from that work, I propose that any consequence has four important dimensions to consider: (a) the *recipients* of consequences, which could range from examinees and educators all the way up to society at large; (b) the *timing* of consequences being triggered, whereby consequences can be due to anticipation of an assessment, the activity of completing an assessment, or the interpretation and use of scores after an assessment; (c) whether consequences are *intended* or *unintended*; and (d) whether consequences are *beneficial* and/or *harmful* from the perspective of each recipient. Arguably, consequences constitute the most important aspect of one's validity and quality considerations. If a test does not achieve what you want it to achieve or causes major problems, it does not matter much if it is accurate; you are not going to use it.

The often-unintended nature of consequences has special implications for us. For a well-formulated validity argument, it should generally be possible to *prospectively* determine what data are needed to test controversial assumptions. However, in the case of assessment consequences, we must cast a "wide net," collecting data that could alert us to effects we had not anticipated. For instance, we might include relatively open-ended sampling of perspectives from many stakeholders—not just examinees.

TAKING A PREVENTION FOCUS: UNDERSTANDING THREATS TO VALIDITY

Since assessment validity investigation and quality evaluation is a logical process, it features certain typical logical "fallacies": common ways that assumptions fail to hold or that unintended influences creep into our interpretations, called threats to validity or validity threats. Just as it is useful to check your thinking carefully against the major validity frameworks, it is useful to review lists of common validity threats and ask whether any might be at play in your assessment context. "Threat"-focused thinking is a prevention-focused parallel to the thinking you applied in outlining your assumptions: the assumptions are what you hope will happen, and the threats are the ways they might not happen.

Threats to validity can be grouped into two basic categories. *Construct-irrelevant variance* ("CIV") is at play when scores are being affected by something *other* than your target attribute. For instance, if you mean to test "diagnostic accuracy," but your case descriptions use slang that is only familiar to people from the northeastern United States, the test could inadvertently be a test of "examinee location." *Construct underrepresentation* ("CU") is when scores only reflect part of the target attribute and are missing other important parts. For instance, if you mean to broadly test "diagnostic accuracy," but your test only features diabetes and hypotension cases, it might fail to reflect how examinees would perform with other common diagnoses. That example reflects *systematic* failure to sample subcategories of a target attribute; you can also underrepresent the attribute simply by sampling too few data points, i.e., without any systematic bias.

Since "validity" and "quality" are distinct concepts, it is useful to also think about "quality" threats for consequences of assessment practices. Again, if a test is very expensive, that does not necessarily threaten its measurement validity, but it does make it hard to implement and therefore of lower overall quality. Table 2.3 lists 58 distinct validity and quality threats, organized according to how they can cause breakdowns in logic within an IUA. Even that long list is not comprehensive, and it is especially not comprehensive for "Decisions & Consequences"; as the field considers consequences more closely, we will likely discover many more common concerns there. However, I hope that carefully reviewing these concerns for your assessment endeavors helps you spot opportunities for improvement.

To end on a positive note, we should recognize that even a somewhat flawed assessment—one for which several threats are realized—might still be suitable for use. There is no easy answer to the question "how valid is valid enough?" or "how good is good enough?" Different purposes require different levels of validity evidence. A national licensing exam with the potential to impact practitioner livelihood and patient safety demands a very high level of evidence to ensure that

Table 2.3 Selected Threats to Assessment Validity and Quality

Inferences and their underlying assumptions	Selected validity/quality threats and general notes CIV = construct-irrelevant variance. CU = construct underrepresentation.
Scoring	
Accuracy of scoring key: Points assigned to examinee behaviors or choices reflect how correct those would be in the real world	• correct answer key based on faulty evidence or incorrect content experts' beliefs (CIV) • correct answer key based on limited sample of evidence or content expertise (CU) • inappropriate limitation of credit to a single "correct" response when multiple responses may be acceptable (CU) • failure to weigh item-level scores appropriately, e.g., to identify non-compensatory items that should trigger an immediate "failure" decision (CU)
Experience and interpretation of stimuli: Items, case descriptions, and/or scenarios and interactions are similarly experienced and interpreted by all examinees	• construct-irrelevant differences in reading ability (CIV) • differences in interpretation of concepts for different cultural groups (CIV) • inconsistent portrayal of scenarios by actors or simulators (CIV) *Inconsistency is especially problematic when it is systematic, e.g., if whenever examinee performance is low, the items/cases become easier or harder*
Interpretation of response options: For selected-response-format assessments: Response options are similarly and correctly interpreted by all examinees For free-response-format assessments: All examinees have a similar, correct understanding of permissible behaviors	• construct-irrelevant differences in reading ability (CIV) • differences in interpretation of concepts for different cultural groups (CIV) • varying familiarity among examinees with simulation-based or computer-mediated environments (CIV)

Inferences and their underlying assumptions	Selected validity/quality threats and general notes CIV = construct-irrelevant variance. CU = construct underrepresentation.
Examinee response process: Examinees' cognitions and behaviors during the assessment are consistent with our theory of how the target attribute leads to responses	• guessing (CIV) • cheating (CIV) • gaming, i.e., taking advantage of known idiosyncrasies in scoring, detecting subtle differences in how correct vs. incorrect responses are phrased in MCQ items, detecting "tells" in actors' behaviors during scenarios that hint at desired behaviors (CIV) • insufficient clarity about the purpose of the assessment, e.g., some examinees thinking a scenario meant to assess leadership is meant to assess medical knowledge (CIV) • insufficient cues to perform, e.g., excessively ambiguous situations (CIV) • overly strong cues to perform, e.g., a situation that makes the correct answer obvious (CU)
Rater response process: Raters' cognitions and behaviors during the assessment are consistent with our theory about how behaviors should be categorized and scored	• rater biases, e.g., excessive leniency, severity, or central tendency; first impression bias; rater drift over time; contrast effects between subsequent examinees (CIV) • insufficient and/or variable rater training (CIV) • unclear coding and scoring rules (CIV) • rater distraction/fatigue (CIV)
Internal structure: Individual items/cases relate to one another as expected, making calculation of total scores (or other composites) suitable	• lack of internal consistency among items that are added to create a composite/total score (CIV—or more specifically, "construct mis-specification"; total scores may reflect two or more underlying constructs, each of which may be a "relevant" construct but which are not *coherent* with one another) *Note that it is not always necessary to assume internal consistency among items/cases*
Generalization	
Item/case sampling: Enough items/cases are sampled to obtain sufficiently consistent scores	• insufficient sampling, especially exacerbated if examinees vary greatly in their ability to respond to specific items or cases, e.g., case specificity in clinical reasoning tasks (CU)
Rater sampling: Enough raters observe examinees to obtain sufficiently consistent scores	• insufficient sampling, especially exacerbated if raters have substantial *biases* rather than random intra-rater variability, e.g., being assigned a "hawk" vs. a "dove" rater (CU)
Occasion sampling: Examinees (and raters, if applicable) complete the assessment on enough occasions to obtain sufficiently consistent scores	• insufficient sampling, especially exacerbated if occasion effects are *systematic* rather than random, e.g., confounding of assignment to testing date with other difficult life events (CU) *Research often fails to investigate this facet; when it does, the occasion facet is often found to be a significant contributor to score unreliability*
Format sampling: Examinees complete the assessment in enough different formats to obtain sufficiently consistent scores	• insufficient sampling, especially exacerbated by systematic examinee variance in format familiarity, e.g., using novel simulation-based formats without familiarizing examinees from foreign countries who had not experienced those in prior educational experiences (CU)

(*Continued*)

Table 2.3 (continued)

Inferences and their underlying assumptions	Selected validity/quality threats and general notes CIV = construct-irrelevant variance. CU = construct underrepresentation.
Interactions among sampled conditions: Sampling of all combinations of measurement possibilities is thorough enough to obtain sufficiently consistent scores	• insufficient sampling of combinations (CU) *Any two or more measurement facets may interact with each other to create inconsistency (including "examinees" as a measurement facet), e.g., rater-by-item (e.g., one rater is harsh on item 1, another is harsh on item 2), rater-by-examinee (e.g., rater 1 rates women harshly, rater 2 rates men harshly), etc.*
Extrapolation	
Suitable construct (or "attribute") definition: The attribute is named according to what it is, e.g., knowledge vs. skill, recognition vs. recall; the attribute is identified correctly as having one or more aspects, i.e., its "factor structure"	• naming an attribute too broadly, e.g., referring to "teamwork" when only "communication" was assessed (CU) • naming an attribute incorrectly, e.g., calling something a "skill deficit" that really reflects lack of knowledge or motivation, etc. (CIV) • treating temporary and malleable "states" of attributes as if they were permanent and immutable "traits" (CU) • inappropriately attributing performance to individuals when it was heavily influenced by group processes, or vice versa (CIV) • mischaracterizing the dimensionality of attributes, e.g., deeming an examinee "adequate" overall as if there was only one attribute at play, when really the examinee is "exceptional" in one subattribute of performance and "deficient" in another (CIV—or more specifically, "construct mis-specification"; a single label may reflect two or more underlying constructs, each of which may be a "relevant" construct but which are not *coherent* with one another)
Individual item/case and response fidelity: Items or cases and their response options correspond well to the real world	• excessively easy or difficult items/cases (CU) • unrealistic items/cases or response options (CU)
Item/case fidelity as a set: The aggregate of items/cases corresponds to the patterns found in the real world and/or intended domains to be sampled	• inaccurate base rates of normal vs. abnormal clinical findings in items/cases (CU) • over- or undersampling of certain conditions or challenges (CU)
Predictive validity: Scores relate positively to the desired attribute's levels in the real world, or to its effects in the real world	• lack of correlation between assessment scores and other measures of the attribute • lack of correlation between assessment scores and outcomes associated with the attribute
Decisions and Consequences	
Decisions: Any pass/fail or other categorization decisions are made with acceptable sensitivity and specificity, and without biases	• low sensitivity and/or specificity • failure to adjust estimates of validity and reliability for the specific decision(s) • little justification for categorization, e.g., remediation interventions would be equally effective and indicated for all, or differential intervention is impossible • limited diagnostic value, e.g., scores identify a problem but fail to suggest likely solutions • inappropriate labeling of examinees, e.g., labeling examinees "deficient" when they are still within reasonable performance expectations • inappropriate examinee interpretations and decisions, e.g., misinterpreting results as evidence one should quit medicine or a certain specialty

Inferences and their underlying assumptions	Selected validity/quality threats and general notes CIV = construct-irrelevant variance. CU = construct underrepresentation.
Learning and teaching effects: The assessment leads to productive learning and teaching behaviors	• unhelpful feedback formatting, e.g., excessive feedback delays, feedback only at an abstract level • unsupportive environment for applying attribute in the real world, aka unsupportive transfer climate • maladaptive learning strategies or attitudes, e.g., "cramming" before a test
Well-being effects: The assessment supports well-being of all involved	• excessive emotional/psychological strain for examinees, educators, etc.
Communicative effects: The assessment correctly portrays the values of the administering institution	• failure to communicate values, e.g., seeming to value readily assessable attributes greatly, while failing to value hard-to-quantify attributes
Costs: Costs can be borne by all stakeholders and are justified by returns	• excessive costs on examinees, including test prep costs, lost time • excessive costs for administrators, given return on investment
Distributive justice: Outcomes associated with the assessment's use are experienced equally by examinees and other stakeholders	• adverse impact or perhaps even bias against certain groups, e.g., lower promotion rate of underrepresented minorities • unfair costs, e.g., only wealthy examinees can afford test prep materials
Procedural justice: The process of assessment is carried out in a fair manner	• lack of effective process for examinees to challenge scores they believe are in error • transparency with examinees about score use, privacy protection and data security, etc.
Interactional justice: Assessment experiences are humane, treating examinees and other stakeholders with dignity and respect	• feedback is delivered without kindness or respect, e.g., without gauging examinee readiness to receive • negative feedback is disclosed in an unnecessarily public way • category labels are overly harsh, e.g., labeling examinees as "failures"
Political harmony: All relevant stakeholders are considered in assessment design, delivery, and evaluation, and are reasonably supportive	• failure to garner understanding and support of a key partner, e.g., educators opposing an assessment and undermining messaging about it
Broader uptake: The assessment is valued broadly and becomes applied in a growing number of contexts	• failure to package assessment to promote usability elsewhere
Unintended effects: The assessment does not result in negative unintended effects, and ideally has positive unintended effects	*(This is by definition difficult to predict specifically)*

its decisions are appropriate and defensible. On the other hand, a local, course-level formative assessment or quiz may well suffice with a less exhaustive appraisal of validity, focusing only on major threats. Chapters 16 (Programmatic Assessment) and 17 (Assessment Affecting Learning) offer additional insights on balancing the (sometimes divergent) purposes of measurement rigor and educational feedback.

CONCLUDING THOUGHTS

Assessment validity and quality considerations in health professions education are central to how we foster effective learning, safe patient care, and the well-being of health professionals. We have an opportunity to more consistently and rigorously use critical thinking, strong conceptual frameworks, and evidence to understand and improve our assessment practices.

Note: Additional material and resources may be available at the UIC AHPE website: https://go.uic.edu/AHPE

REFERENCES

American Educational Research Association, American Psychological Association, Joint Committee on Standards for Educational, Psychological Testing (US), & National Council on Measurement in Education. (2014). *Standards for educational and psychological testing.* Washington, DC: American Educational Research Association.

Borsboom, D., Mellenbergh, G.J., & van Heerden, J. (2004). The concept of validity. *Psychological Review, 111*(4), 1061.

Cizek, G.J. (2012). Defining and distinguishing validity: Interpretations of score meaning and justifications of test use. *Psychological Methods, 17*(1), 31.

Cook, D.A., Brydges, R., Ginsburg, S., & Hatala, R. (2015). A contemporary approach to validity arguments: A practical guide to Kane's framework. *Medical Education, 49*(6), 560–575.

Cook, D.A., & Hatala, R. (2016). Validation of educational assessments: A primer for simulation and beyond. *Advances in Simulation, 1*(1), 31.

Cook, D.A., & Lineberry, M. (2016). Consequences validity evidence: Evaluating the impact of educational assessments. *Academic Medicine, 91*(6), 785–795.

Cook, D.A., Zendejas, B., Hamstra, S.J., Hatala, R., & Brydges, R. (2014). What counts as validity evidence? Examples and prevalence in a systematic review of simulation-based assessment. *Advances in Health Sciences Education, 19*(2), 233–250.

Cortina, J.M. (1993). What is coefficient alpha? An examination of theory and applications. *Journal of Applied Psychology, 78*(1), 98.

Downing, S.M. (2003). Validity: On the meaningful interpretation of assessment data. *Medical Education, 37*(9), 830–837.

Hatala, R., Gutman, J., Lineberry, M., Triola, M., & Pusic, M. (2018). How well is each learner learning? Validity investigation of a learning curve-based assessment approach for ECG interpretation. *Advances in Health Sciences Education,* 1–19.

Kane, M.T. (2013). Validating the interpretations and uses of test scores. *Journal of Educational Measurement, 50*(1), 1–73.

Messick, S. (1995). Validity of psychological assessment: Validation of inferences from persons' responses and performances as scientific inquiry into score meaning. *American Psychologist, 50*(9), 741.

Schmitt, N. (1996). Uses and abuses of coefficient alpha. *Psychological Assessment, 8*(4), 350.

Shadish, W.R., Cook, T.D., & Campbell, D.T. (2002). *Experimental and quasi-experimental designs for generalized causal inference.* (William R. Shedish, Thomas D. Cook, Donald T. Campbell, eds.). Boston: Houghton Mifflin.

St-Onge, C., Young, M., Eva, K.W., & Hodges, B. (2017). Validity: One word with a plurality of meanings. *Advances in Health Sciences Education, 22*(4), 853–867.

van der Vleuten, C.P. (1996). The assessment of professional competence: Developments, research and practical implications. *Advances in Health Sciences Education, 1*(1), 41–67.

3

RELIABILITY

Yoon Soo Park

INTRODUCTION

Reliability refers to the *consistency* of scores or decisions from assessments (Lord & Novick, 1968). We often think of reliability in lay terms, as consistency or dependability of actions in everyday activities—for example, your friend or your car may be reliable, because you can depend on them. Assessment reliability is conceptualized in a similar manner. When a learner passes an assessment, we would expect the same "pass" decision to be replicated on a retest (assessment scores with good reliability), providing confidence and trustworthiness of the assessment. However, if the learner were to "fail" the retest, then the assessment may not be reliable. Reproducibility or dependability of scores is a key characteristic of assessment reliability. Given this conceptualization, reliability can be captured in multiple ways—it can refer to the consistency between occasions, items, raters, or stations. As such, reliability can be measured differently depending on the context, giving rise to different reliability statistics available to educators and researchers.

In this chapter, we describe the theory and practical application of reliability for health professions education (HPE). We discuss differences between reliability statistics. Each reliability index is described with (1) foundational concepts, (2) illustrative examples, and (3) implications for HPE. We focus on commonly used approaches for reliability estimation and the psychometric inferences that underlie these methods.

We begin with classical test theory (CTT), which provides the theoretical foundation and assumptions underlying measurement and error. CTT forms the basis for reliability estimation. Using CTT, we describe common test-based reliability indices:

1. test-retest reliability;
2. split-half reliability; and
3. internal-consistency reliability (Cronbach's alpha).

Reliability between raters are presented with the following inter-rater reliability statistics:

1. exact agreement;
2. kappa; and
3. intraclass correlations.

We discuss similarities and differences between these reliability indices—*when* to use which statistic and *how* they inform the validity of assessment scores. In addition, we present composite score reliability when reliability indices from multiple assessments are combined.

Reliability plays a central role in educational measurement and social science research. Reliable data are fundamental to effective assessment practices and comprise an essential element of validity. Although reliability and validity are often treated as distinct and separate aspects or indicators of data quality, they are in fact inextricably linked. Perhaps the most succinct description of this relation is conveyed by the observation that reliability is a necessary but insufficient condition for validity (Feldt & Brennan, 1989). Assessment scores may be consistent (reliable), but not accurate (valid). Think of raters who have high agreement, but are also very lenient, giving everyone high passing marks regardless of their poor performance. It becomes obvious that if scores are unreliable, they will also lack validity for use toward interpretation. In this chapter, we provide the reader with meaningful ways of understanding, evaluating, and applying information about reliability.

THEORETICAL FRAMEWORK FOR RELIABILITY

Test scores and assessment data are reliable to the degree to which they can be replicated or reproduced. While all educational measurements contain some level of measurement error, the particular types of assessments used in health professions education and in social sciences more broadly are prone to measurement error.

An Analogy

To illustrate the concept of error, consider the following situation. You and a friend are having a video conference over the Internet. There are many factors contributing to the quality of sounds transmitted—the speed of your computer, fluctuation in Internet speed and bandwidth, and even perhaps the background noise in your office. These factors contribute to the quality of conversation you have with your friend. The types of sounds that you hear during this meeting can be classified as distractors (random background sound or weak Internet connection) or your friend's words (meaningful sound or information). The proportion of your friend's remarks that you hear and could interpret could range from 0 (weak Internet connection completely prevented any meaningful conversation) to 1.0 (clearly understood every word communicated). The closer you are to 1.0 on this scale, the more likely to give a trustworthy and reliable account of the conversation.

Similarly, one could look at assessment data in this same way; it contains two sources of variation—random error or noise, and systematic information. The reliability of assessment data increases as it contains less random error.

CLASSICAL TEST THEORY (CTT)

Reliability is based on the fundamental assumption known as classical test theory (Lord & Novick, 1968):

$$\text{Observed Score } (X) = \text{True Score } (T) + \text{Error} (e) \tag{3.1}$$

This simple formula encompasses an assumption that assessment scores (observed score, X) are a function of some latent "true" score (T) and measurement error (e). This implies that measurement error (noise) is an inevitable aspect of assessments. In CTT, reliability is defined as the ratio between "true variance" $\sigma^2(T)$ and "total variance" $\sigma^2(X) = \sigma^2(T) + \sigma^2(e)$. This is captured in Equation (3.2):

$$reliability = \frac{\sigma^2(T)}{\sigma^2(X)} = \frac{\sigma^2(T)}{\sigma^2(T) + \sigma^2(e)} \tag{3.2}$$

Underlying this statement is the question—what proportion of data is useful information rather than noise?

Illustrative Example

Let's consider the following *hypothetical example*. You administer a quiz to your class with the following descriptive statistics: Test Mean (average) = 65 and Standard Deviation (SD) = 5. Here, the standard deviation is the $\sigma(X)$ in Equation (3.2). To derive total variance, we simply square this value, which yields $\sigma^2(X) = 25$. Figures 3.1a and 3.1b illustrates this example, with Mean = 65 and Variance = 25 (derived by squaring the SD of 5).

We know from CTT that True Variance is a subset of the Total Variance of 25:

$$\text{Observed Variance} = \text{True Variance} + \text{Error Variance}$$
$$25 = \text{True Variance} + \text{Error Variance} \tag{3.3}$$

Let's say hypothetically that using some statistical approach, you are able to identify the error variance as 10. Then, using Equation (3.3), we know that True Variance would be 15 (= Total Variance – Error Variance = 25 – 10). As such, reliability would be as follows:

$$\text{Reliability} = 15/25 = 15/(15+10) = 0.60.$$

Therefore, if we can determine either the true variance or the error variance, we can calculate reliability. This is the foundational principle of CTT. There are many different reliability estimation formulas available to health professions educators for specific situations; these formulas are all based on principles of CTT.

Implications

In CTT, systematic variation is solely attributable to differences in true scores. However, in practice, there are other sources of systematic variation, such as rater or measurement bias. For example, a scale that consistently registers 10 pounds heavier than the object's true weight produces a systematic rather than a random source of error. Systematic measurement error will not be detected in reliability analyses, but it will negatively impact the interpretability of the measure, and hence its validity. Chapter 2 provides a comprehensive discussion of validity and systematic error. Chapters 7 to 12 provide recommendations for decreasing systematic error for various types of testing formats. In the ensuing sections, we review commonly used reliability statistics of two types: those that look at error variance due to the test itself (for example, due to the number or qualities of test items), known as test-based methods, and those that focus on error variance related to the rater or person scoring the exam.

RELIABILITY INDICES: TEST-BASED METHODS

We present three reliability statistics for test-based methods: (1) test-retest reliability, (2) split-half reliability, and (3) internal-consistency reliability. Test-retest reliability and split-half reliability are rarely used in health professions education. However, they inform the basis for internal-consistency

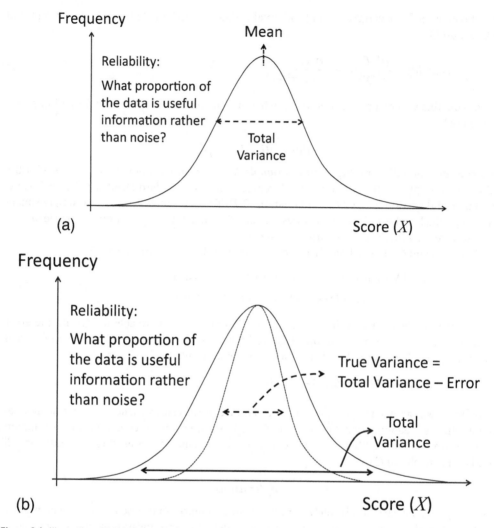

Figure 3.1 Illustration of total variance

Note: The illustration on the top (Figure 3.1a) shows the distribution of a hypothetical assessment with mean = 65 and SD = 5. To derive the total variance, we simply square the SD. The illustration on the bottom (Figure 3.1b) shows that the true variance is a subset of the total variance.

reliability, which is widely used. For each reliability statistic, we present a conceptual definition, an illustrative example (see figures within each section), and implications for reliability interpretation.

1. Test-Retest Reliability

Conceptual Basis for Test-Retest Reliability

The idea of test-retest reliability is perhaps the most basic when thinking about the replication of test scores and decisions—if I administer the same test on multiple occasions, do I get the same score assuming nothing else occurred? Test-retest reliability evaluates the error associated with administering a test at two different times. Conceptually, it is simple to do: (1) give a test at Time 1, (2) give the same test at Time 2, and (3) calculate the correlation (r) between the two scores.

ID	Time 1	Time 2
1	62	86
2	50	69
3	47	69
4	54	69
5	18	47
6	40	65
7	57	69
8	50	56
9	57	60
10	50	65

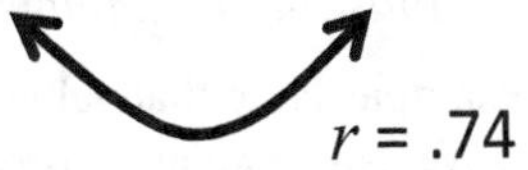

$r = .74$

Figure 3.2 Illustrative example—test-retest reliability

Note: In Figure 3.2, the covariance between assessment scores at Time 1 and Time 2 is 92.50. The standard deviations for scores at Time 1 and Time 2 are 12.33 and 10.18. Following Equation (3.4), this yields test-retest reliability (correlation) of 0.74 (= 92.50 / [12.33 × 10.18]).

How does test-retest reliability relate to CTT? If you recall, reliability is conceptualized as the proportion between true score variance and total variance (see Equation [3.2]). Mathematically, the formula for correlation is the ratio of shared variability between two scores (covariance) and the total variance between the two scores (product of standard deviation [SD] from the two scores). See Equation (3.4). In this regard, the shared variability is viewed as the "true variance."

$$\text{Reliability} = (\text{True Variance})/(\text{Total Variance})$$
$$\text{Test-Test Reliability} = (\text{Covariance of Test 1 and Test 2})/$$
$$(\text{SD of Test 1} \times \text{SD of Test 2})$$

(3.4)

Illustrative Example: Test-Retest Reliability

Figure 3.2 illustrates this example. Scores from ten learners are provided across Time 1 and Time 2. To calculate reliability, we simply calculate the correlation of scores between these two time points.

Implications: Test-Retest Reliability

Historically, the concept of consistency across occasions was the first attempt at measuring reliability. In HPE, test-retest reliability has limited use; learner performance changes over time, regardless of how long or short the interval between testing occasions. This is known as *maturation effect*. There are additional sources of error, including random fluctuations in performance, uncontrolled testing conditions, and other internal factors that can bias the quality of scores (response process validity evidence, see Chapter 2). Moreover, there is also the logistic challenge of arranging repeated testing sessions for individuals.

Obtaining accurate estimates with this approach rests upon the dubious assumption that examinees do not remember information from earlier testing sessions. As such, the test-retest method of estimating reliability is of only theoretical and conceptual interest. Regardless, test-retest reliability still provides the conceptual foundation for understanding most other methods of estimating reliability. In the ensuing sections, we present reliability estimation for single test administrations through split-half reliability and internal-consistency reliability.

2. Split-Half Reliability

Conceptual Basis for Split-Half Reliability

The idea of spit-half reliability is based on the motivation to estimate reliability using a single test administration—what if we treat halves of one test as parallel (equivalent) test forms? For example, if we have ten items administered in a single test, we can treat scores from the first and latter halves as two separate tests and correlate their scores, as we have done for test-retest reliability.

Illustrative Example: Split-Half Reliability

Figure 3.3 shows this example. Note that values "0" and "1" correspond to incorrect and correct responses, respectively. We can calculate scores from the first five items (items A1 to A5) and correlate these scores with the last five items (items B1 to B5), which yields a split-half reliability of .48.

$r = .48$

Item Total: A   **Item Total: B**

ID	A1	A2	A3	A4	A5	B1	B2	B3	B4	B5
1	1	0	0	0	0	0	0	0	0	1
2	1	0	0	0	0	0	1	0	0	1
3	1	0	0	0	0	0	1	1	0	1
4	1	0	0	0	0	0	1	0	1	1
5	0	1	0	0	0	0	1	1	0	1
6	1	1	1	0	0	1	0	1	0	1
7	1	1	1	0	0	0	1	1	0	1
8	1	1	1	0	0	1	1	0	1	0
9	1	0	0	0	0	0	0	0	0	0
10	0	1	0	0	0	0	0	0	0	0

Figure 3.3 Illustrative example—split-half reliability

Note: Split-half reliability takes the correlation between the two halves of the test. In this example, scores from the first five items are correlated to the latter half.

Implications: Split-Half Reliability

A central question for split-half reliability is how to split the test into meaningful halves. One may use the first half and the last half as in Figure 3.3. Another possibility is to use the odd versus even numbered items from the test; one may even create groups of items based on domains of content measured and use that as the basis for splitting the test into halves. However, similar to test-retest reliability, there are many conceptual challenges for using split-half reliability in health professions education due to the complexity of content assessed. One may not necessarily create a meaningful half based on the assessment. As such, split-half reliability is also seldom used in health professions education. Prompted by this challenge, psychometricians have struggled with the same question: how can reliability be calculated from a single test administration and yet yield meaningful estimates? One solution is to split the test in every possible half and then to aggregate their score estimates in a meaningful manner. This is the basis for the next reliability calculation: internal-consistency reliability.

3. Internal-Consistency Reliability: Cronbach's Alpha

Conceptual Basis for Internal-Consistency Reliability

Internal-consistency reliability is based on the idea to calculate the average correlation across all possible splits in a single test. The most widely used internal-consistency reliability statistic is the coefficient alpha, also known as Cronbach's alpha. Like other measures of reliability, it represents the proportion of systematic or true score variance in the total test score variance. Consider each item in the test as an attempt to measure an underlying ability or construct such as knowledge of biochemistry. Cronbach's alpha reflects how strongly the responses to the different items on the test all depend on examinee ability in biochemistry. Greater shared variance or correlations among the items results in higher coefficient alpha values; this indicates closer alignment around the common underlying construct (Traub, 1997).

Cronbach's alpha takes the idea that true variance is the difference between total variance and error variance, where error variance is attributed to variability in items. Equation (3.5) shows the relationship between CTT and Cronbach's alpha:

$$\text{Reliability} = (\text{True Variance})/(\text{Total Variance})$$
$$\text{Cronbach's alpha} = (\text{correction factor}) \times$$
$$\left[1 - (\text{Error Variance/Total Variance})\right]$$
$$= \left[\# \text{Items}/(\# \text{Items} - 1)\right] \times \tag{3.5}$$
$$\left[1 - (\text{Sum of Item Variance/Total Score Variance})\right]$$

As shown in Equation (3.5), there is a correction factor that controls for the number of items administered.

Illustrative Example: Internal-Consistency Reliability

Let's look at an illustrative example as shown in Figure 3.4 with 12 items administered to learners.

Note that values "0" and "1" correspond to incorrect and correct responses, respectively. To calculate Cronbach's alpha, we need to calculate the total score variance, which is the variance associated with the total scores by student (see "Total" column). This is 5.64 in Figure 3.4. We also need to calculate the item variance, which is the variance associated with each item. For example, item variance for item 1 is 0.08. The sum of item variance is the sum across the item variances, which is 2.35. These are the components needed to calculate Cronbach's alpha = 0.64 = (12/11) × [1 − (2.35/5.64)].

Learner	i1	i2	i3	i4	i5	i6	i7	i8	i9	i10	i11	i12	Total
1	1	1	0	1	1	0	0	1	1	0	0	0	6
2	1	1	0	1	0	0	0	0	1	0	0	0	4
3	1	0	1	1	1	1	1	1	1	0	1	1	10
4	1	1	1	1	1	0	1	1	1	1	0	1	10
5	1	1	1	1	1	1	0	1	0	1	1	0	9
6	0	1	1	1	1	1	1	1	0	0	0	1	8
7	1	0	1	1	1	1	1	1	1	0	1	1	10
8	1	1	1	1	0	1	0	0	1	0	0	1	7
9	1	0	1	1	1	1	0	1	1	0	0	0	7
10	1	1	0	1	1	1	1	1	0	0	0	1	8
11	1	1	0	0	1	0	0	0	0	0	0	0	3
12	1	1	0	1	0	0	0	0	0	1	0	0	4
Total	11	9	7	11	9	7	5	8	7	3	3	6	86
Item Variance	.08	.19	.24	.08	.19	.24	.24	.22	.24	.19	.19	.25	2.35

Figure 3.4 Illustrative example—internal-consistency reliability (Cronbach's alpha)

Note: Total number of items = 12
Sum of item variance = 2.35 (Error Variance)
Total score variance = 5.64 (Total Variance)
Cronbach's alpha = (correction factor) × [1 − (Error Variance/Total Variance)]
= [# Items/(# Items—1)] × [1 − (Sum of Item Variance/Total Score Variance)]
= 0.64 = (12/11) × [1 − (2.35/5.64)]

Most statistical software allows calculation of Cronbach's alpha. A Cronbach's alpha of 0.64 indicates that 64% of the observed variation in total scores is due to variation in examinee ability (true score). Or conversely, it also implies that 36% of observed score variation is due to random error rather than examinee ability. Random error in this example is primarily derived based on item variation. In Chapter 4 (Generalizability Theory), we cover situations when sources of error are due to multiple factors such as raters, items, and stations, such as in an objective structured clinical examination.

Implications: Internal-Consistency Reliability

Reliability coefficients of less than 0.50 are not uncommon for very short tests and quizzes. Whether this alpha indicates a sufficient level of reliability depends upon how the test will be used. Downing (2004) and Nunnally (1978) note that educational measurement professionals generally suggest the following interpretive guidance for Cronbach's alpha:

- 0.90 or higher is needed for very high-stakes tests (e.g., licensure, certification exams);
- 0.80–0.89 is acceptable for moderate-stakes tests (e.g., end-of-year summative exams in medical school, end-of-course exams); and
- 0.70–0.79 would be acceptable for lower-stakes assessments (e.g., formative or summative classroom-type assessments created and administered by local faculty).

Although many in-course or classroom-type educational assessments have reliability estimates below 0.70, there may still be a sound rationale for using test score information with relatively low levels of reliability. For example, test scores with a reliability coefficient below 0.70 might be useful as one component of an overall composite score.

As shown in Equation (3.5), the number of items plays an important role in the derivation for Cronbach's alpha. This is an important concept for reliability—in general, adding more items increases reliability. Similarly, adding more raters or adding scores from multiple assessments (composite scores) yields an enhanced total score reliability (Park, Lineberry, Hyderi, Bordage, Xing, & Yudkowsky, 2016). These concepts will be discussed later in this chapter.

RELIABILITY INDICES: RATERS

Up to this point, the focus has been on assessment instruments producing data that can be objectively scored as correct (1) or incorrect (0). However, many educational assessments within the health professions education are conducted through structured observations and the rating of performance (Chapter 9). In this section, we discuss commonly used inter-rater reliability statistics in health professions education: (1) % exact agreement, (2) kappa, and (3) intraclass correlation (Park, Hyderi, Bordage, Xing, & Yudkowsky, 2016).

Conceptual Basis for Inter-Rater Reliability

Most inter-rater reliability estimates in health professions education are based on the concept of agreement—how well do scores assigned by a rater agree with scores assigned by another rater? In this regard, there are three inter-rater reliability statistics that are useful (Park, Hyderi et al., 2016):

- exact agreement: proportion of agreement between raters;
- kappa: proportion of agreement between raters taking into account chance agreement; and
- intraclass correlation (ICC): agreement between raters taking into account the degree of variability (magnitude of difference), in addition to correcting for chance agreement.

Exact agreement simply takes the crude proportion of agreement between raters. For example, if seven out of ten ratings are in complete agreement between raters, the exact agreement statistic would be 70%. Now, if the rating instrument were based on a four-point rating scale, there is a 25% chance that raters could agree. Kappa corrects for this chance agreement. ICC takes the correction further by taking into account variability in ratings across raters. For example, if Rater 1 assigned a "3" and Rater 2 assigned "4," the difference in their rating is one point. This is different if Rater 1 assigned a "1" and Rater 2 assigned "4," the difference being three points. ICC takes such difference into account (one-point different versus three-point difference between raters). In contrast, exact agreement and kappa are primarily concerned with absolute agreement.

Illustrative Example: Inter-Rater Reliability

Let's consider an example in Figure 3.5 with ten learner observations conducted by two faculty raters using a four-point global rating scale.

The column Exact Agreement is marked "1" if the raters are in agreement; the column is marked "0" if they are in disagreement. Since there are five observations with agreement, the exact agreement is 50%. Kappa is 0.31, taking into account the chance agreement. ICC comes to 0.42. Most statistical software packages allow calculation of these statistics.

Implications: Inter-Rater Reliability

Similar to internal-consistency reliability estimates, there are no clear rules on what ranges of inter-rater reliability constitutes an acceptable level. In particular, for exact agreement, this statistic becomes more complex, with larger numbers of scoring categories. For example, achieving greater exact agreement on a nine-point milestones scale is more difficult than a binary "yes/no" scale. You are more likely to agree on a binary scale than a nine-point scale. As such, a direct comparison of exact agreement statistics for varying numbers of scoring categories should be avoided.

Learner	Rater 1	Rater 2	Exact Agreement	Absolute Difference
1	3	4	0	1
2	2	3	0	1
3	2	4	0	2
4	1	3	0	2
5	4	4	1	0
6	2	2	1	0
7	2	2	1	0
8	3	3	1	0
9	4	3	0	1
10	4	4	1	0

Figure 3.5 Illustrative example—exact agreement, kappa, and intraclass correlation

Note: Raters observed learners using a four-point rating instrument.
"Exact Agreement" is coded "1" when Rater 1 and Rater 2 scores agree.
"Absolute Difference" is the difference in scores between Rater 1 and Rater 2.
Exact Agreement = 50%. (There are five ratings where Rater 1 and Rater 2 agree.)
Kappa = 0.31. (Correcting for chance agreement, kappa is 0.31.)
Intraclass correlation = 0.42. (Correcting for chance agreement and weighting the degree of difference between raters.)

For kappa, Landis and Koch (1977) provide guidelines: < 0 as indicating no agreement, 0–0.20 as slight, 0.21–0.40 as fair, 0.41–0.60 as moderate, 0.61–0.80 as substantial, and 0.81–1 as almost perfect agreement. For ICC, Fleiss, Levin, and Paik (2004) provide guidelines as less than 0.40 as poor, 0.40–0.75 as fair to good, and over 0.75 as excellent. Researchers argue that these guidelines are somewhat arbitrary. However, they provide useful guidelines for practitioners. ICC sparked the notion that you could begin to estimate various sources of rater error and was the foundation for generalizability theory, which will be discussed in greater detail in Chapter 4.

An important note for inter-rater reliability is the difference between scoring accuracy versus scoring consistency. Raters can be consistent, but not accurate. Two inaccurate raters can have high agreement and two accurate raters can disagree. As such, it is important to distinguish these differences.

STANDARD ERROR OF MEASUREMENT (SEM)

To gain a better sense of an assessment's reliability, one can also calculate the standard error of measurement (SEM) and form confidence intervals for an obtained score (see Chapter 5 on test statistics for further discussion on interpretation). SEM can be derived using the formula in Equation (3.6).

$$\text{Standard Error of Measurement (SEM)} = SD \times \sqrt{1 - reliability} \qquad (3.6)$$

SEM provides the precision of assessment scores, by building confidence intervals as Assessment Score ± SEM. The following illustrative example clarifies this application.

Illustrative Example

Let's assume that you have two candidates with different test scores:

- Learner A: 81%
- Learner B: 83%

The overall class average was 80% (SD = 5%). The test reliability based using Cronbach's alpha was 0.85. Based on these results, might promotions committees make high-stakes decisions that favor Learner B over Learner A? To answer this question, SEM can be helpful.

In this example, $SEM = 5 \times \sqrt{1 - 0.85} = 5 \times \sqrt{0.15} = 1.94$

We can build confidence intervals for Learner A and Learner B as follows:

- Learner A: 81% ± 1.94: (79.1, 82.9)
- Learner B: 83% ± 1.94: (81.1, 84.9)

The two learner's scores overlap, indicating that within measurement error, their assessment scores are not different.

Implications

SEM can be multiplied by 1.96 to obtain the 95% confidence intervals; multiplying by 1.65 would yield the 90% confidence interval. However, in practice, educators often use ±1 SEM to construct the 68% confidence interval, as this yields a more practical degree of measurement intervals. Using larger confidence intervals in education would make score comparisons more challenging.

SEM should not be confused with standard error of the mean, which is a different statistic. Standard error of the mean is used to describe the confidence interval assuming no measurement error. For example, if one were to report the descriptive statistics associated with the number of cars in major cities, standard error of the mean should be used, as there is no measurement error in counting cars (as opposed to assessments or psychological constructs that deal with latent constructs with underlying measurement error, a key assumption in CTT).

HOW TO INCREASE RELIABILITY

For educators and practitioners, there are three main options to increase the reliability of an assessment:

1. adding more test items (or raters, stations, or other assessment components);
2. conducting item analysis and removing, revising, or replacing items that do not work well (see Chapter 5), which will improve the overall quality of items; and
3. combining scores from multiple assessments to form composite scores.

In this section, we focus on adding more items through the application of the Spearman-Brown formula. We also discuss how to combine scores to form composite scores (Park, Lineberry et al., 2016; Kane & Case, 2004).

PROJECTIONS IN RELIABILITY: SPEARMAN-BROWN FORMULA

If the reliability of an assessment is low, an option is to increase the number of test items. The Spearman-Brown formula can be used to estimate the likely impact on reliability of a lengthened test (see also Chapter 5).

Equation (3.7) shows the Spearman-Brown formula; Equation (3.8) shows a rearrangement of the formula.

$$r^* = \frac{N(r)}{1 + (N-1)(r)} \tag{3.7}$$

$$N = \frac{r^*(1-r)}{r(1-r^*)} \qquad (3.8)$$

The values correspond to the following:

- N: Factor of increasing/decreasing the test length
- r: Reliability of original test
- r^*: Spearman Brown predicted reliability

Illustrative Example

A 30-item test with test-retest reliability of 0.65 is lengthened to 90 items (three-fold increase in test length). Using these values, we can insert them to the Spearman-Brown Formula:

$$r^* = \frac{N(r)}{1+(N-1)(r)} = \frac{3(.65)}{1+(3-1)(.65)} = \frac{1.95}{2.3} = .85$$

Here, $N = 3$, $r = .65$, and r^* is the predicted reliability. If the test length were tripled from 30 to 90 items, the reliability would be 0.85. Alternatively, if we know our current reliability, say 0.65, and want to know by what factor we need to increase our test length to achieve a reliability of 0.85, we can use Equation (3.8) to yield a factor of 3.

Implications

The Spearman-Brown formula can be a powerful tool to make inferences on projected reliability estimates. However, it makes the assumption that the test characteristics remain consistent. For example, knowing that tripling the test length would increase reliability does not simply mean adding poor-quality items. Consideration for validity of test items should be central to adding or modifying items (see Chapter 2).

COMPOSITE SCORES AND COMPOSITE SCORE RELIABILITY

In health professions education, instructors often need to generate composite summary scores based on multiple diverse measures. For example, a course grade might be derived by summing written test scores assessing knowledge achievement and ratings of clinical performance. Given that the final grade is usually the most important and consequential score awarded for a course, it may be important to accurately assess its reliability. Composite score reliability is a special topic that may require a specialized software to conduct the analysis (Park, Lineberry et al., 2016; Kane & Case, 2004). The Appendix provides detailed illustrative examples with accompanying formulas. Interested readers should refer to that section for further details.

Illustrative Example

Assume that you have three assessments that are combined with weights derived by expert faculty judgment (see Figure 3.6).

In this example, you are weighting rotation evaluations scores, written assessment scores, and objective structured clinical examination (OSCE) scores with 37%, 30%, and 33% weights, respectively. These assessments also have varying reliability estimates ranging from 0.50 to 0.60 and have inter-assessment correlations that range between 0.40 and 0.65. The bottom diagram in Figure 3.6 shows the range of composite score reliability estimates by weighting the rotation evaluation scores differently. For example, if we weight rotation evaluations at 50% (assuming evenly splitting the weights for OSCE = 25% and written exam = 25%), we achieve a composite score reliability of .75. Increasing the weight for rotation evaluations to 35% (with even weights

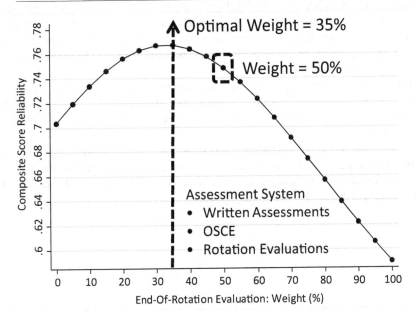

Assessments	Weight	Reliability
Rotation Evaluations	37%	.58
Written Exam	30%	.60
OSCE	33%	.50

Figure 3.6 Illustrative example—composite score reliability

Note: Top figure shows Weight, Reliability, and Correlation between Assessments; the bottom figure shows the relationship between weights and composite score reliability.

for OSCE and written exam at 32.5%), we achieve optimal reliability of .77. Increasing the weight beyond 35% lowers composite score reliability.

Implications

Combining scores requires educational rationale, which is used to determine the magnitude of weights applied to each component. These factors have important validity implications beyond reliability, affecting the consequential validity. There are several approaches available for optimizing weights to maximize composite score reliability. In this section, we used Kane's approach to composite score reliability. A multivariate generalizability theory approach is also a widely used method (see Chapter 4).

SUMMARY

This chapter illustrated concepts of reliability and their use in different contexts and showed how reliability can help determine the adequacy and validity of assessment data for particular uses. We provided a conceptual discussion of reliability and its relationship to variance, and then moved toward a more precise formulation of reliability through a discussion of its role in CTT. Each concept was also demonstrated with examples from health professions education.

Assessment scores usually contain error (noise) that limits our ability to accurately measure an examinee's ability or performance. Reliability analysis allows educators to quantify error and facilitates the correct interpretation and use of scores containing random measurement error. To provide a conceptual framework for reliability analysis, CTT was introduced as a method for partitioning total test score variance into two components: (1) true score and (2) error. It was emphasized that the notion of replication provides the necessary framework for representing reliability. Applications of reliability are discussed with respect to measurement error. Measurement error deals with the degree to which scores are precise. Unreliable assessment scores yield larger measurement error, making scores less precise. Strategies to improve reliability were discussed with respect to adding more items.

We discussed methods for estimating reliability with examples. We provided guidelines and implications on the use of test-based reliability statistics and inter-rater reliability statistics. In addition, approaches to improve reliability were presented based on the Spearman-Brown formula and composite scores.

As we noted earlier in this chapter, reliability is one component of the validity argument. As such, the reliability of an assessment should be taken into context when determining the use and interpretation of assessment scores for making summative decisions (Chapter 5, Statistics of Testing) and to affect learning (Chapter 17, Assessment Affecting Learning).

APPENDIX

Supplement—Composite Scores and Composite Score Reliability

Assume that an institution combines scores from three assessments using predetermined weights:

- Working group process (WGP) evaluation: 37% of final grade
- HPI written exam: 30% of final grade
- Standardized patient (SP) exam: 33% of final grade

OBJECTIVE

The course director asks the following questions:

- What is the reliability of the composite score?
- How would I calculate composite scores for my students?

WHAT WE KNOW

Reliability of three assessments. We know that the reliabilities of the three tests are as follows:

- WGP evaluation: 0.58
- HPI written exam: 0.80
- SP exam: 0.50

Correlations between assessments. Using student performance data, we calculated the degree of association between the assessments (using correlations):

- WGP evaluation and HPI written exam: 0.40
- WGP evaluation and SP exam: 0.50
- HPI written exam and SP exam: 0.65

Sample student scores. As an example, scores from three "fake" students are provided below to demonstrate calculating the composite scores.

Student	WGP Evaluation (37%)	HPI Exam (30%)	SP Exam (33%)
1	96.0	78.0	82.0
2	80.0	72.0	86.5
3	96.0	52.0	71.8

Note: Values in parentheses represent assessment specific weight.

This document will provide a step-by-step guide to calculate composite score reliability and composite scores for the three students. Calculations used in this example are based on the following reference:

Kane, M., & Case, S.M. (2004). The reliability and validity of weighted composite scores. *Applied Measurement in Education, 17*(3), 221–240.

I. CALCULATING THE COMPOSITE SCORE RELIABILITY

The reliabilities of the three assessments range between 0.50 and 0.80. Combining assessments generally increases the reliability when a composite score is generated.

Step 1: Calculate the squared sum of the weights associated with each assessment. The reason these squared weights are added is that we are summing weighted variances (width of the score distribution for a particular assessment), which have a mathematical property that requires them to be squared.

$$\left(\text{weight of assessment 1}\right)^2 + \left(\text{weight of assessment 2}\right)^2 + \left(\text{weight of assessment 3}\right)^2$$
$$= 0.37^2 + 0.30^2 + 0.33^2$$
$$= 0.335$$

Step 2: Calculate the weighted sum of the correlations.

$$\left(2 \times \text{product of weights from assessments 1 and 2} \times \text{correlation of assessments 1 and 2}\right) +$$
$$\left(2 \times \text{product of weights from assessments 1 and 3} \times \text{correlation of assessments 1 and 3}\right) +$$
$$\left(2 \times \text{product of weights from assessments 2 and 3} \times \text{correlation of assessments 2 and 3}\right)$$
$$= \left(2 \times 0.37 \times 0.30 \times 0.40\right) + \left(2 \times 0.37 \times 0.33 \times 0.50\right) + \left(2 \times 0.30 \times 0.33 \times 0.65\right)$$
$$= 0.340$$

Step 3: Take the sum of value from Step 1 and Step 2. This is the "total" variance of the composite score.

$$= \text{Step 1} + \text{Step 2} = 0.335 + 0.340$$
$$= 0.675$$

Step 4: Calculate the product of the reliability with the squared weights of the assessment and take their sum.

$$\left(\text{reliability of assessment 1}\right) \times \left(\text{weight of assessment 1}\right)^2 +$$
$$\left(\text{reliability of assessment 2}\right) \times \left(\text{weight of assessment 2}\right)^2 +$$
$$\left(\text{reliability of assessment 3}\right) \times \left(\text{weight of assessment 3}\right)^2$$
$$= \left(0.58 \times 0.37^2\right) + \left(0.80 \times 0.30^2\right) + \left(0.50 \times 0.33^2\right)$$
$$= 0.205$$

Step 5: Sum the result in Step 4 with Step 2. This is the "true" variance of the composite score.

$$= \text{Step 4} + \text{Step 2} = 0.205 + 0.340$$
$$= 0.545$$

Step 6: Divide the result from Step 5 by the result in Step 3. Recall that by definition, reliability is the proportion of variability accounted by the "true" score variance.

$$\left(\text{true score variance in Step 5}\right)/\left(\text{total score variance in Step 3}\right) = 0.545/0.675$$
$$= 0.807 \approx 0.81$$

Based on these calculations, **the composite score reliability of the three assessments is 0.81**. Combining scores from the three assessments has sufficient reliability.

II. CALCULATING THE COMPOSITE SCORES OF THE THREE EXEMPLAR STUDENTS

Calculating the composite scores of students cannot simply be derived by taking their weighted sum. We need to standardize the scores using z-scores. Standardization allows all three assessments to have the same mean and variance. Using z-scores simplifies complexities in calculation, because the mean is set to equal 0, and the variance is set to equal 1 (same for standard deviation, which equals 1; standard deviation is the square root of variance).

Step 1: Standardize the scores to z-scores. To calculate the z-score, use the following formula:

$$z\text{-score} = (\text{score} - \text{class average for the assessment})/(\text{standard deviation})$$

For example, if John received a score of 80, and the class average was 75 with a standard deviation of 5 points, John's z-score is $1 = (80 - 75) / 5$. Below are the z-scores for the three students:

Student	Evaluation (37%)	HPI Exam (30%)	SP Exam (33%)
1	1.751	0.772	0.915
2	0.842	0.583	1.103
3	1.751	0.050	0.579

Step 2: Take the weighted sum of each assessment z-score:

Student 1: $(1.751 \times 0.37) + (0.772 \times 0.30) + (0.915 \times 0.33) = 1.181$

Student 2: $(0.842 \times 0.37) + (0.583 \times 0.30) + (1.103 \times 0.33) = 0.850$

Student 3: $(1.751 \times 0.37) + (0.050 \times 0.30) + (0.579 \times 0.33) = 0.854$

Step 3: Divide the weighted sum of z-scores from Step 2 by the standard deviation of the composite score. Recall that we calculated the variance of the composite score in Part I, Step 3, so we can just take its square root to get the standard deviation.

$$\text{Standard deviation of composite score} = \sqrt{(\text{Variance of composite score})}$$
$$= \sqrt{(0.675)} = 0.821$$

Composite score of student 1: $1.181/0.821 = 1.439$

Composite score of student 2: $0.850/0.821 = 1.035$

Composite score of student 3: $0.854/0.821 = 1.040$

Step 4: The z-scores can be converted to percentiles by looking at a z-table (easily accessible online).

Student	Weighted Score (Using Traditional Method)	Composite Score	Difference
1	86.0	92.5	6.5
2	79.7	85.0	5.3
3	74.8	85.1	10.3

Note: The traditional method simply takes the weighted sum of the assessment scores. The "difference" takes the difference between the composite score and the weighted score.

Results indicate that there are differences between the composite scores derived in this example exercise and the traditionally weighted method. This *may* alter decisions on scores reported to students.

Note: Additional material and resources may be available at the UIC AHPE website: https://go.uic.edu/AHPE

REFERENCES

Downing, S.M. (2004). Reliability: On the reproducibility of assessment data. *Medical Education, 38,* 1006–1012.

Feldt, L.S., & Brennan, R. (1989). Reliability. In R.L. Linn (Ed.), *Educational measurement* (3rd ed., pp. 105–146). New York: Palgrave Macmillan.

Fleiss, J.L., Levin, B., & Paik, M.C. (2004). *Statistical methods for rates and proportions.* Hoboken, NJ: Wiley.

Kane, M., & Case, S. (2004). The reliability and validity of weighted composite scores. *Applied Measurement in Education, 17*(3), 221–240.

Landis, J.R., & Koch, G.G. (1977). The measurement of observer agreement for categorical data. *Biometrics, 33,* 159–174.

Lord, F.M., & Novick, M.R. (1968). *Statistical theories of mental test scores.* Reading, MA: Addison-Wesley.

Nunnally, J.C. (1978). *Psychometric theory* (2nd ed.). New York: McGraw-Hill.

Park, Y.S., Hyderi, A., Bordage, G., Xing, K., & Yudkowsky, Y. (2016). Inter-rater reliability and generalizability of patient note scores using a scoring rubric based on the USMLE Step-2 CS format. *Advances in Health Sciences Education, 21*(4), 761–773.

Park, Y.S., Lineberry, M., Hyderi, A., Bordage, G., Xing, K., & Yudkowsky, R. (2016). Differential weighting for subcomponent measures of integrated clinical encounter scores based on the USMLE Step-2 CS examination: Effects on composite score reliability and pass-fail decisions. *Academic Medicine, 91,* S24–S30.

Traub, R.E. (1997). Classical test theory in historical perspective. *Educational Measurement: Issues and Practice, 16*(4), 8–14.

4

GENERALIZABILITY THEORY

Clarence D. Kreiter, Nikki L. Zaidi, and Yoon Soo Park

INTRODUCTORY COMMENTS

This chapter provides a brief introduction to many important aspects of generalizability (G) theory. Despite the brevity, we attempt to provide the learner an overview of the basic concepts and procedures used in both univariate and multivariate G theory. The primary objective of this chapter is to provide the background needed to comprehend common applications of the theory in health professions education. To achieve this goal, we demonstrate G theory concepts with simulated and real assessment data that were created and selected for its instructional value. Computational methods and equations are presented only when they promote the learner's conceptual understanding of G theory. For readers interested in studying the technical aspects of the theory, we have attempted to use notation and terminology that are consistent with Brennan's more comprehensive and authoritative text: *generalizability theory* (Brennan, 2001). This chapter will allow the learner to apply and interpret most common applications of G theory.

All topics covered in this chapter are presented from a practical applications perspective. To achieve this, we include only limited background regarding the mathematical foundations of the theory. The three appendices at the end of the chapter do, however, provide a description of the analysis of variance (ANOVA)-based statistical foundations along with other technical information.

BACKGROUND AND OVERVIEW

In classical test theory (CTT; see Chapter 3), we present *reliability*—the consistency or reproducibility of assessment scores—for multiple-choice tests or global ratings by raters. However, imagine an assessment with multiple factors contributing to variability of assessment scores, including different numbers of items, raters, stations, among others. When assessments become more complex, the traditional CTT framework cannot be used. A more comprehensive approach to reliability estimation is needed—this is the motivation for G theory, which allows estimation and analysis of more complex assessments, such as objective structured clinical examinations, rotation evaluations, and other performance-based assessments that are common in health professions education.

As discussed in Chapter 3, CTT assumes that an observed score is composed of two components, a "true score" and random error. A shorthand way of representing this concept is:

$$Observed\ Score = True\ Score + Error \qquad (4.1)$$

The CTT expression for reliability as:

$$Reliability = True\ Score\ /\ (True\ Score + Error) \qquad (4.2)$$

Similar to CTT, G theory also assumes that the variance of an observed score can be partitioned (decomposed) between true score variance and error variance. However, G theory differs from CTT in allowing *multiple* sources of error to be examined, and hence expands the CTT equation:

$$Observed\ Score = True\ Score + (Error_1 + Error_2 + Error_3 \ldots) \qquad (4.3)$$

And the expression for reliability as:

$$Reliability = True\ Score\ /\ (True\ Score + Error_1 + Error_2 + Error_3 \ldots) \qquad (4.4)$$

In conceptualizing score variance within two broad categories (true score and error), G theory shares a common theoretical framework with CTT. However, G theory differs dramatically from CTT in the details related to estimating the variance components associated with both the true score and error.

G theory is unique in its use of variance estimates to calculate multiple reliability-like coefficients for specific measurement applications. CTT estimates only one source of error in each analysis; therefore, for measurement processes that generate scores averaged over more than one dimension (or *facet*), CTT reliability will provide a less informative estimate of reliability than can be obtained with G theory.

While CTT recognizes that different sources of error exist in measurements, it requires different research designs to estimate each error source independently. For example, if a measurement process uses raters to assess examinee performance across multiple clinical cases, classical methods might calculate an inter-rater reliability coefficient (either within or across cases), an "inter-case" reliability coefficient, or an internal consistency alpha statistic on checklist or rating items within a case—each reflecting a different source of error. However, it would be difficult to meaningfully integrate these different CTT measures to globally assess reliability or to estimate and report the relative importance of each source of error.

G theory allows simultaneous estimation of each source of error in a single analysis. This allows the researcher to forecast reliability for varying *conditions of measurement* by characterizing how accurately an obtained score estimates a hypothetical average score. This average score is conceptualized to be the mean score obtained across many replications of a multi-faceted measurement process. In G theory, this average score, or *universe score*, is similar to a "true score" in CTT and is defined in relation to all identified *facets* of the measurement process. In G theory, the facets of a measurement process specify important aspects regarding the conditions of measurement.

The generalizability, or *dependability*, of a measure as defined in G theory is conceptually very similar to the concept of reliability in CTT. It is, however, more targeted, as it refers to the *accuracy* of generalizing from a single score an examinee obtains on a particular assessment to the average score that the same examinee would achieve if we could repeatedly assess that examinee across all of the conditions of measurement. To better understand the concepts associated with the facets and the conditions of measurement, it is useful to now introduce a hypothetical performance assessment with synthetic data to demonstrate the concepts and procedures of G theory. It should be noted that the small, computer-generated hypothetical data set used here was designed for instructional purposes. In practice, obtaining stable and meaningful statistical estimates of the effectiveness of a measurement procedure would require a much larger data set.

THE HYPOTHETICAL MEASUREMENT PROBLEM—AN EXAMPLE

Data used in this example represent results from a hypothetical measurement problem where a medical education researcher is asked to report on the reliability of assessment scores from a piloted version of an objective structured clinical examination (OSCE; for more about OSCEs see Chapter 9). The researcher is also asked to make recommendations for structuring a larger, operational version of the assessment. To help answer these questions, global ratings of 10 examinees' video-recorded performances on a five-station OSCE have been provided. The (simulated) scores, displayed in Table 4.1, represent ratings by two expert physician raters independently rating the 10 examinees' performances on a five-point scale.

CTT methods could have been used to calculate an inter-rater or inter-station reliability coefficient; however, it would be difficult to simultaneously estimate true score variability and the variance associated with each source of error. Since CTT cannot provide the estimates needed to make an informed recommendation regarding the optimal measurement design, the researcher uses G theory to address the measurement problem.

DEFINING THE G STUDY MODEL

Before analyzing the information presented in Table 4.1, the researcher must first define the G study measurement model. Before doing so, it is important to provide some formal definitions for the conditions of measurement, or how the data were collected, along with the notational conventions used to represent model specifications. First, we must define what we mean by an *object of measurement*. The object of measurement is defined as the element of the sample that the examination is designed to assess. In most assessment applications, the object of measurement is the examinee, commonly referred to as the person (p). After identifying the object of measurement, the facets within a G study are identified by default as the other sources of variation in the G study model. A *facet* represents a dimension, or source of variation, across which the researcher wishes to generalize.

Reflecting on the conditions of measurement of this OSCE, the researcher observes that the same two expert raters rated all 10 examinees on each of the five stations, and that the exam was designed to assess students' clinical skills. With this information, the researcher can define import-

Table 4.1 Data for the Example OSCE Measurement Problem

Learner	Rater 1					Rater 2				
	Station 1	Station 2	Station 3	Station 4	Station 5	Station 1	Station 2	Station 3	Station 4	Station 5
1	5	4	4	4	4	4	3	3	3	3
2	4	3	3	3	3	3	2	2	3	2
3	4	3	4	2	2	3	2	4	3	3
4	4	3	3	3	2	4	2	3	3	4
5	5	4	4	5	4	4	4	3	4	4
6	3	3	4	4	4	2	2	3	4	3
7	4	3	5	3	3	4	3	5	4	4
8	3	4	3	4	3	1	2	2	3	3
9	3	1	1	3	4	3	2	2	3	3
10	3	2	3	4	3	3	1	2	4	3

ant aspects of the G study model. First, since the exam was designed as a measure of examinee performance, as opposed to rater or station performance, the researcher can conclude that the examinee (p) is the object of measurement. The notational convention in the majority of G studies is to represent persons, the object of measurement, with the small letter "p". Once the object of measurement has been identified, the researcher can further assume that the remaining conditions of measurement, raters and stations, represent facets in the G study measurement model. In our example problem, we have two facets—raters and stations. To represent the model with notation, "r" and "s" denote raters (r) and stations (s) respectively. It should be noted that there might be other important measurement facets, or influences related to the scores obtained in Table 4.1; however, the researcher does not have information characterizing these other influences.

Again, considering our example problem, every examinee (p) experienced every station (s) and is rated by the same two raters (r) on each station. The shorthand way of expressing this concept in generalizability terminology is to say all conditions of measurement are completely *crossed*. The notation for the *crossed* concept is the symbol "×". So, with these simple notational conventions, we can write a symbolic expression that summarizes the G study model as [$p \times s \times r$]. Hence, our G study model is a persons-*crossed*-with-stations-*crossed*-with-raters design. Not all G study models are completely crossed. For example, it would be possible to conduct an OSCE, similar to the one described in the example problem, using a different pair of raters for each station. In G theory terminology, this is called a *nested* design and is represented by the symbol ":". For instance, had the ratings been collected using two different raters for each station, we would have represented the G study design as [$p \times (r : s)$]. In G theory terminology, this would be a persons-*crossed*-with-raters-*nested*-within-stations design. There will be additional discussions of design variations throughout this chapter.

All G study models must define whether the facets are *random* or *fixed*. A facet is considered *random* when observed values of the facet within the G study are regarded as a sample from a much larger population. In G theory, this larger population is considered the *universe of admissible observations*, and observations from this sample are considered interchangeable. In our example problem, both raters and stations are considered *random* variables. Hence, in G theory terminology, we would define our G study model from the example problem as being a *random model*. The reason we consider stations as *random* is that our interest is not focused solely on the five stations observed. Rather, the goal of the measurement process is to generalize from performance on the five stations to performance on a *universe* of similar stations from which the five stations are sampled. In the example problem, the same argument applies to raters. The two expert physician raters employed in the pilot exam are considered a sample from a population of potential expert physician raters we might use or consider acceptable to rate performance. For example, if no special rater training of the physician raters was provided, the population of acceptable raters might reasonably be defined as academic physicians at US medical schools. However, if the two academic physician raters in the study received special rater training, we would need to modify our definition of the rater universe as academic physicians who received that special training. A facet is regarded as fixed when all conditions of a facet are observed in the G study, or when the researcher does not wish to generalize beyond the levels of the facet used in the G study. An example of a fixed facet will be presented later in the chapter.

OBTAINING G STUDY RESULTS

Now that the basic G study model has been presented, the next step in the G study is to obtain results. *Variance components* (VCs) represent the primary output of a G study analysis. VCs are estimates of the magnitude of variability of each effect in the G study model. The model in the example problem has three main effects: the object of measurement—persons (p), and the two facets—stations (s) and raters (r). In addition, as in ANOVA, there are also interactions. So, in

Table 4.2 G Study Results for Example Problem [$p \times s \times r$]

Effect	df	Variance Component	Percent Variance
p	9	.137	15.6
s	4	.053	6.0
r	1	.057	6.5
ps	36	.267	30.5
pr	9	.118	13.4
sr	4	.034	3.9
psr/e	36	.211	24.1

Note: p = examinee; s = station; r = rater.

addition to p, s, and r, there are four interactions effects: ps, pr, sr, and psr/e (the "e" will be discussed later in the next section). Therefore, in the example problem, the G study will estimate a total of seven VCs (p, s, r, ps, pr, sr, psr/e). A description of these effects and how to interpret them is presented shortly. The statistical procedures for the estimation of the VCs are presented in Appendix 4.1.

Table 4.2 displays the G study output for the data displayed in Table 4.1. The VCs in Table 4.2 can be calculated using GENOVA software (Crick & Brennan, 1982), which is specifically designed for conducting G study and decision (D) study analyses. Similar VC results can be derived with SPSS or SAS (see Appendix 4.3 for code); however, these programs provide less information than GENOVA. For R users, the VarComp package can be used to estimate VCs. In Stata, the "xtmixed" command or the "gstudy" ado-file package (obtained from the user-group library) can be used to estimate variance components.

INTERPRETING G STUDY RESULTS

The first column of Table 4.2 lists each of the effects estimated in the G study, the *main* effects (p, s, r) and the *interaction* effects (ps, pr, sr, psr/e). The second column displays the degrees of freedom. The third column of Table 4.2 displays the VC values for each of the seven effects estimated. The fourth column provides the percentage of variance represented by each VC.

In the first row of Table 4.2, we observe that 15.6% of the variance in an examinee's score from a single rater on a single OSCE station is attributable to systematic differences between persons (p). This is the object of measurement variance and is similar to "true" score variance in CTT. The ratio definition of reliability provided in Equation (4.4) suggests that the larger the percentage of variance accounted for by examinees (p), the greater the reliability. The second row of Table 4.2 displays the systematic variance attributable to station and reflects the degree to which stations have different means. The station (s) effect accounts for 6% of the total observed variance in scores; this implies that there were small to moderate differences in the level of difficulty between stations in our sample. The third row shows the variance associated with the systematic effects of rater (r), and it reflects the difference in raters' overall mean scores across stations and examinees. In the example problem, the small to moderate proportion of variance related to the systematic effects of raters (6.5%) suggests that the mean difference between raters is not large; or stated another way, the two raters were similar in their overall level of stringency.

Rows 4–7 in Table 4.2 list the interaction effects. The fourth row in that table displays the person-by-station (ps) interaction. This indicates the degree to which stations tend to rank order persons (examinees) differently. This represented the largest percentage of variance (30.5%) and suggests that an examinee's rank order would change considerably depending on which station(s)

Table 4.3 Verbal Description of Sources of Variance in the Example Problem

Effect	Description
Person (p)	"True score" variance for the examinee (e.g., the object of measurement)
Station (s)	Systematic effect due to variability in station difficulty
Raters (r)	Systematic effect due to raters' leniency/stringency
Person-station (ps)	Inconsistencies in examinees' performance from one station to the next
Person-rater (pr)	Inconsistencies in raters' assessment of an examinees' skill
Station-rater (sr)	Inconsistencies in station difficulty by rater
Residual (psr/e)	Three-way interaction between person, station, and rater. Also error not included in the model (e)

were sampled. This variability in individuals across stations is also commonly understood to represent "case specificity." This case specificity may be a result of variability among individuals' level of knowledge or skillset that is germane to a specific station. The person-by-rater (pr) interaction accounted for 13.4% of the total variance and indicates that there was moderate agreement between raters in the scores they assigned to an examinee at a given station. The station-by-rater (sr) interaction produced the smallest observed variance (3.9%), indicating that the level of station difficulty changed little depending on which rater assigned the ratings at a particular station. The residual (psr/e) is a confounded measure of the triple interaction of person (p), station (s), and rater (r), along with error (e) not modeled in the $[p \times s \times r]$ design; this accounted for a large percentage of variance (24.1%). Table 4.3 provides a verbal description of the effects described by each VC.

It is instructional here to consider what VCs would be estimated in a G study analyzing a $[p \times (r{:}s)]$ design as commonly encountered in many OSCE exams. As in the crossed design, the nested design allows us to estimate three main effects: p, s, and r:s. Although the rater effect is now designated as the rater-nested-within-station effect (r:s), its interpretation is same as in the crossed design. For the interaction effects, it is possible to estimate only two interactions: ps and pr:s. The ps VC is interpreted in the same way as in the fully crossed design. However, the pr:s VC is different from the pr VC estimated in the fully crossed model. The pr:s interaction effect, being the highest order interaction, will include residual error and hence is not interpreted in the same fashion as the pr VC from the fully crossed design. It should also be noted that in the $[p \times (r{:}s)]$ design, raters rate only one station. This means that the rater-by-station (rs) VC cannot be estimated separately, and it is therefore included as part of residual error in the $[p \times r{:}s]$ design.

CONDUCTING THE D STUDY

In the description of our example problem, it was noted that the researcher was asked to not only characterize the reliability of the scores from the pilot test, but also to make recommendations for how an operational version of the test might best be structured. A *decision* (D) study can provide reliability estimates not only for the scores collected in the actual G study, but also for alternate assessments that employ different designs and sample sizes. Hence, a D study can address questions related to optimal test design.

The structure of the G study determines which designs a D study can address. Completely crossed G study designs allow the estimation of the maximum number of VC effects, and also maximizes the number of possible D study designs. This is because a D study requires VCs from the G study to calculate estimated reliability coefficients for various designs. In the example problem, the D study could estimate not only the reliability of the assessment with the observed conditions of measurement (a completely crossed random model with two raters and five stations), but it could also estimate the reliability of other OSCE designs using any number of raters and stations and variations in design. For example, estimates from the crossed random model could be used to estimate reliability for a partially nested design. In our example problem, if each of the five stations was rated by a different pairing of raters, this would have resulted in a person-crossed-with-raters-nested-within-stations ($p \times r{:}s$) design. This particular design is common in real-world applications of repeated measurement processes such the OSCE and the multiple mini-interview (MMI) because it is often impractical to assign the same raters to all stations. Using a series of D studies to examine various designs can help the researcher determine how best to structure an operational version of an assessment.

Before proceeding further, it is useful here to discuss D study notation. In the G study model of the example problem, we employed small letter notation to represent the facets. The small letter notation is a way of indicating that in the G study analysis, estimated effects are for one rating on a single station. However, in a D study, we are interested in representing average ratings across a sample of conditions, and capital letters are used to indicate this. For this reason, our notational system for the D study model employs capital letters to express the D study design. For instance, a D study model, which is similar to the design in our example measurement problem but perhaps with a different number of stations and raters, is represented as $[p \times S \times R]$.

The D study can generate two types of reliability-like coefficients: a generalizability coefficient (G or $E\rho^2$) and a measure of dependability (Phi or Φ). The G coefficient is sensitive to relative error and is useful for expressing the reproducibility of examinee rankings. The dependability measure, commonly referred to as Phi, expresses the absolute reproducibility of a score and reflects the degree to which an obtained score is likely to change upon replication of the measurement process. In considering a complete replication of the OSCE measurement procedure as documented in our example problem (i.e., a sample of five different stations and two different raters), a Phi will reflect how closely a replication is likely to reproduce an examinee's final score. The G coefficient, on the other hand, will estimate how consistently we can rank examinees upon replicating the measurement process. Because of this distinction, the Phi coefficient is useful for answering questions related to criterion-referenced testing, while a G coefficient is more informative for norm-referenced testing applications.

$$G = \left(E\rho^2\right) = \frac{\sigma^2(p)}{\sigma^2(p) + \sigma^2(\delta)} \tag{4.5}$$

$$\text{Phi} = \left(\Phi\right) = \frac{\sigma^2(p)}{\sigma^2(p) + \sigma^2(\Delta)} \tag{4.6}$$

where:
  $\sigma^2(p)$ = the variance associated with person;
  $\sigma^2(\delta)$ = the sum of relative error variances; and
  $\sigma^2(\Delta)$ = the sum of absolute error variances.

Absolute error variance (Δ) includes all sources of error except the object of measurement. Relative error (δ) includes only those sources of error that will impact examinee rank order, and in our example problem does not include s, r, or sr VCs in the denominator. Hence, the variation in station difficulty (6% of the total variance), variation in rater stringency (6.5% of the total variance), and the station-rater interaction (3.9% of the total variance) will govern the difference between Phi and G, as represented in Equations (4.5) and (4.6).

This implies that for all D study designs, absolute error will always be greater than or equal to relative error. Hence, Phi (Φ) will always be less than or equal to G ($E\rho^2$). Appendix 4.2 provides additional detail regarding the VCs and sources of error that are included as part of absolute and relative error calculations.

INTERPRETING THE D STUDY

Table 4.4 represents a D study for our example OSCE assessment data in which G and Phi are estimated based on varying numbers of raters and stations. In interpreting a D study, it is often helpful to graphically display the results as shown in Figure 4.1. When the G coefficients from Table 4.4 are graphed across levels of the two facets (raters and stations), several important outcomes become apparent. First, modest gains in reliability are observed by using more than two raters. On the other hand, increasing the number of stations substantially increases reliability. For example, with two raters, increasing the number of stations from one to five increases the G coefficient by 0.266. Also, this D study suggests that the addition of stations beyond five continues to produce practically important gains in the estimated reliability. A summary of how the number of raters and stations impacts the dependability of scores is displayed as Phi (Φ) values in the last column of Table 4.4. Although Phi is not graphically presented in Figure 4.1, the pattern is much the same for Phi and G in our example problem. Phi values, however, are somewhat smaller com-

Table 4.4 D Study Results for Example Problem [$p \times S \times R$]

Number of Raters	Number of Stations	G ($E\rho^2$)	Phi (Φ)
1	1	.187	.156
1	5	.391	.323
1	10	.453	.372
2	1	.241	.206
2	5	.507	.438
2	10	.588	.510
3	1	.267	.230
3	5	.562	.497
3	10	.653	.582

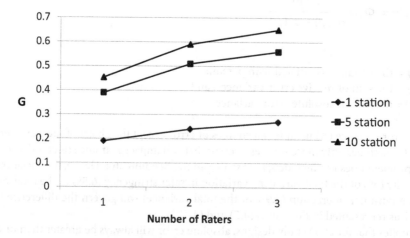

Figure 4.1 Graphic depiction of D study G coefficients

pared to G coefficients because the Phi calculations include additional sources of error (*s*, *r*, and *sr*) in the denominator.

All measurement processes include unwanted sources of error. Therefore, an individual's score is never a "true" reflection of the person's attributes, skills, or knowledge. The error terms used to calculate a G or Phi reflects an estimate of how much relative or absolute error is likely to arise from various sources. We can also use these estimates of error to calculate a standard error of measurement (SEM) which conveys how much observed scores are likely to vary upon repeating the measurement process. One advantage of SEMs over G or Phi is that SEM is expressed in the same metric as the score scale, reflecting the expected standard deviation of score outcomes upon replication of the measurement process. As in CTT, the SEM can be used to calculate confidence intervals around obtained scores (see Chapter 3).

There is broad G study literature regarding standardized patient (SP)-based OSCEs and OSCE-like admissions assessments (e.g., MMI). Van der Vleuten and Swanson (1990) provide a useful summary of major findings in the SP literature. They note that in most SP studies, the primary source of measurement error is due to variation in examinee performance from station to station (*ps* variance). Eva, Rosenfeld, Reiter, and Norman (2004) report similar conclusions for the MMI, in which variance attributable to the candidate-station (*ps*) interaction is much greater than variance attributable to other sources of error. This *ps* variance is often referred to as "content specific" or "case specific" variance (i.e., examinee or candidate performance in one context is often a poor predictor of performance in another context).

G AND D STUDY MODEL VARIATIONS

To obtain meaningful results, it is essential that the researcher accurately specify G and D study models. This section briefly discusses two additional measurement examples and considers commonly encountered G and D study model variations. Our example OSCE problem presented a two-facet [$p \times s \times r$] random model design. However, many commonly encountered models utilize just one facet. For example, a typical multiple-choice test can be modeled as a simple persons (*p*)-crossed (×)-with-items (*i*) one-faceted random model design [$p \times i$]. A [$p \times i$] G study design yields estimates for three effects: *p*, *i*, and *pi*; and the G coefficient for this design is calculated as:

$$G = \left(E\rho^2 \right) = \frac{\sigma^2(p)}{\sigma^2(p) + \sigma^2(pi)/n_i} \tag{4.7}$$

$$\text{Phi} = (\Phi) = \frac{\sigma^2(p)}{\sigma^2(p) + \sigma^2(i)/n_i + \sigma^2(pi)/n_i} \tag{4.8}$$

where n_i equals the number of items. When n_i is equal to the number of items used in the G study, the G coefficient is equivalent to Cronbach's coefficient alpha (or KR 20) for the observed data used in the G study. The Phi for the multiple-choice test example is presented in Equation (4.8).

To demonstrate a fixed facet within a nested G study, consider a written examination employing two formats (*f*)—multiple-choice (MC) and true-false (TF). Since it is logically impossible for an item to be in both formats, the reader should recognize first that for an examination employing both formats (MC and TF), items must be nested within format (*i:f*). Second, the two formats do not represent a sample from an infinitely large population of possible formats; therefore, the MC and TF formats are the only two formats of direct interest in this study. Given that the two observed levels of format are not a sample from a larger population of formats, and that the two formats represent the only two formats of interest, format (*f*) in this example is considered a fixed rather than a random facet. This implies that the model is *mixed* since it contains both a random

Design	Facet				
Crossed	Rater	A		B	
	Station	1	2	1	2
Nested	Rater	A & B		C & D	
	Station	1	2	3	4
Confounded	Rater	A	B	C	D
	Station	1	2	3	4

Figure 4.2 Illustrated examples of crossed, nested, and confounded designs

facet (items) and a fixed facet (format). Hence, the G study design would be a persons (p)-crossed ($\times$)-with-items (i)-nested (:)-within-format (f) *mixed* model design [$p \times (i{:}f)$].

Confounding is a common problem encountered by researchers utilizing data from clinical assessments. *Confounding* occurs when a single, different condition of each facet is combined with another facet. To illustrate the nature of crossed, nested, and confounded data, Figure 4.2 shows an example of crossed, nested, and confounded data collection designs. It should be noted that the confounded design in this figure illustrates a case where a single different rater is associated with each OSCE station. Since there is only one rater per station, a generalizability analysis of data structured in this way would not allow the researcher to estimate the independent effects of raters and stations. Rather, a G study could provide only an estimate of the combined effects of rater and station error.

UNBALANCED DESIGNS

Unbalanced designs are another commonly encountered condition of measurement within naturalistic clinical assessment settings. For example, it is often the case that a different number of raters or observations of clinical performance are associated with each person. As we will discuss in the next section, unbalanced data may also arise when there is an unequal number of levels in a nested facet. If there is a large amount of assessment data available, one approach for analyzing such data is to select a stratified random sample of data to achieve a balanced data set such that each person has the same number of observations. But, of course, this discards some data. Alternately, there are a number of statistical approaches available for estimating VCs with unbalanced data; however, there is no clear logical basis for selecting one approach over the other, and each will produce a somewhat different estimate. When a G study contains unbalanced data within a fixed facet, multivariate generalizability is an efficient and straightforward technique for addressing this type of unbalanced design. We will introduce a multivariate approach within an unbalanced design in the next section.

In summary, this section briefly discussed modeling concepts of just four G study designs ([$p \times i$], [$p \times (i{:}f)$], [$p \times s \times r$], and [$p \times (r{:}s)$]). Even though variants of G study models grow rapidly with the addition of facets, nesting, and mixed model conditions, these four models provide the reader with the building blocks and core concepts to understand most commonly encountered applications of G theory in health science education research. While it is beyond the scope of this chapter to provide the reader with an exhaustive list of models, the reader is encouraged to reference texts offering a wider presentation of models and design considerations (Brennan, 2001; Shavelson & Webb, 1991; Norman 2003).

MULTIVARIATE GENERALIZABILITY

Up to this point, we have focused exclusively on univariate G theory. We discussed how G studies estimate VCs that can be used to calculate reliability-like coefficients for measurement procedures that yield a single summary score for each examinee. In this section, we broaden the application of G theory to include multivariate generalizability (MVG) procedures that can be used when the measurement process yields multiple summary scores for each examinee. In general, MVG can be usefully applied whenever an assessment generates multiple measures that describe distinct aspects of an examinee's performance. For example, an SP-based OSCE that uses both communication and clinical reasoning items within each station might naturally prompt an interest in generating summary scores for each of these two performance dimensions; or, as the instructional example will introduce, when students receive grades reflecting two or more distinct phases of a health science professions education program. When receiving grades in different phases of the curriculum, an educator might find it useful to generate a grade point average (GPA) for each type of educational experience. While univariate G theory focuses exclusively on the use of VCs, MVG also produces covariance and universe score correlations that reflect on the relationships between the multiple measures.

We will use as an MVG instructional example, a study by Kreiter and Ferguson (2016) that analyzed grades from didactic and clinical instruction. In that study, students were presented with didactic courses during the first two years of their medical education and experienced clinical courses during their third year. Grades were awarded for each course, and a course occurred either during the didactic or clinical phase of the curriculum. The researchers were interested in understanding the measurement characteristics of GPAs calculated from within and across the two types (t) (didactic and clinical) of courses. The researchers first employed a univariate mixed-model G study that regarded course grades (g) as nested within the fixed facet type (t) ($p \times g{:}t$) (note: for consistency, the notation used here is somewhat different than that used in the research paper). Table 4.5 shows the results from the univariate G study analyzing 20 grades (14 didactic and six clinical) for 1,101 students. While there is important information conveyed in this univariate study, examining the grade data in this way did not provide the variance estimates needed to calculate and compare the reliabilities of the individual GPAs that were computed from within each of the two levels of type (t), and most importantly, did not provide sufficient information about the relationship between the two types of grades. In addition, it should be noted that this data was unbalanced, in that a different numbers of grades (14 and six grades) were nested within the two types. Addressing this in a univariate model required that the researchers select, somewhat arbitrarily, one of several statistical methods for accommodating the unbalanced nature of the data. However, MVG is another strategy for dealing with this unbalance design and gaining a more complete perspective of this data. The MVG analysis of this data is discussed next.

Before demonstrating how MVG addressed this grading data, it is necessary to provide some background on multivariate concepts and their notation. As this example demonstrates, an MVG

Table 4.5 Univariate Mixed Model [$p \times (g{:}t)$] G Study

Effect	df	VC	% Total
p	1,100	.19150	30
t	1	.00001	0
$g{:}t$	18	.00450	1
pt	1,100	.05604	8
$pg{:}t$	19,800	.39228	61

Note: p = person; t = type; g = grade.

design has a univariate G study counterpart containing a fixed facet (a mixed model). Instructionally, it is useful to use the univariate model as a starting point for understanding and representing the MVG design. In the mixed-model univariate grading example, type (t) had two levels (didactic and clinical), implying that the MVG analysis will have two summary scores for each student. Representing the fact that each student (p) had two unique sets of grades (g) in this MVG model requires special notation. To indicate that each person (p) has scores for each level of type (t), we use the symbol "•". Therefore, a solid circle (•) associated with a facet indicates that there are observations for each level of the multivariate variable (the fixed facet), and it is represented here as "p•". On the other hand, in our example, grades (g) are nested within type (t), and this is signified with the symbol "○". So, the notation to represent the complete MVG model in this research study on grading is (p• × g○).

It is important to notice that since the univariate model counterpart in our example has two levels of the fixed facet (type; t), our MVG model will have a univariate (p × g) design associated with each of these two levels. In this case each p × g design is linked (•) by the fact that students (p) receives scores for both types of courses. The MVG output for this data is displayed in Table 4.6.

Interpreting MVG results differs from the univariate context in that the MVG results include universe score correlations and covariances. Table 4.6 displays the results of the MVG grading study in a matrix format. The VCs are reported on the diagonals of each of the three matrices (p, g, pg), and these VCs are interpreted in the same way as the results from two individual univariate p × g studies. In this analysis, the proportion of variance attributable to student (p) was considerably higher for didactic courses (43% of total variance) than for clerkship courses (25%). The *covariance* between the two types of courses is reported in the lower off diagonal cell of the p matrix as cov = 0.16625. This is a measure of the relationship between didactic and clinical grades. However, for interpretation purposes, the universe score correlation in the upper off-diagonal cell of matrix p is easier to interpret. The universe score correlation is similar to the CTT "true score" correlation we encountered in Chapter 5. The magnitude of this correlation coefficient ($r = 0.798$) suggests that there is a strong positive relationship between the constructs measured by grades

Table 4.6 Multivariate G Study (p• × g○) With Two Levels (Didactic and Clinical)

Effect	VC and CoV[†] Didactic [%]	Corr[*] and VC Clinical [%]
p	.28671 [43%]	.79815*
	.16625[†]	.15132 [25%]
g	.00337 [1%]	
		.00741 [1%]
pg	.37419 [56%]	
		.43930 [74%]

* universe score correlation; † covariance.

earned in the didactic courses and those assigned in the clinical courses. Since grades are not linked across levels of the multivariate variable (type), the bottom two matrices (g, pg) in Table 4.6 do not contain covariance information. The VCs in the p and pg matrices are interpreted in the same way as in the univariate ($p \times g$) analyses. The 2×2 matrices in Table 4.6 is a reflection of the fact that the fixed facet (the multivariate variable) had two levels. The size of the MVG matrix will always be equal to the number of scores (i.e., levels of the fixed facet) obtained for the object of measurement (p).

The MVG output, like that shown in Table 4.6, can serve a number of useful functions in health professions education assessments. In D studies, the VCs can be used to estimate the reliability of subscores given various conditions of measurement. They can also provide researchers with an estimate of the reliability of composite scores given any number of items, ratings, or weights applied to the subscores and can help determine which composites will yield acceptable generalizability. In more advanced applications, the results of an MVG analysis can provide key validity evidence by unveiling the relationship between universe scores and error variances.

ADDITIONAL CONSIDERATIONS

Because this is a short introduction, we could not provide a complete treatment of G theory. We will briefly outline some additional topics and concerns that researchers who use G theory should consider.

G theory is highly flexible but does rely on some key assumptions. First, data should be interval or clearly ordinal. This allows for clear interpretation of VCs. Second, all effects in a G study model are assumed to be uncorrelated. This assumption, however, is sometimes violated when dealing with repeated observations of a fixed task or assessment practice—especially when measurements are taken within short period of time. Finally, there are two main statistical approaches to G theory—ANOVA methods and maximum likelihood (ML) procedures. While ANOVA methods do not impose distributional assumptions, ML assumes normality of the score effects.

Applying and interpreting G theory analyses requires special considerations. First, VCs are subject to sampling variability; therefore, researchers should consider the accuracy and stability of the VC estimates in relation to sample size and sample variability. Standard error (SE) of estimates can be helpful in this regard, but researchers should also consider the nature and size of the facet and person samples employed. In practice, it is not uncommon to observe a very small sample of certain facets that have not been selected in a true random fashion. It is also the case that G studies typically require more than 30 examinees (p) to yield reasonably stable estimates. Since conclusions are only as credible as the sample used to estimate the VCs, the sample should accurately reflect the intended universe (i.e., population parameters).

Second, while negative error variances are conceptually impossible, they do occur in applications of G theory. Negative estimates are generally a result of either sampling error (e.g., small sample from large universe) or a misspecified model (e.g., important facet(s) not modeled). Negative variance components are usually set to zero (Shavelson & Webb, 1991). Alternatively, one advantage of ML over ANOVA estimation is that ML procedures provide variance components that cannot be negative (Shavelson & Webb, 1991).

Third, an incomplete understanding of error sources can lead to misinterpretations. It is important to note that many real-world studies involve hidden facets, which are created when there is only one sampled condition of a facet in a G study (Brennan, 2001). For example, if all OCSE measurements were rated by a single rater, "rater" might become a hidden facet. This is because any variance associated with the rater would be confounded with the station variance components. Researchers often disregard these hidden facets, despite the fact that they can result in misleading interpretations.

Finally, while this chapter exclusively considered examples where the individual person (p) is the object of measurement, G theory is well suited for analyzing the means across persons (e.g., class means), with (p) then serving as a facet.

FINAL CONSIDERATIONS

G theory provides a method for examining a wide array of both simple and complex measures. A thorough consideration of G and D study results can provide a better understanding of the measurement process and how to improve it. Through the facilitation of insights regarding validity and reliability, G theory methods provide social scientists with a powerful research tool. The reader is encouraged to explore more advanced demonstrations of the theory to gain an appreciation of G theory's many applications to health science education and implications for validity.

APPENDIX 4.1

Statistical Foundations of a Generalizability Study

To understand the derivation of the VC, it is necessary to briefly review methods employed in ANOVA. In ANOVA, *sums of squares* (SS) characterize the distribution of scores around a mean. For example, the total SS in our example problem can be computed as:

$$\sum_p \sum_s \sum_r (X_{psr} - \overline{X})^2 \tag{4.9}$$

where:

   Σ is the summation operator;

   X_{psr} is a rating for a single person on one station by a single rater; and

   $\overline{X}$ is the grand mean across all raters, stations, and persons.

Hence, the total SS in our example problem is simply the sum of the squared difference of each rating subtracted from the overall mean. The three summation operators (Σ) in Equation (4.9) simply indicate this sum is performed across all persons (p), stations (s), and raters (r). To continue with this example, the SS for stations (s) can be calculated using Equation (4.10).

$$SS_{(s)} = n_p n_r \sum_s (\overline{X}_s - \overline{X})^2 \tag{4.10}$$

This equation contains just one summation operator, indicating the sum is across just stations. Hence, Equation (4.10) indicates that the SS for stations equals the sum of the squared differences between each stations mean and the grand mean, multiplied by the number of persons (n_p) and raters (n_r). A derivation for the SS for each SS follows similar notation and techniques. It is beyond the scope of this chapter to provide the complete derivation of all SS; however, an in-depth treatment of ANOVA estimation methods is provided in Kirk's *Experimental Design* (Kirk, 1982).

    Table 4.7 displays the ANOVA results from the data set in Table 4.1. In the first column is the source of the variance, and the second column displays the degrees of freedom (*df*) for that source

Table 4.7 ANOVA Table [$p \times s \times r$]

Effect	*df*	Sum-of-Squares (SS)	Mean Square (MS)	Expected Mean Square (EMS)
p	9	24.36	2.71	$\sigma^2(psr) + n_s\sigma^2(pr) + n_r\sigma^2(ps) + n_s n_r \sigma^2(p)$
s	4	8.56	2.14	$\sigma^2(psr) + n_p\sigma^2(sr) + n_r\sigma^2(ps) + n_p n_r \sigma^2(s)$
r	1	4.00	4.00	$\sigma^2(psr) + n_p\sigma^2(sr) + n_s\sigma^2(pr) + n_p n_s \sigma^2(r)$
ps	36	26.84	.75	$\sigma^2(psr) + n_r\sigma^2(ps)$
pr	9	7.20	.80	$\sigma^2(psr) + n_s\sigma^2(pr)$
sr	4	2.20	.55	$\sigma^2(psr) + n_p\sigma^2(sr)$
psr	36	7.60	.21	$\sigma^2(psr)$

of variance. Dividing the SS (column 3) by the degrees of freedom yields the mean squares (MS) displayed in the fourth column of Table 4.7.

The fifth column of Table 4.7 expresses the expected mean squares (EMSs) in terms of variance components (σ^2), and the number of raters (n_r), stations (n_s), and persons (n_p) sampled. The EMSs describe the composition of the MSs, or what elements of variance comprise a MS obtained from a sample. The MS values in Table 4.7 are for the sample data in Table 4.1. It is important to note that because the MSs are calculated on a sample, only in the case of the *psr* interaction will the sample MS act as an estimator of the population VC ($\hat{\sigma}^2$) (the "^" symbol over the σ^2 indicates that it is an estimate of the population variance). As shown in the fifth column of Table 4.7, for MS values calculated from a sample, the MS includes both the effect of interest and also other interactions. An estimate of a population VC is derived algebraically, solving in reverse for each VC using observed sample MSs. For example, as indicated in the last row of Table 4.7, for the triple interaction effect (*psr*), the MS from the sample directly estimates the population VC for the psr effect. Therefore, by using this MS (*psr*) as an estimated variance component for $psr(\hat{\sigma}^2(psr))$ in the double interaction (*ps, pr,* and *sr*) EMS equations, simple algebra permits one to isolate the estimated population VCs ($\hat{\sigma}^2$) for each of the double interactions (e.g., $\hat{\sigma}^2(sr) = (0.55 - 0.21)/10 = 0.034$). Deriving the estimated population VCs ($\hat{\sigma}^2$) for the three main effects ($\sigma^2(p), \sigma^2(s), \sigma^2(r)$) is only slightly more complicated. For example, the VC for persons can be estimated by inserting the MSs from Table 4.7 into Equation (4.11). Similar equations exist for estimating each population VC with observed sample MS values. Brennan (2001) provides a complete description of the rules and methods used for estimating population VCs from MSs obtained from a sample. Fortunately, specialized statistical software (GENOVA, SAS, and SPSS), examples of which are shown in Appendix 4.3, is capable of computing estimated VCs for the user, and in practice, researchers are not required to manually derive VC estimates.

$$\hat{\sigma}^2_{(p)} = \frac{MS_{(p)} - MS_{(ps)} - MS_{(pr)} + MS_{(psr)}}{n_s n_r} \tag{4.11}$$

APPENDIX 4.2

Statistical Foundations of a Decision Study

This appendix presents the logical and technical background for understanding the ratios used to compute G and Phi coefficients. Again, employing the design used in the example problem, let's consider what the ratio for the G coefficient would be using various numbers of raters and stations. Equation (4.12) expresses the D study G coefficient as a ratio of VCs. Equation (4.13) expresses the D study Phi as a ratio of VCs. Estimated VCs can be used in Equations (4.12) and (4.13) to provide D study reliability estimates. The reader is encouraged to verify the results reported in Table 4.4 by using Equations (4.12) and (4.13) with the appropriate sample sizes and the VC estimates from Table 2.2. It should be noted that the denominator for the Phi (Equation [4.13]) contains all sources of error, whereas the denominator for G (Equation [4.12]) contains just the error sources impacting examinee rankings. The reader should additionally recognize that Equations (4.12) and (4.13) are simply a more detailed version of Equations (4.5) and (4.6) respectively.

$$G = E\rho^2 = \frac{\sigma^2(p)}{\sigma^2(p) + \sigma^2(ps)/n_s + \sigma^2(pr)/n_r + \sigma^2(psr)/n_s n_r} \tag{4.12}$$

$$\text{Phi} = \Phi = \frac{\sigma^2(p)}{\sigma^2(p) + \sigma^2(s)/n_s + \sigma^2(r)/n_r + \sigma^2(ps)/n_s + \sigma^2(pr)/n_r} \\ + \sigma^2(sr)/n_s n_r + \sigma^2(psr)/n_s n_r \tag{4.13}$$

For each D study design, there is an associated pair of G and Phi equations similar to Equations (4.12) and (4.13) but unique to the D study design. By inserting the appropriate values for n_r and n_s, the number of raters and stations, Equations (4.12) and (4.13) are appropriate for all [p × S × R] designs with any number of stations and raters. However, if the researcher would choose to examine other designs, such as a [p × (R:S)] design for example, a different D study equation would apply. A more detailed treatment of these equations can be found in G theory texts (Brennan, 2001; Shavelson & Webb, 1991). One of the primary strengths of G theory relates to the fact that it is easy to use G study results to calculate G and Phi for designs different from that employed in the G study.

APPENDIX 4.3

Software Syntax for Estimating Variance Components From Table 4.1 Data

SPSS SYNTAX FOR ESTIMATING VARIANCE COMPONENTS FROM TABLE 4.1 DATA

```
VARCOMP
Score BY Examinee_id Rater_id Station_id
/RANDOM = Examinee_id Rater_id Station_id
/METHOD = SSTYPE(3)
/DESIGN = Examinee_id Rater_id Station_id
Examinee_id*Station_id Examinee_id*Rater_id
Rater_id*Station_id
/INTERCEPT = INCLUDE.
```

SAS SYNTAX FOR ESTIMATING VARIANCE COMPONENTS FROM TABLE 4.1 DATA

```
PROC MIXED data=gdata method=REML;
CLASS Examinee_id Rater_id Station_id;
MODEL score =;
random Examinee_id Rater_id Station_id
Examinee_id*Station_id Examinee_id*Rater_id
Rater_id*Station_id;
run;
```

GENOVA SYNTAX FOR ESTIMATING VARIANCE COMPONENTS FROM TABLE 4.1 DATA

```
GSTUDY (p x r x s)—random model
OPTIONS RECORDS 2
EFFECT * P 10 0
EFFECT + R 2 0
EFFECT + S 5 0
FORMAT (10F2.0)
PROCESS
5 4 4 4 4 4 3 3 3 3
4 3 3 3 3 3 2 2 2 3 2
:
:
FINISH
COMMENT
DSTUDY
DEFFECT $ P
DEFFECT R 2
DEFFECT S 5
ENDDSTUDY
FINISH
```

Note: Additional material and resources may be available at the UIC AHPE website: https://go.uic.edu/AHPE

REFERENCES

Brennan, R.L. (2001). *Generalizability theory*. New York: Springer-Verlag.

Crick, J.E., & Brennan, R.L. (1982). *GENOVA⁺–A generalized analysis of variance software system* (Version 3.1). [Computer software]. Iowa City, IA: University of Iowa. Retrieved from www.education.uiowa.edu/casma/GenovaPrograms.htm.

Eva, K.W., Rosenfeld, J. Reiter, H.I., & Norman, G.R. (2004). An admissions OSCE: The multiple mini-interview. *Medical Education*, 38(3), 314–326.

Kirk, R.E. (1982). *Experimental design: Procedures for the behavioral sciences* (2nd ed.) Brooks: Cole Publishing.

Kreiter, C.D., & Ferguson, K.J. (2016). An investigation of the generalizability of medical school grades. *Teaching and Learning in Medicine*, 28(3), 279–285.

Norman, G.R. (2003). Generalizability theory. In D.L. Streiner & G.R. Norman (Eds.), *Health measurement scales: A practical guide to their development and use* (3rd ed., pp. 153–171). New York: Oxford University Press.

Shavelson, R.J., & Webb, N.M. (1991). *Generalizability theory: A primer*. Newbury Park, CA: Sage.

van der Vleuten, C.P.M., & Swanson, D.B. (1990). Assessment of clinical skills with standardized patients: State of the art. *Teaching and Learning in Medicine*, 2(2), 58–76.

5

STATISTICS OF TESTING

Steven M. Downing, Dorthea Juul, and Yoon Soo Park

INTRODUCTION

This chapter discusses statistics commonly utilized in testing. Since this book focuses primarily on tests and other types of measures that result in quantitative data, some statistics are inevitable. Many of the tools used to evaluate tests and other measures used in health professions education require the application of some basic quantitative methods or statistics applied to testing.

As in other chapters, this treatment of statistics in testing is general and applied, avoiding statistical proofs and theoretical explanations and derivations. All of the statistics discussed in this chapter are based on classical measurement theory (CMT; see Chapter 3 and Chapter 4). Another measurement theory, principally item response theory (IRT), is used extensively in large-scale testing but is not discussed in this chapter (see Chapter 19 for an introduction to IRT). The purpose of this chapter is to give the reader an overview of some commonly used statistical techniques and their purpose and rationale, together with examples of their computation and use.

USING TEST SCORES

Assessments in health professions education generally yield quantitative data. Thus, it is important to consider some basic uses of such data, including the types of scores and score scale properties, and correlation and some of its special applications in assessment. In this chapter, we present fundamental statistical formulas that are useful in health professions education settings.

Basic Score Types

Test or assessment data can be expressed as many different types of scores or on many different types of score scales. Each type of score or score scale has its advantages and disadvantages, and each has certain properties that must be understood in order to properly and legitimately interpret the scores. This section notes some basic information about various types of scores and score scales commonly used in health professions education. Table 5.1 summarizes various types of scores used in assessment and their characteristics.

Table 5.1 Types of Scores

Score	Definition	Advantages	Limitations
Raw Scores	Count of number correct; raw ratings	Straightforward; simple to compute, understand, interpret	No relative meaning; need to know total number of items, prompts, points
Percent-Correct Scores	Percentage of raw number correct	Simple to compute; widely used and understood	Cannot be used with all statistical calculations; may be misleading
Standard Scores	Linear transformed score in SD units	Easily computed and explained relative score; linear transformation; useful in all statistics	May not be familiar to all users
Percentiles	Score rank in distribution	Commonly used and reported; easily computed; traditional score	Easily misunderstood, misused; not useful in statistical calculations; non-equal intervals; often misinterpreted
Equated Scores	Score statistically adjusted to maintain constancy of meaning, score scale	Interchangeability of scores on different test forms, from different administrations	Complex statistical calculations; complex assumptions

Number Correct Scores or Raw Scores

For all assessments that are scored dichotomously as right or wrong, such as written achievement tests, the most basic score is the *number correct score*. The number correct or raw score is simply the count of the number of test items the examinee answered correctly. The number correct score or raw score is useful for nearly all types of statistical analyses, score reporting to examinees, and research analyses. The raw score is basic and fundamental, and it is therefore useful for nearly all testing applications.

Percent-Correct Scores

Raw scores are frequently converted to or transformed to *percent-correct scores* in health professions education settings. The percent-correct score is a simple linear transformation of the raw or number-correct score to a percentage, using Equation (5.1):

$$\text{Percent-correct score} = (\text{raw score }/\text{number of items}) \times 100 \tag{5.1}$$

The percent-correct score is a linear transformation, which means that the raw scores and percent-correct scores correspond one-to-one and the basic shape of the underlying distribution does not change. Generally, if percent or percent-correct scores are reported and used, the raw score upon which the percent-correct score is based should also be reported. (Percent scores can be misused and can be misleading in some applications, especially when they are presented as the only data.) Also, percent-correct scores do not work properly with all statistical formulas commonly used to evaluate tests (such as the Kuder-Richardson formula 21 [KR 21] used to estimate scale reliability), so it is usually best to use raw scores or linear standard scores in most statistical calculations.

Derived Scores or Standard Scores

Several types of derived or linear standard scores are used in assessment applications. The linear standard score scale is expressed in the standard deviation (SD) score units of the original score distribution. The basic linear standard score, the z-score, has a fixed mean of 0 and an SD of 1 and is computed by the following formula in Equation (5.2):

$$z\text{-score} = (x - \text{mean})/\text{SD} \qquad (5.2)$$

where:

  x = raw score;
  mean = mean of the raw score distribution; and
  SD = standard deviation of the raw score distribution.

Table 5.2 gives an example of 10 raw scores and their transformation to z-scores with a further transformation to T-scores, which are defined as having a fixed mean of 50 and an SD of 10. Some researchers prefer T-scores because they eliminate negative values and also eliminate a mean score equal to zero, which the z-score transformation yields (some learners may be discouraged to receive a negative score, for example).

$$T\text{-score} = 10 \times z\text{-score} + 50 \qquad (5.3)$$

As shown in Equation (5.3), the T-score formula is 10 multiplied by (z-score) plus 50, but a standard score can be created with any mean and SD. Simply multiply the z-score by a desired SD and add the desired mean score to this quantity (SD × (z-score) + desired mean).

The main advantage of these types of derived or standard scores is that they put score data in the metric of the standard deviation of the original raw scores and maintain the exact shape of the original score distribution. For example, if the original raw scores are skewed to the right (which means that more students score to the high side of the mean than the low side of the mean), the standard score will have exactly the same shape as the original scores. This is a desirable characteristic for most scores that are computed in assessment settings. Other advantages of standard scores such as z- and T-scores is that they can be used in all other statistical calculations such as correlations, t-tests, and ANOVA, plus they can provide easily interpretable absolute and relative score information.

Table 5.2 Raw Scores, z-scores, and T-scores

Raw Score	z-score	T-score
41.00	−.30921	46.91
45.00	−.07584	49.24
50.00	.21587	52.16
55.00	.50758	55.08
60.00	.79929	57.99
74.00	1.61608	66.16
18.00	−1.65108	33.49
20.00	−1.53440	34.66
55.00	.50758	55.08
45.00	−.07584	49.24
Mean = 46.3 (SD = 17.1)	Mean = 0; SD = 1	Mean = 50; SD = 10

Normalized Standard Scores

It is possible to carry out another type of score transformation that normalizes or forces the transformed distribution of scores to be normally distributed or to follow the normal curve. These *normalized standard scores* are sometimes used by large testing agencies for research purposes, but they are rarely used in health professions education classrooms or reported at the local university level, since there is little benefit to normalizing scores for these ordinary applications. Standard scores, such as z- and T-scores, are not normalized scores, since such derived scores maintain the exact shape of the underlying raw score distribution. Simple z- and T-scores should therefore not be referred to as normalized scores.

Percentiles

Percentiles or percentile ranks are a favorite type of standard score in health professions education. Percentiles have several slightly different definitions, but generally a percentile refers to a score below which that percentage of examinees falls on some distribution of scores.

Percentiles are an inherently relative score with some benefits and many limitations. The advantage of percentiles is that they are commonly reported and easily computed. Most users think they understand the proper interpretation of percentiles or percentile ranks, yet they are frequently misunderstood or misinterpreted.

Percentiles usually have very unequal intervals so that, for instance, the five-point interval between the 50th and 55th percentiles is most likely not the same as the five-point interval between the 90th and 95th percentile. For example, for a student to increase her test score from the 90th to the 95th percentile typically requires answering many more items correct than to move from the 50th to 55th percentile because of unequal intervals on the percentile scale. Also, if the underlying raw score distribution upon which percentiles are based is normally distributed, then percentile ranks can be used to make familiar standard score-type of interpretations such as "84 percent of scores fall below +1 SD above the mean score." If the underlying score distribution is non-normal or skewed, as most classroom test score distributions are, this interpretation may be incorrect.

Also, percentiles have limited usefulness in other statistical calculations. For example, one cannot legitimately compute correlations with percentiles or use percentiles in inferential statistics, such as t-tests or ANOVA. Percentiles may be used only to report the rank of the examinee with respect to whatever reference group is used for percentile calculation. Percentiles may be misunderstood by some users as simple percent-correct scores, which is an incorrect interpretation.

Because of all these limitations, caution is urged in using and reporting percentiles or percentile ranks. Linear standard scores, such as z- or T-scores or their variants, are preferred because there are many fewer limitations for these types of scores, and there may be less potential for misinterpretation, misuse, or misunderstanding. Standard scores can be used in almost all statistical calculations, including correlations, inferential statistics, and so on. In addition, standard scores indicate relative standing using the standard deviation units of the underlying distribution. Generally, derived scores such as z- or T-scores are considered to have equal-interval properties, making the absolute (as opposed to relative) interpretation of these scores more straightforward.

Corrections for Guessing (Formula Scores)

One of the persistent controversies in educational measurement concerns the use of so-called "corrections for guessing" or "formula scores" (e.g., Downing, 2003a, and Chapter 7). These formula scores attempt to compensate for random guessing on selected-response test items, such as multiple-choice items, by either rewarding non-guessing behavior on tests or by penalizing guessing behavior. Generally, neither approach works very well and may in fact be somewhat harmful. Since the tendency to guess on selected-response items is a psychological characteristic that varies across a group of examinees, any attempt to control or compensate for presumed guessing is likely to create some error in the measurement. In fact, since the tendency to guess is a psychological construct that certain bold examinees may exhibit even if they are directed not to guess and are threatened with loss of fractional score points, the so-called "corrections for guessing" may add construct-irrelevant variance (CIV) to the scores. CIV, as noted in Chapter 2, is the measurement of some construct other than that which is intended to be measured by the assessment.

Generally, formula scoring or corrections for guessing are not recommended. Simple raw scores or derived or standard scores, in addition to percent-correct scores, are typically sufficient. The best defense against random guessing in selected-response test items is to present well-written items in sufficient numbers to reduce any ill effect of random guessing on the part of some examinees.

Equated Scores

Most high-stakes large-scale testing programs use and report an *equated standard score*. This score may look similar to standard scores such as *z*-scores or some variant of the *z*-score, but these equated scores can be interpreted differently than linear standard scores and are considerably more complex than simple linear standard scores. Equated scores statistically adjust the average difficulty of test scores up or down slightly in order to hold constant the exact meaning of the measuring scale over time and over various administrations of the test. If this statistical adjustment is carried out properly, equated scores maintain the same meaning over time and test forms and can be legitimately compared and interpreted across different test administrations and different time periods of test administration. In statistical jargon, if the test scores are successfully equated, it is a matter of indifference which test form (at which test administration) the examinee takes, because the resulting scores are on the same scale (Kolen & Brennan, 2014). Test score equating is beyond the scope of this chapter (see Chapter 19 for some conceptual explanations based on IRT). The major consideration to note here is that equated scores, such as those reported by large-scale testing agencies like the National Board of Medical Examiners, the Medical Council of Canada, and the Educational Testing Service permit more complex interpretations of scores than the simple *z*- and *T*-scores discussed here. Conversely, simple *z*- or *T*-scores can be interpreted as invariant with respect to mean difficulty, as are equated scores, only when the groups tested have approximately equal levels of ability, which rarely occurs in practice.

Composite Scores

The term *composite score* refers to a summary score that reflects multiple component scores. Commonly, a composite score is a total score (or grade) which is formed by adding scores from multiple scores generated during a course. For instance, a total composite score may be formed by adding together (and possibly differentially weighting) various individual component test or assessment scores for a class or a clerkship. A simple example of a composite score is a total score that is formed by averaging differentially weighted individual test scores collected during a semester-long class in which several different tests are administered to students. Instructors decide how much to weight each individual test score (and inform students of these weights) and then apply these policy weights to test scores prior to summing in order to form an overall composite score upon which the final grade is determined.

In order to ensure that the weights for each individual component score are exact, it is best to transform each component score to a linear standard score, using the mean and standard deviation of that score distribution, prior to multiplying by the assigned policy weight. If scores are not standardized, the effective weighting may be quite different from the weight applied to the raw scores, since the test score distribution with the larger standard deviation will contribute more weight to the final composite score than component scores with a lower standard deviation.

For composite scores in more complex settings, such as clerkships or other performance settings in health professions education, scores often display widely different scales with widely different variances, so it is especially important to standardize component scores prior to weighting and summing to a composite. Each individual component score should first be transformed to a standard score, then multiplied by the desired weight (as determined by some rational, judgmental, or empirical process), and then summed or averaged to a final composite (which might be transformed to some other metric for convenience). Prior studies in health professions education (e.g., Corcoran, Downing, Tekian, & DaRosa, 2009; Nassar, Park, & Tekian, 2017; Park et al., 2016; and Park et al., 2017) provide good examples of using composite scores in health professions education settings (see Chapter 3's Appendix for a comprehensive review of composite score calculation based on Kane's method [Kane & Case, 2004]).

The determination of the reliability of the composite score is a special topic in reliability. In order to estimate the reliability of the composite score accurately, it is necessary to take into account the reliability of each individual component score and the weight assigned to that component. Several methods, such as the stratified alpha coefficient, are available to properly estimate the reliability of the composite score. If the differential policy weights are not considered, the reliability of the composite score will be underestimated.

CORRELATION AND DISATTENUATED CORRELATION

Correlation coefficients are central to many statistical analyses used in assessment research. For example, correlation is a primary statistical method used in validity and reliability analyses and also for test item analysis. Various specialized types of correlation coefficients are used in test analysis and research, but all have the Pearson product-moment correlation as their basis. All correlations track the co-relationship between two variables, showing both the strength and the direction of any relationship. Correlation coefficients range from −1.0 to +1.0, with both extremes indicating a perfect relationship between the variables. A perfect negative correlation is just as strong a predictor as a perfect positive correlation. With a negative correlation, of course, the variables move in exactly opposite directions, such that as one variable increases the other variable decreases. In some test analyses that use correlation coefficients, such as the item discrimination index used in item analysis, it would be rare if the correlation of the item score (0,1) and the total test score were to reach ±1.0.

Correlation coefficients are attenuated or decreased by measurement error. For example, the correlation between test scores on two different tests, administered to the same examinees, is often used as one source of validity evidence for the test scores. However, we know that the observed correlation is lower than the "true" correlation because unreliable measures reduce (attenuate) or disguise the underlying relationship between the variables. If we could know the perfectly reliable scores (the true scores) from one or both tests, we could correlate these so-called true scores and understand the true relationship between the underlying traits that the two tests measure.

Classical measurement theory allows us to estimate this true score correlation or, as it is often called, the disattenuated correlation coefficient. The disattenuated correlation formula is presented in more detail in the Appendix of this chapter. This simple formula shows that the observed correlation is divided by the square root of the product of the reliability of each test. If the reliability of only one of the two tests is known, typically 1.0 is used for the value of the unknown reliability, since this will be the most parsimonious or conservative assumption. Obviously, the lower the reliabilities of the measures, the more correction will be observed in the disattenuated correlation coefficient.

The disattenuated correlation is a useful theoretical tool that is often reported in research studies, because it helps to elucidate the underlying or true relationship between test or assessment scores and criterion scores. It is important to emphasize that in actual practice, the errors of measurement, for example, the unreliability of the predictor test scores and/or the unreliability of some criterion measure, should be included in the validity coefficients, since this represents the state of nature and the actual or observed correlation of the two variables in the real-world setting. Disattenuated correlation coefficients should be clearly labeled as such and always reported together with the observed correlations upon which they are based.

ITEM ANALYSIS

Item analysis is a quality control tool for tests, providing quantitative data at the item level as well as some important summary statistics about the total test. Item analysis should be used extensively for selected-response tests such as multiple-choice tests but can (and should) also be utilized for observational rating scale data, ratings used in performance assessment simulations, and so on. Careful review of item analysis data can help to improve the reliability and consequently the validity of scores generated by instruments.

Item analysis data is frequently used to complete a key validation step prior to final scoring (Paniagua & Swygert, 2016; Lane, Raymond, Haladyna, & Downing, 2016; also see Chapter 7). Items that were keyed incorrectly can be rekeyed, and poorly performing items can be deleted from the final scoring. Some scoring programs may not have that option, and in that case multiple answers, possibly all of them, are scored as correct, although this may result in a slightly lower reliability estimate for the test.

Item analysis data, which represent the history of past performance of an item, should be stored in an item bank or other secure file for development of future tests. These data can then be used to improve the quality and clarity of test items and other types of rating scale prompts when they are administered again.

In its most basic form, item analysis represents counts (and percentages) of examinee responses to the options that make up a selected-response item. In order to evaluate the performance of the item or rating scale prompt, these counts are usually further evaluated in terms of groups of high-scoring examinees and low-scoring examinees with various statistics computed to summarize the item discrimination (how well the test item differentiates between high- and low-scoring students).

Item Analysis Report for Each Test Item

Table 5.3 presents a detailed annotated example of typical item analysis data for a single test item. The top portion of the table gives the text of the multiple-choice item. The middle portion of the table presents the item analysis data followed by a description of each entry of the item analysis data. Software used to calculate item analyses differ in style, format, and some of the specific statistics computed, but all are similar to the one displayed in Table 5.3. Common data entries for most item analyses are test item number or other identifier, indices of item difficulty and item discrimination, option performance usually grouped by examinee ability, and a discrimination index for each option of the test item.

Looking at the detail in Table 5.3, under the heading of "Option Statistics," note a breakdown of how examinees responded to each MCQ option. The MCQ options are listed as A to E, and "Other" refers to those who omitted or failed to answer this item. The column labeled "Total" is the total proportion marking each option. The keyed correct option or answer is indicated, and its total is used to calculate the "Prop. Correct" for this test item. The "Low" and "High" groups refer to the lowest scoring 27% and the highest scoring 27% of examinees on the total test, with the numbers in the columns indicating the proportion of examinees in each group who selected each option. (Using the lowest and highest 27% of examinees is the minimum group size needed in order to maximize the reliable difference between these two extreme score groups, because we can be fairly certain that there is no overlap in group membership between the upper and lower 27% proficiency groupings.)

Table 5.3 Item Analysis Example

Where it is an absolute question of the welfare of our country, we must admit of no considerations of justice or injustice, or mercy or cruelty, or praise or ignominy, but putting all else aside must adopt whatever course will save its existence and preserve its liberty.
This quote is most likely from which of the following?

A. Niccolo Machiavelli
B. Attila the Hun
C. King Henry VIII
D. Vlad the Impaler
E. Napoleon Bonaparte

Item Statistics			Option Statistics				
Prop.[1] Correct	Disc.[2] Index	Point[3] Biser.	Option[4]	Total[5]	Low[6]	High[7]	Point[8] Biser.
.70	.30	.27	A[*9]	0.70	0.55	0.85	0.27
			B	0.05	0.08	0.01	−0.14
			C	0.02	0.03	0.02	−0.01
			D	0.13	0.18	0.07	−0.13
			E	0.10	0.16	0.04	−0.15
			Other	0.00	0.00	0.00	0.00

Guide to Item Analysis Statistics
1. Proportion Correct (*p*-value): The total proportion (percentage) of examinees who marked the item correct. In this example, the *p*-value or item difficulty is 0.70, indicating that 70% of all examinees who attempted this question marked it correct.
2. Discrimination Index (*D*): This discrimination index is the simple difference between the percentage of high and low group of examinees who mark the item correct. In this example, $D = (0.85 - 0.55) = 0.30$.
3. Point Biserial Correlation/Discrimination Index (r_{pbis}): Correlation between the item score (0,1) and the total score on the test.
4. Option: The item options (1–5 or A–E). Other refers to missing data or blanks.
5. Total: Total proportion (percent) marking each option or alternative answer.
6. Low (Group): Proportion marking each option or alternative answer in the lowest scoring group of examinees on the total test. In this case, the group of examinees scoring in the lowest 27% of the total score distribution.
7. High (Group): Proportion marking each option or alternative answer in the highest scoring group of examinees on the total test. In this case, the group of examinees scoring in the highest 27% of the total score distribution.
8. Point Biserial Discrimination Index: This is the r_{pbis} for each option of the item, including the correct option. Note that, for the keyed correct option, the r_{pbis} is the same as noted in #3.
9. *Answer Key: The keyed correct answer.

Item Difficulty

Item difficulty refers to the proportion of examinees who answer an item correctly (also referred to as proportion correct or *p*-value; not to confuse with statistical significance), and it is the most basic essential information to evaluate about the performance of a test item. This index is usually expressed as a proportion or percent, such as 0.60, which means that 60% of the test-takers answered the item correctly. (This index might more accurately be called an item easiness index since it reflects proportion correct, but it is usually referred to as an item difficulty index.)

Item Discrimination

Effective test items differentiate high-ability examinees from low-ability examinees. (Ability means achievement proficiency in this context.) This is a fundamental principle of all educational measurement and a basic validity principle. For example, an achievement test in head and neck anatomy purports to measure this achievement construct in a unified manner. Theory posits that those students who are most proficient in the content should score higher than students who are less proficient or who have learned less of the content tested. For this particular construct, the best criterion variable available is probably the total score on this particular test of head and neck anatomy. It follows that highly proficient students should score better on individual test items than less-proficient or -accomplished students. This logic describes the basic conceptual framework for item discrimination.

Item discrimination is the most important information to evaluate the performance of the test item, because the level of discrimination reflects the degree to which an item contributes to the measurement objective of the test.

Discrimination Indices

Several different statistics are used as discrimination indices for tests. The most basic discrimination index is given by the simple difference in proportions of examinees in a high-scoring group who get the item correct and those in a low-scoring group who get the item correct. This index (D) is easily computed and can be interpreted like all other discrimination indices, such that high positive values are best and very low, 0, or negative values are always undesirable. See Note 2 in Table 5.3 for an example of D.

As an example, if 77% of a high-scoring examinee group gets an item correct, but only 34% of a low-scoring group of examinees gets the item correct, the simple discrimination index (D) is equal to $77 - 34 = 43$. A D of 43 (usually expressed as $D = 0.43$) indicates strong positive discrimination for this test item and shows that this particular item sharply differentiated between high and low achievers on this test. The D index should be interpreted like all other item discrimination indices such that a minimum acceptable value is about +0.20. While the D index provides useful interpretation of item discrimination, it is no longer widely used. The point-biserial correlation presented in the ensuing section has now become the new standard for item discrimination.

Point Biserial Correlation as Discrimination Index

Special types of correlation coefficients are also used as item discrimination indices for test item analyses. The point biserial (r_{pbis}) index of discrimination is the correlation between student performance on the item (that is, getting the item correct or incorrect, where 1 = correct and 0 = incorrect) and performance on the entire test. As in all correlation, the (theoretical) values of the point biserial index of discrimination can range from -1.0 to $+1.0$, indicating the strength of statistical relationships. (Because one variable in the correlation is dichotomous, the upper and lower bound of this type of correlation is usually not actually ±1.0.) Practically, point biserial correlations of about 0.45 to 0.65 or so are considered very high. See Note 3 in Table 5.3 for an example.

A simple quantitative illustration of item discrimination calculation for a single test item is given in Table 5.4. This example shows how 10 students score on one test item. The middle column describes how each of these 10 students scored on this particular test item, with a 1 indicating that the student got the item correct and a 0 indicating that the student got the item incorrect. The third column gives the total score on this test. In this example, student 1 answered this item correctly and scored 41 on the total test. The discrimination index (r_{iT}) for this item equals +0.14. This shows the correlation between the item scores $(1, 0)$ and the total score on the test for this group of examinees and indicates that this item positively differentiated high- and low-scoring examinees.

What Is Good Item Discrimination?

High positive discrimination is always better than low or negative discrimination, but how high is high? Typically, large-scale standardized test developers expect effective items to have point biserial discrimination indices of at least +0.30 or higher, but for locally developed classroom

Table 5.4 Correlation of Test Item Score With Score on the Total Test

Student	Item Score (Right-Wrong)	Score on Total Test
1	1	41
2	0	45
3	0	50
4	1	55
5	0	60
6	1	74
7	1	18
8	0	20
9	1	55
10	0	45

Note: Correlation between item score (1 = right, 0 = wrong) and score on total test is r_{iT} = +0.14. This low correlation of the item and total scores indicates a low (but positive) item discrimination for this single test item.

tests, discrimination indices in the mid- to high +0.20s are expected. At minimum, all discrimination indices should be a positive number, especially if there are any stakes involved in the assessment. (Negatively discriminating test items add nothing to the measurement and may detract from some of the important psychometric characteristics of the overall test and reduce the validity of the test scores.)

General Recommendations for Item Difficulty and Item Discrimination

Table 5.5 presents an overview of some general recommendations for ideal item difficulty and discrimination for most classroom achievement tests. All of these recommended values should be interpreted in terms of the purpose of the examinations, the types of instructional settings, the stakes associated with the tests, and so on. These recommended values for item difficulty and discrimination represent ideals. For most classroom settings, especially those with a more "mastery" instructional philosophy, these recommendations will be too stringent and may have to be realistically adjusted downward somewhat.

These recommendations are based on theory, which suggests that the most informative test items are those of middle difficulty that discriminate highly. For most achievement tests, we would like most items to be in this middle range of average item difficulty with high discrimination. These are the Level I items noted in Table 5.5. The next best item statistical characteristics are those noted as Level II items: somewhat easier items than Level I but with fair discrimination. Level III and Level IV items are either very easy or hard with low item discrimination. These are the least effective items psychometrically, but it is certainly possible that such items measure important content and should therefore be used (if absolutely necessary) to enhance the content-related validity of the test scores.

In interpreting the recommendations in Table 5.5, both item difficulty and item discrimination should be considered, although item discrimination may be more important than difficulty (if you have to choose between the two parameters). It should be noted that item difficulty and item discrimination are not totally independent. Middle-difficulty items have a better chance of discriminating well because of higher expected variance, but very easy items and very difficult items sometimes have high discrimination indices as an artifact of their extreme difficulty. Since

Table 5.5 Item Classification Guide by Difficulty and Discrimination

Item Class	Item Difficulty	Item Discrimination (Point Biserial)	Description
Level I	0.45 to 0.75	+0.20 or higher	Best item statistics; use most items in this range if possible
Level II	0.76 to 0.91	+0.15 or higher	Easy; use sparingly
Level III	0.25 to 0.44	+0.10 or higher	Difficult; use very sparingly and only if content is essential; rewrite if possible
Level IV	<0.24 or >0.91	Any discrimination	Extremely difficult or easy; do not use unless content is essential

Source: Adapted from Haladyna (2004)

few examinees fall into the category groups for very hard or very easy items, a change of a few examinees can change the discrimination index greatly, but this may be an artifact of the small numbers of examinees in ability groups.

Item Options

The ideal item is one in which each distractor (incorrect option) is selected by at least some students who do not know the content tested by the question. An incorrect option that fails to attract any examinees is a dysfunctional distracter and adds nothing to the item or the test (psychometrically). The correct or best answer option should have a positive discrimination index (the higher the better); of course, this is the discrimination index for the item. Incorrect options (the wrong answers) should have negative discrimination indices, because the less able examinees should choose the incorrect answers at higher frequency than the more able examinees.

Number of Examinees Needed for Item Analysis

Treat any item difficulty or item discrimination index cautiously if the statistics are based on a test administration with fewer than 100 examinees or so. About 200 examinees are needed to have stable item analysis statistics. However, even for small samples ($n \leq 30$) the results may still provide some useful guidance for item improvement. Usually some information is better than no information for improving a test, realizing that the statistics based on small numbers are unstable and may change at the next administration of the item. (In statistical terms, the smaller the sample size on which an item analysis is based, the greater the sampling error and the larger the standard errors around the sample statistics.)

Note that all item analysis data based on classical measurement theory are sample dependent: all item difficulty and discrimination statistics are confounded with the ability or proficiency of the particular sample of examinees. If the sample of examinees is large and if the range of student ability is fairly consistent for each administration of the test, item difficulty and discrimination values are likely to be stable over time.

SUMMARY STATISTICS FOR A TEST

Table 5.6 illustrates an example of summary statistics computed as part of a complete item analysis. These statistics are for a total test with all terms defined in the last column of the table.

These statistics describe the overall performance of the test and provide validity evidence useful for test score interpretation. They provide guidance for using scores to make judgments about

Table 5.6 Example of Summary Item Statistics for Total Test

		Definition of Terms
N of items	35	Number of items
N of examinees	52	Number of examinees
Mean raw score	26.56	Mean number-correct raw score
SD	2.89	Standard deviation, number-correct raw score
Variance	8.36	Variance, number-correct raw score (= SD^2)
Minimum	21.00	Minimum, number-correct raw score
Maximum	32.00	Maximum, number-correct raw score
Median	27.00	Median, number-correct raw score
Reliability	0.35	Internal consistency reliability: KR 20 or Alpha
SEM	2.33	Standard error of measurement
Mean difficulty	0.76	Mean proportion/percent correct
Mean r_{pbis} discrimination	0.08	Mean point biserial item discrimination
Mean biserial	0.13	Mean biserial item discrimination

examinees and also provide useful information about the performance of the test. This summary (Table 5.6) presents the total number of examinees and the total number of test items and the mean raw score (number correct score) with its standard deviation and variance (SD^2), along with the minimum, maximum, and median raw scores. These data give an overview of the shape of the score distribution and describe generally where on the distribution most examinees scored. The mean item difficulty, together with the two mean item discrimination indices, give us additional information about how hard or easy the items were on average and how well they discriminated. The reliability coefficient is the Kuder-Richardson formula 20 (KR 20 or Cronbach's alpha), which is an index of the internal consistency of the measuring scale, indicating the precision of measurement. The standard error of measurement is computed from the reliability coefficient and shows the precision of measurement on the raw score scale.

USEFUL FORMULAS

The Appendix presents some useful formulas together with examples using synthetic data. These formulas can be found in any basic educational measurement text, such as Crocker and Algina (2008) and Thissen and Wainer (2001). These four formulas are frequently used in assessment settings and can be hand calculated using readily available data. If computer software is unavailable, these formulas can provide some useful information about assessments and assist health professions educators in evaluating assessment data and planning future assessments.

A formula is provided to estimate the internal consistency reliability of a test when only the mean of test scores, the variance (SD^2), and the total number of test items are known. The Kuder-Richardson formula 21 (KR 21) typically underestimates the more precise Kuder-Richardson formula 20 (KR 20) slightly, but it can be computed by hand from the limited data available. The KR 20 is usually generated by computer software (within item analysis software) because it is computationally complex, using item-level data to estimate the variances used in the calculation.

The standard error of measurement (SEM) is an important statistic that is computed from the reliability coefficient and the standard deviation of scores. Most item analysis software applications compute the SEM, but it is easily computed by hand if software is unavailable. The SEM can be used to calculate confidence intervals around observed test scores and indicates the precision of measurement and the amount of measurement error in scores, expressed in the metric of the standard deviation of the test scores.

The Spearman-Brown (S-B) prophecy formula is used to estimate the expected increase or decrease in test reliability resulting from increasing or decreasing the number of test items. The S-B formula assumes that items that are added or subtracted from a test are more or less identical to the original items with respect to content, item difficulty, and item discrimination.

The formula for the disattenuated correlation coefficient or the correction for attenuation of a correlation coefficient is also presented in the Appendix and was discussed in the text above. With all the cautions for its use noted above, the disattenuated correlation coefficient estimates the correlation of true scores (in classical measurement theory) and answers the theoretical question, "What is the estimated correlation between the two variables, usually test scores or assessment ratings, if the scores or ratings were perfectly reliable?" The disattenuated correlation coefficient should be reported only together with the observed or actual correlation coefficient and should always be clearly labeled as the disattenuated correlation coefficient or the correction for attenuation.

ITEM RESPONSE THEORY

The approaches to analyzing test data presented in this chapter are based on classical test theory (CTT). Item response theory (IRT) is an alternative measurement model that addresses the confounding of examinee ability and item difficulty inherent in CTT, in which estimates of person ability depend on the difficulty/easiness of the specific items encountered, and item difficulty depends on the ability (or lack thereof) of the examinees. IRT provides statistical procedures for estimating ability and difficulty independently. However, IRT has assumptions that can make it challenging to apply in the classroom or school setting, with the main obstacle being the requirement for a sample size of at least 100. Because of this constraint, CTT methods are commonly used for local tests, and IRT methods are used, often in conjunction with CTT methods, for situations that require constructing multiple test forms for large numbers of examinees and to support computer adaptive testing.

See Chapter 19 for an expanded overview of the IRT approach. Downing (2003b) and De Champlain (2010) also provide useful introductions to IRT, comparing the approaches with classical test theory, and Tavakol and Dennick (2013) provide a guide for using Rasch analysis for analyzing data from a knowledge-based examination.

SUMMARY

This chapter has summarized some of the basic statistics used for assessment. Raw scores, the basic number-correct scores that generally serve as the fundamental scoring unit, were discussed. Standard scores, which express assessment scores in the metric of the standard deviation of the raw score scale, were generally recommended as more useful than percentiles. The fundamentals of classical item analysis and summary test score analysis were discussed, and item analysis was recommended for all assessments in health professions education as a basic tool to improve assessments. Finally, several statistical formulas that are frequently used in evaluating assessments were presented, such that the reader can easily compute many of the basic evaluative test statistics.

APPENDIX

Some Useful Formulas With Example Calculations

KUDER-RICHARDSON FORMULA 21 RELIABILITY ESTIMATE

Use: An estimate of the internal consistency reliability if only the total number of test items, mean score, and standard deviation (SD) are known. Note raw scores, not percent-correct scores, should be used for these calculations.

Note that the KR 21 usually slightly underestimates the more precise KR 20 reliability, but the KR 20 requires computer software for calculation:

$$KR\ 21 = \frac{K}{K-1}\left[1 - \frac{M(K-M)}{K(Var)}\right]$$

where:
K = number of test items (raw number of items);
M = raw score mean; and
Var = raw score variance (SD^2).

Example: A basic science test has 50 test items, with a mean score of 36.5 and a standard deviation of 10. What is the KR 21 reliability estimate for this test?

$$\begin{aligned}
KR\ 21\ Reliability &= \frac{50}{50-1}\left[1 - \frac{36.5(50-36.5)}{50(100)}\right] \\
&= \frac{50}{49}\left[1 - \frac{36.5(13.5)}{5000}\right] \\
&= 1.0204\left[1 - \frac{492.75}{5000}\right] \\
&= (1.0204)\times(1-0.09855) \\
&= (1.0204)\times(0.90145) \\
&= 0.92
\end{aligned}$$

STANDARD ERROR OF MEASUREMENT (SEM)

Use: To form confidence bands (CIs) around the observed score indicating the range of scores within which the "true score" falls, with known probability:

$$SEM = SD \times \sqrt{1 - Reliability}$$

where:
SD = standard deviation of the test; and
Reliability = reliability estimate for the test.

Example: A test of 100 items has a mean of 73 and an SD of 12, with a KR 20 reliability of 0.89. What is the standard error of measurement?

$$SEM = 12 \times \sqrt{1 - .89}$$
$$= 12 \times \sqrt{.11}$$
$$= 12 \times 0.33$$
$$= 3.96$$

If a student has a raw score of 25 on this test, what is the 95% confidence interval for his true score?

$$95\% \ CI = X \pm 1.96 \ (SEM)$$
$$= 25 \pm 1.96 \ (3.96)$$
$$= 25 \pm 7.76$$
$$= 17.24 \leq \text{True Score} \leq 32.76$$

SPEARMAN-BROWN PROPHECY FORMULA

Use: To estimate the reliability of a test that is longer (or shorter) than a test with a known reliability:

$$\text{SB reliability of longer test} = \frac{Kr}{1 + (K-1)r}$$

where:

K = number of times test is lengthened (or shortened); and

r = reliability of original test.

Example: A test of 30 items has a reliability of 0.35. What is the expected reliability if the test is lengthened to 90 items?

$$\text{SB Reliability} = \frac{3(0.35)}{1 + (3-1)0.35}$$
$$= \frac{1.05}{1 + 0.70}$$
$$= \frac{1.05}{1.70}$$
$$= 0.62$$

DISATTENUATED CORRELATION: CORRECTION FOR ATTENUATION

Use: To estimate the "true score" correlation between two variables; to estimate the (theoretical) correlation between two variables if one or both variables were perfectly reliable. The disattenuated correlation coefficient (theoretically) removes the attenuating effect on the correlation coefficient due to random errors of measurement or unreliability:

$$\text{Disattenuated Correlation} = R_{tt} = R_{xy} / \sqrt{(R_{xx} * R_{yy})}$$

where:

R_{tt} = estimated disattenuated correlation coefficient;

R_{xy} = the observed correlation coefficient between variables X and Y;

R_{xx} = the reliability of variable (test) X; and
R_{yy} = the reliability of variable (test) Y.

Example: Tests A and B correlated 0.48. The reliability of Test A is .70 and the reliability of Test B is .51. What is the disattenuated correlation between Test A and Test B?

$$R_{tt} = .48 / \sqrt{(.70 * .51)}$$
$$= .48 / \sqrt{.357}$$
$$= .48 / .597$$
$$= 0.80$$

If both Tests A and B were perfectly reliable, the expected true score correlation is 0.80. The disattenuated correlation should be reported only in conjunction with the observed correlation and the estimate of reliability for both measures.

Note that if the reliability for only one of the two measures is known, set the unknown reliability to 1.0 for this calculation.

Note: Additional material and resources may be available at the UIC AHPE website: https://go.uic.edu/AHPE

REFERENCES

Corcoran, J., Downing, S.M., Tekian, A., & DaRosa, D.A. (2009). Composite score validity in clerkship grading. *Academic Medicine, 84,* S120–S123.

Crocker, L., & Algina, J. (2008). *Introduction to classical and modern test theory.* Mason, OH: Cengage Learning.

De Champlain, A.F. (2010). A primer on classical test theory and item response theory for assessments in medical education. *Medical Education, 44,* 109–117.

Downing, S.M. (2003a). Guessing on selected-response examinations. *Medical Education, 37,* 670–671.

Downing, S.M. (2003b). Item response theory: Applications of modern test theory in medical education. *Medical Education, 37,* 739–745.

Haladyna, T.M. (2004). *Developing and validating multiple-choice test items* (3rd ed.). Mahwah, NJ: Lawrence Erlbaum Associates.

Kane, M., & Case, S.M. (2004). The reliability and validity of weighted composite scores. *Applied Measurement in Education, 17*(3), 221–240.

Kolen, M.J., & Brennan, R.L. (2014). *Test equating, scaling, and linking: Methods and practices* (3rd ed.). New York: Springer-Verlag.

Lane, S., Raymond, M.R., Haladyna, T.M., & Downing, S.M. (2016). Test development process. In S. Lane, M.R. Raymond, & T.M. Haladyna (Eds.), *Handbook of test development* (2nd ed., pp. 3–18). New York: Routledge.

Nassar, H.M., Park, Y.S., & Tekian, A. (2017). Comparison of weighted and composite scores for pre-clinical dental learners. *European Journal of Dental Education, 22*(3), 143–208.

Paniagua, M.A., & Swygert, K.A. (Eds.). (2016). *Constructing written test questions for the basic and clinical sciences.* Philadelphia: National Board of Medical Examiners.

Park, Y.S., Hyderi, A., Heine, N., May, W., Nevins, A., Lee, M., Bordage, G., & Yudkowsky, R. (2017). Validity evidence and scoring guidelines for standardized patient encounters and patient notes from a multisite study of clinical performance examinations in seven medical schools. *Academic Medicine, 92,* S12–S20.

Park, Y.S., Lineberry, M., Hyderi, A., Bordage, G., Xing, K., & Yudkowsky, R. (2016). Differential weighting for sub-component measures of integrated clinical encounter scores based on the USMLE Step 2 CS Examination: Effects on composite score reliability and pass-fail decisions. *Academic Medicine, 91,* S24–S30.

Tavakol, H., & Dennick, R. (2013). Psychometric evaluation of a knowledge based examination using Rasch analysis: An illustrative guide: AMEE Guide No. 72. *Medical Teacher, 35,* e838–e848.

Thissen, D., & Wainer, H. (Eds.). (2001). *Test scoring.* Mahwah, NJ: Lawrence Erlbaum Associates.

6

STANDARD SETTING

Rachel Yudkowsky, Steven M. Downing, and Ara Tekian

INTRODUCTION

A standard determines whether a given score or performance is good enough for a particular purpose (Norcini & Guille, 2002). The term "standard setting" refers to a process used to create boundaries between categories such as pass | fail or honors | proficient | needs remediation. Standard setting is "central to the task of giving meaning to test results and thus lies at the heart of validity argument" (Dylan, 1996). Establishing credible, defensible, and acceptable passing or cut-off scores for examinations in health professions education can be challenging (Norcini & Shea, 1997; Norcini & Guille, 2002; Friedman, 2000; Chapman, 2014; Karam, Park, Tekian, & Youssef, 2018). There is a large literature of standard setting, much of which is devoted to empirical passing score studies and comparisons of various standard-setting methods that are appropriate for selected-response tests or performance tests used in K–12 educational settings (Cizek, Bunch, & Koons, 2004; Cizek, 2006, 2012; Norcini, 2003; Livingston & Zieky, 1982). This chapter will discuss key issues and decisions regarding standard setting, identify ways to assess the quality and consequences of resulting standards, and address special situations such as combining standards across subtests, setting standards for performance tests, and multiple-category cut scores. At the end of the chapter, we provide detailed instructions for conducting seven standard-setting methods commonly used in health professions settings: Angoff, Ebel, Hofstee, borderline group, contrasting groups, body of work, and patient safety methods.

A cut score is an operational statement of policy and values. All standard-setting methods require judgment; the object of a standard-setting exercise is to capture the opinions of expert judges in order to inform a policy decision of "how much is enough" for a given purpose. There is no single correct or best method to set standards for an examination; nor is there a single correct or "true" cut score that must be discovered. All standards are, to some extent, arbitrary. Thus standard setting can best be viewed as "due process"—a procedure to be followed to ensure that the cut score is not capricious; that it is reasonable, defensible, and fair.

Standards can be categorized as either relative (norm-based) or absolute (criterion-based). Relative standards identify a group of passing and failing examinees *relative* to the performance of some well-defined group; the cut score or standard will depend on the performance of the specific group tested—for example, the bottom 5% of the class, or those who score more than two standard deviations below the mean of first-time test-takers. Relative standards are most appropriate when a rank ordering of learners is needed in order to distribute limited resources: for example, to give "honors" grades to the top 10% of the students in a surgery clerkship, to select top-scoring applicants for entry to dental school, or to identify pharmacy students most in need of remedial tutoring before progressing to the next stage of training. The placement of the cut score will depend on the resources available.

Absolute or criterion-based standards are based on a predetermined level of competency that does not depend on the performance of the group—for example, a score of 70%. Absolute standards reflect a desired level of mastery; the criterion stays the same whether all students pass or none do. In health professions education, the purpose of most examinations is to confirm mastery of a domain of knowledge or skill, so in the past decades most professional schools in the US have moved to the use of absolute standards.

EIGHT STEPS FOR STANDARD SETTING

Hambleton and Pitoniak (2006) divide the process of setting absolute or criterion-based standards into six critical steps: selecting a method, preparing performance category descriptions, forming a standard-setting panel, training panelists, providing feedback to panelists, and evaluating and documenting the validity of the process. In this chapter, we will use a modification of their scheme, slightly elaborated to include eight steps (see Box 6.1). We will discuss the key issues involved in each of these steps in turn.

Step 1: Select a Standard-Setting Method

There is no "gold standard" for a passing score. There is no perfect passing score "out there" waiting to be discovered. Rather, the passing score is whatever a group of content expert judges determine it is, having followed a systematic, reproducible, absolute, and unbiased process. The key to defensible and acceptable standards is the implementation of a careful, systematic method to collect expert judgments, preferably a method that is based on research evidence. Different standard-setting methods will produce different passing scores; different groups of judges, following exactly the same procedures, may also produce different passing scores for the same assessment. Such facts are troubling only if one expects to discover the perfect or "gold standard" passing score. Process is the key concept, remembering that *all passing scores are ultimately policy decisions*, which are inherently subjective (Ebel, 1972; Norcini, 2003).

Box 6.1 Eight Steps for Standard Setting

Step 1: Select a standard-setting method
Step 2: Select judges
Step 3: Prepare descriptions of performance categories
Step 4: Train judges
Step 5: Collect ratings or judgments
Step 6: Provide feedback and facilitate discussion
Step 7: Evaluate the standard-setting process
Step 8: Provide results, consequences, and validity evidence to final decision makers

Source: Modified from Hambleton and Pitoniak (2006)

Methods for setting standards can be described broadly as either test-based or examinee-based. In *test-based methods* such as the Angoff (Angoff, 1971) and Ebel (Ebel, 1972) methods described at the end of this chapter, judges review test items or prompts and estimate the expected level of performance of a borderline examinee (one just at the margin between two categories) on a given task. The patient safety method (Yudkowsky, Tumuluru, Casey, Herlich, & Ledonne, 2014) similarly reviews performance test items (e.g., checklist items), to determine those that must be performed correctly to accomplish patient safety or other critical goals. In *examinee-based methods*, represented by the borderline group (Livingston 1982), contrasting groups (Livingston & Zieky, 1982; Burrows, Bingham, & Brailovsky, 1999; Clauser & Clyman, 1994) and body of work (Kingston & Tiemann, 2012) methods, judges categorize the performance of individual examinees, either through direct observation, review of proxies of their behavior such as performance checklists, or review of examinee products such as chart notes written after a standardized patient encounter. In these methods, the scores of examinees in different performance categories are utilized in order to generate the final cut score. Finally, *compromise methods* such as the Hofstee method (Hofstee, 1983) combine features of absolute and relative standards, asking judges to estimate both acceptable passing scores and acceptable fail rates.

At the end of this chapter we describe these seven methods—Angoff, Ebel, Hofstee, borderline group, contrasting groups, body of work, and patient safety—all of which are potentially useful for establishing defensible and practical standards for examinations in the health professions. Choice of method depends on the purpose of the assessment, the desired inferences regarding examinees in different performance categories, type of assessment data, feasibility, resources available, and the preferences of decision makers at a given site.

Step 2: Select Judges

For the absolute methods discussed here, the choice of content expert judges is crucial. The passing scores established are only as credible as the judges and the soundness of the systematic methods used (Norcini & Shea, 1997; Norcini, 2003). Content expertise is the most important characteristic of judges selected for the standard-setting exercise. Judges must also know the target population well, understand both their task as judges and the content materials used in the performance assessment, be fair, open-minded, and willing to follow directions, be as unbiased as possible, and be willing and able to devote their full attention to the task. In some settings, it may be important to balance the panel of judges with respect to demographic variables, such as ethnicity, gender, geography, and subspecialization. For most methods and settings, 5–6 independent judges might be considered minimum, with 10–12 judges the maximum. Practical considerations must often play a major role in judge selection, the numbers of judges used, the venues for standard-setting exercises, and the exact manner in which the procedures are implemented.

Step 3: Prepare Descriptions of Performance Categories

Standard setting results in one or more cut scores that divide the distribution of scores into two or more performance categories or levels such as pass | fail or basic | proficient | advanced. Judges must have a clear idea of the behaviors expected in each of the categories. What behaviors characterize graduating medical students who are ready for supervised practice as residents? How does an "advanced"-level nursing student differ from a "proficient" student in the context of a pediatric rotation? Performance categories are narrative descriptions of the minimally acceptable behaviors required in order to be included in a given category. The cut points represent the boundaries between these performance categories on the exam score distribution. The performance category descriptions may be generated by the same judges who will set the cut points, or by a different group of persons familiar with the curriculum and the examinees.

Step 4: Train Judges

It is essential that every standard-setting judge fully understand the relationship between passing scores and passing rates. The passing *score* is the score needed to pass the performance test, often expressed as a percent-correct score. The passing *rate* is the percentage of students who pass the test at any given passing score (sometimes expressed as the failure rate). The higher the passing score, the lower the passing rate. If standard-setting judges confuse these two statistics, their judgments will confuse the passing score and become a threat to the validity of the standard.

Most absolute standard-setting methods pivot on the idea of the borderline or minimally competent student or examinee. This concept originated with Angoff's original work on absolute passing scores (Angoff, 1971). The cut score separating those who pass from those who fail corresponds to the point that exactly separates those who know (or can do) just enough to pass from those who do not know enough (or cannot do enough) to pass. The borderline examinee is thus one who is right on the border between two performance categories (see Figure 6.1).

The definition of borderline examinee is straightforward, but operationalizing this definition can be challenging. Asking judges to describe borderline students they have known and how they differ from clearly passing or clearly failing students (or other categories to either side of the border) imparts a clear understanding of what it means to be "borderline" and facilitates group consensus prior to beginning the standard-setting work.

Step 5: Collect Ratings or Judgments

Different standard-setting methods vary in the particular judgments each requests, and in how these are collected. See the detailed instructions for each of the methods provided at the end of this chapter. Quality control and documentation of collection processes are essential to provide "response process"-type evidence for the validity of the standards obtained. The procedures described in this chapter are examples of only one particular way to implement each method. Every setting is unique, and minor (or major) modifications to these standard-setting procedures may be required in some settings.

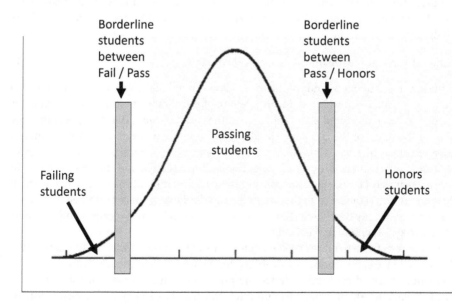

Figure 6.1 Borderline students

Step 6: Provide Feedback and Facilitate Discussion

Many of the test-based methods include an iterative procedure in which outlier ratings are discussed and justified, performance data may be provided, and consequences (failure rates based on the judgments at that stage) may be revealed. The item rating procedure is then repeated, and judges may choose to revise their ratings but are not required to do so. The cycle may be repeated one or two times. Iterative procedures tend to create more of a consensus among judges, but do not necessarily substantively change the resulting cut score (Stern, Friedman Ben-David, Norcini, Wojtczak, & Schwarz, 2006). Some educators forgo discussions and iterations for local examinations that are low to medium stakes.

Some judge panels wish to know, from time to time throughout the process, what passing score and/or passing rate they have established thus far in the process. Again, this is a matter for professional judgment, and we take the position that, in general, more data is better than less data for all judgments. Some test professionals, those who are of a more purist philosophy with respect to standard setting, will disagree with providing feedback to judges during the process.

Step 7: Evaluate the Standard-Setting Procedure

No matter which standard-setting method you choose, some evaluation of the resulting standard is appropriate. Is your cut score acceptable to your stakeholders? If not, is it because the test was not appropriately constructed, because your curriculum did not prepare students for the exam, or because your standard-setting judges did not have (or use) information about the actual performance of the students?

Judges can provide information about whether they were sufficiently trained for the procedure, their ability to make the requested judgments, and their confidence in the resulting cut scores. Positive answers to these questions from judges chosen for their content expertise provide an additional measure of credibility to the standards. Judges could be surveyed at two points—after training and after the entire procedure is complete. A sample survey is shown in Table 6.1.

Formal approaches to assessing the psychometric characteristics of standards can assist in the evaluation of the standard-setting results. Generalizability coefficients can provide a measure of the reliability of the judgments and D studies can suggest the number of judges needed to achieve a reliable standard. The standard error of the mean (SE Mean) passing score is the standard deviation (SD) of the passing score judgments across all judges, divided by the square root of the number of judges (n), as shown in Equation (6.1):

$$\text{Standard Error of the Mean Cut Score} = (\text{SD of cut score})/\sqrt{n} \tag{6.1}$$

Computing the lower and upper bounds of the mean allows us to build a 95% confidence interval around the cut score (Cut Score ± [2 × SE Mean]). Solving for n allows an estimate of the number of judges needed to reach a desired standard error of the mean. Jaeger (1991) suggests that the standard error of the mean of the cut score should be no more than one-fourth of the standard error of measurement of the test. Cohen, Kane, and Crooks (1999), perhaps more realistically, suggest that there is little impact if the SE of the cut score is less than half of the SE of the test. In a similar vein, Meskauskas (1986) suggests that the standard deviation of the judgments be small (no more than one-fourth) compared to the size of the standard deviation of examinee test scores. These recommendations may be difficult to achieve at a local level with typically small numbers of judges (Yudkowsky, Downing, & Wirth, 2008).

Kane (1994) suggests three main sources of evidence to support the validity of standards. *Procedural evidence* includes explicitness, practicability, implementation, feedback from the judges, and documentation. *Internal evidence* includes the precision of the estimate of the cut scores (such as the SE Mean above), intra-panelist and inter-panelist consistency, and decision consistency. *External evidence* includes comparison to other standard-setting methods, comparisons to

Table 6.1 Standard-Setting Feedback Questionnaire for Judges

After Orientation and Training:

1. How clear is the purpose of the test and the nature of the examinees?	Very clear	Clear	Not clear
2. How clear are the characteristics of a borderline examinee?	Very clear	Clear	Not clear
3. How clear is the rating task to be performed?	Very clear	Clear	Not clear

After the Completion of the Standard-Setting Exercise:

4. How difficult was it to provide ratings?	Very difficult	Difficult	Not difficult
5. Was sufficient time provided for the rating task?	Too much time	Right amount of time	Not enough time
6. Was sufficient time provided for discussion?	Too much time	Right amount of time	Not enough time
7. How useful was the performance data provided?	Very useful	Useful	Not useful
8. Do you think the final passing scores are appropriate for the examinees?	Too high	Just right	Too low
9. How confident are you in appropriateness of the cut scores?	Very confident	Confident	Not confident

Comments:

other relevant criteria such as similar tests, and the reasonableness of the cut scores in terms of pass/fail rates.

Step 8: Provide Results, Consequences, and Validity Evidence to Final Decision Makers

In the final analysis, standards are set not by content experts (judges) but by policy decision makers. They must consider the recommended cut scores, the consequences of applying these scores in terms of pass/fail rates, and evidence as to the credibility of the cut scores before reaching a decision whether to accept the recommendations. The consequences of different types of classification errors must be considered, especially in high-stakes situations such as licensing or certification exams. False negative decisions are those in which someone who is qualified is categorized as "fail"; false positive decisions are those in which someone who is not qualified is categorized as "pass." A false positive error, licensing some unqualified practitioners, may pose patient safety risks; a false negative decision will result in a qualified practitioner being denied a license and may result in some patients being denied access to care. One way to minimize such errors is to increase or decrease the cut score by one standard error of measurement of the test, depending on the type of error deemed most salient (Clauser, Margolis, & Case, 2006). In practice, an adjustment of the cut score by policy makers occurs with some frequency, but purists may find this practice unsavory, despite its legitimacy and practicality.

At times, especially if no performance data were provided to the judges, the recommended standards may be unacceptably high; in that case the options are (1) to reconvene the panel of judges and ask them to repeat the exercise with performance data; (2) to convene a different panel of judges, and/or use a different standard-setting method; or (3) to otherwise adjust the standards to be more acceptable. Since different standard-setting methods are likely to produce different cut scores, some educators recommend using more than one method and taking a mean across the different methods to increase the credibility of the final cut score (Wayne, Barsuk, Cohen, & McGaghie, 2007).

SPECIAL TOPICS IN STANDARD SETTING

Combining Standards Across Components of an Examination: Compensatory vs. Non-Compensatory Standards

Some assessments include several distinct components or stations—for example, a written test that includes separate sections on physiology, pharmacology, and pathology, a performance test composed of a series of standardized patient encounters, or a clerkship grade that encompasses a written exam, end-of-rotation faculty evaluations, and an OSCE. Can good performance on one component compensate for poor performance on another? If so, the overall standard can consist of the simple average of standards across encounters or components (compensatory scoring). Component scores (and standards) can be differentially weighted if desired—in the case of the clerkship grade, for example, the written test can comprise 50% of the final grade, with the faculty evaluations and OSCE each contributing another 25%. Component scores should be transformed to linear standard scores before weighting (see Chapter 3 on reliability and Chapter 5 on statistics of testing). Alternatively, a whole-test method such as Hofstee can be used to set a single cut score for the entire battery (Schindler, Corcoran, & DaRosa, 2007).

In some cases, however, a non-compensatory approach may be more appropriate, to ensure that learners reach a minimum level of competence in several crucial but different domains. In this case, standards must be set separately for each domain, and examinees must pass each component separately. Each component must include a sufficiently large sample of student behavior in order to be reliable, since very small samples of items—containing large sampling error—may result in incorrect decisions. Setting multiple hurdles to be passed will inevitably increase the failure rate.

In clinical cases, faculty often feel very strongly that a few crucial items must be accomplished for the student to pass, regardless of overall score. These items should be discussed at both the scoring and standard-setting stages of exam planning.

Setting Standards for Performance Tests

Performance tests allow for direct observation of a particular competency in a contrived or simulated environment (see Performance Tests, Chapter 9). An objective structured clinical examination or OSCE is a common example of a performance test, in which examinees rotate through a series of stations, each presenting a particular challenge. If content experts such as faculty observe and rate the performance of the examinees, examinee-based methods such as the borderline group or contrasting groups methods can be used. These methods are convenient and simple to implement; faculty are very comfortable with making judgments about an individual performance, and all judgments are made in the course of the exam so no additional faculty time is needed. If experts are not scoring the exam (for example, when standardized patients provide checklist scores), methods involving judgments about the test items or test content (Angoff, Ebel, Hofstee) can be used.

The use of item-based methods such as Angoff to set standards for standardized patient cases, while very common, has been challenged on the basis that items within a case are not mutually independent (Ross, Clauser, Margolis, Orr, & Klass, 1996; Boulet, de Champlain, & McKinley, 2003). One solution is to have judges work on the case level instead of the item level, estimating the total number of items a borderline examinee would obtain on the case (Norcini, 2003, Stern et al., 2006). An additional strength is that a case-based standard-setting approach is consistent with recommended methods of reliability estimation.

See Chapter 9 for additional discussion of standard setting in the context of performance tests.

Setting Standards for Clinical Procedures

The checklists used to assess procedural skills such as phlebotomy or lumbar puncture are often unique in that (1) they cover the *entire* set of behaviors needed to accomplish the procedure (rather than a sampling of salient items), and (2) the checklists are public—students are expected to use the checklist to learn and practice the procedure, effectively comprising a mastery learning setting. Certain items on the checklist may be essential for patient safety. While in general pass/fail decisions should never be based on a single item because of the possibility of rater errors, in the interest of patient safety judges may require that an error on even one of these core items will trigger a retest on that procedure. The patient safety method and mastery testing approaches (see Chapter 18) are most appropriate for this purpose.

Setting Standards for Oral Exams, Essays, and Portfolios

Standards for oral exams, essay papers, and portfolios can be set using methods that combine expert global (holistic) judgments with analytic scoring methods (e.g., borderline group or contrasting groups), or using whole test (Hofstee) or body of work methods for collections of items. Clear and explicit performance category descriptors or rubrics can provide benchmarks for initial scoring purposes as well as for later standard-setting efforts.

Setting Standards in Mastery Learning Settings

Standards for mastery tests will generally reference the *well-prepared* student rather than the *minimally competent* student. Most of the methods described here can be adapted for mastery settings. See Chapter 18 for a discussion of standard setting in mastery learning curricula.

Multiple Category Cut Scores

Setting cut scores for multiple categories (e.g., honors | pass | fail or expert | proficient | beginner) can be done using the same methods as for dichotomous pass/fail standards. The performance category descriptions provided to the judges must clearly differentiate the behaviors expected at each level. Other features of the pass-fail standard-setting process may have to be modified somewhat to permit multiple outcome categories.

The accuracy of distinguishing cut score categories (e.g., pass | fail; high honors | honors; expert | proficient | needs remediation) is related to the reliability of the assessment scores and other characteristics of the data, such as the shape of the distribution of the scores, the location of the cut score(s), and the true base rates in the population (Clauser et al., 2006). In general, the higher the reliability of the assessment scores and the lower the standard errors of measurement, the better classification accuracy can be expected. For example, Wainer and Thissen (1996) shows that at a reliability of 0.50, one can reasonably expect scores to vary by at least one standard deviation (SD) unit for about one-third of those tested. Even for relatively high reliabilities of 0.80, about 11% of students will have score changes of 1 SD or more.

False positive and false negative classification errors will occur more frequently when multiple cut points are used. In general, as expected, false negatives increase as the passing score increases and false positives decrease as pass scores are raised. The costs of false positives and false negatives must be considered as standard-setting policies and procedures are selected and applied.

Setting Standards Across Institutions

Faculty at different schools setting standards for the same exam using the same standard-setting method are very likely to come up with different cut scores. For example, faculty at five medical schools in the UK used the Angoff method to set passing scores for the same six OSCE stations and came up with widely varying cut scores; a student with a given level of competency might pass at one school and fail at another (Boursicot, Roberts, & Pell, 2006; see also Ward et al., 2018, for a similar experience in Australia). If uniform standards are desired across schools, standard-setting teams should include members across the participating schools as well as external experts, if appropriate. Groups should be encouraged to reach consensus on the characteristics of minimally competent (borderline) students before beginning the exercise. If several (mixed) groups are convened, a single cut score can be obtained by taking the mean across groups. Stern et al. (2006) used the Angoff method creatively in a pilot study to set international standards for medical schools in China. In this study, the concept of the "borderline school" was used to define school-level outcome standards.

SEVEN METHODS FOR SETTING PERFORMANCE STANDARDS

The Angoff Method

The Angoff method (Angoff, 1971) was the first of the absolute methods and thus has the longest history of successful use, even in high-stakes testing situations. In this method, content experts make judgments about every item, so it is fairly easy to defend the resulting passing scores.

Angoff Standard-Setting Procedures

There are five steps in implementing an Angoff standard-setting exercise:

1. The standard-setting judges discuss the characteristics of a borderline examinee and note specific examples of borderline students.
2. Judges come to a consensus agreement on the qualities of the borderline examinee, with specific examples in mind.
3. Each judge estimates the performance of the borderline examinee for each performance prompt, item, or rating (0% to 100%).
4. These judgments are recorded (usually by a non-judge recorder or secretary).
5. Judgments are then systematically combined (totaled and averaged) to determine a passing score on the performance test.

Item Review and Rating

Judgments are made at the item level. The item review begins with one of the judges reading the first item. First, the reader and then the other judges on the panel give their estimate of how well a borderline candidate will score on that item; judges rotate clockwise for each new item. Each judge's estimate (judgment) is recorded on a recording sheet or a computer spreadsheet. For each item, the judges answer one of the following two equivalent questions:

1. How many individuals in a group of 100 borderline examinees *will accomplish* this item correctly? (0% to 100%),

OR

2. What is the probability that one borderline examinee *will accomplish* this item correctly? (0 to 1.0)

Note that the Angoff question asks judges to estimate how well students *will* perform, not how well they *should* perform. The difference between "will" and "should" needs to be emphasized. If the judgments for an item differ by 20% or more, those judges who provided the high and low scores may lead a discussion of their ratings for that item. Throughout the process, judges can modify their ratings or judgments. The review and rating of prompts continues until the entire checklist has been completed. When setting standards for lengthy local or low-stakes tests, judges may review together a subset of 5–10 items to develop a shared mental model of the task and the performance of the borderline examinee and complete the rest of the ratings independently.

Absent data about actual examinee performance, content-expert judges frequently set unrealistically high passing scores. Summary data such as the mean and standard deviation of exam scores or scores on a standardized patient case will help to calibrate judges as to the difficulty of the test for real students. Alternately, more specific data may also be presented, such as the proportion of the total group of students who get each item correct. Proponents of iterative procedures generally withhold item-level performance data until the second iteration; this to discourage judges from basing their judgments formulaically on the performance of the average student, which would convert their judgment into one that is norm-based rather than criterion-based.

One way to help judges maintain a focus on the *importance* of the item in addition to its *difficulty* is to ask judges to rate the relevance of each item as essential, important, acceptable, or unimportant before providing the Angoff judgment. In effect, this creates a method that is a cross between the Angoff and Ebel methods (see Ebel method below). The relevance judgments also provide an additional layer of content validity evidence.

Table 6.2 shows the Angoff ratings for a 10-item performance examination rated by seven Angoff judges. The case passing score (percent) is the simple average of passing scores for all items.

A variant of the Angoff method, called the extended Angoff procedure, can be used with a rating scale rather than a dichotomous item (Hambleton & Plake, 1995). Each judge independently estimates the rating that a borderline student will get on each item. For example, if the student is being rated on a five-point scale, a borderline student might be expected to achieve a rating of "3" on item 1 and of "4" on item 2. Calculate the mean rating for each item across all judges and average over items to obtain the raw passing rating score.

Table 6.2 Sample Angoff Ratings and Calculation of Angoff Passing Score

Item	Rater 1	Rater 2	Rater 3	Rater 4	Rater 5	Rater 6	Rater 7	Mean
1	0.80	0.87	0.85	0.90	0.80	0.95	0.85	0.86
2	0.70	0.75	0.80	0.85	0.75	0.85	0.75	0.78
3	0.50	0.63	0.55	0.60	0.65	0.60	0.60	0.59
4	0.70	0.68	0.70	0.70	0.65	0.70	0.70	0.69
5	0.75	0.70	0.80	0.85	0.70	0.85	0.80	0.78
6	0.60	0.65	0.80	0.75	0.65	0.85	0.80	0.73
7	0.50	0.58	0.55	0.60	0.70	0.90	0.60	0.63
8	0.70	0.78	0.75	0.75	0.65	0.80	0.70	0.73
9	0.45	0.50	0.50	0.45	0.43	0.55	0.45	0.48
10	0.60	0.69	0.65	0.65	0.65	0.70	0.70	0.66
							Sum[1]	**6.93**
							Pass Score[2]	**69.30%**

Notes:
[1] Raw Passing Score = sum of item means = 6.93.
[2] Percent Passing Score = 100% * (sum of item means/number of items) = 100% * (6.93 / 10) = 69.30%.

The Ebel Method

The Ebel method (Ebel, 1972) requires judges to consider both the difficulty of the item and its relevance. This method gives standard-setting judges more information about the test and its individual items, but also requires more work and time of the judges than some other methods.

Ebel Standard-Setting Procedures

There are two major tasks required to implement an Ebel standard-setting procedure:

1. prepare a matrix of item numbers categorized by relevance and difficulty and
2. estimate the proportion of borderline examinees who will succeed on the type of item in each cell in this matrix.

Item difficulty is determined by calculating the average difficulty (percent correct) for each item, based on actual data from an administration of the exam to a (representative) group of examinees. Difficulty ranges (easy, medium, hard) are arbitrarily determined, but should have some rational basis in the empirical data.

Relevance ratings (essential, important, acceptable) for each item must be obtained from judges (see #6 below). It is customary for the same judges used to give the final Ebel ratings to carry out the relevance ratings, but this is not essential. Also, since some time is needed to carry out various computations and to create rating forms once the relevance ratings are obtained, it may be necessary to divide the Ebel standard-setting exercise into two separate sessions. A different group of judges could carry out relevance ratings, if circumstances warrant.

Here is a summary of steps to accomplish an Ebel standard-setting exercise:

1. Familiarize the judges with the content of the test, performance cases, and/or the checklists or rating scales.
2. Discuss specific definitions of the relevance categories used: "essential, important, and acceptable." For example, "essential to good patient care—if this item is not accomplished, the patient's health is at risk."
3. Have each judge rate each item as *essential, important,* or *acceptable*.
4. Compute summary statistics (average across judges) for the relevance ratings of each item.
5. Compute mean item difficulty (proportion correct) for each item or prompt of each case or station, based on actual performance data.
6. For each case, prepare a matrix of items sorted by relevance and difficulty (see Table 6.3).

Table 6.3 Sample Ebel Ratings and Calculation of Passing Score

	Matrix of Checklist Item Relevance by Difficulty			
Item Relevance	**Easy (.80 – .99)**	**Medium (.45 – .79)**	**Hard (0 – .44)**	**Weighted Mean**
Essential	Items # 4, 5 93% correct[1]	Item # 1 81% correct	Item # 3 63% correct	$(2 \times .93) + .81 + .63 = 3.30$
Important	Item # 2 89% correct	Item # 10 76% correct	Item # 9 59% correct	$.89 + .76 + .59 = 2.24$
Acceptable	N/A	Item # 7 62% correct	Items # 6, 8 42% correct	$.62 + (2 \times .42) = 1.46$

Raw Passing Score = sum of weighted means = 3.30 + 2.24 + 1.46 = 7.0 raw points.
Percent Passing Score = 100% * (sum of item means/number of items) = 100% * (7.0 / 10) = 70%.

[1] In this example, for items rated as essential and easy, 93% correct represents the mean judgment of all the Ebel judges.

7. Lead the judges in a discussion of borderline student performance.
8. Reach some common understanding of the characteristics of the borderline examinee.
9. Ask each judge to provide an answer to the following question for each set of items designated by a cell in the matrix: "If a borderline student had to perform a large number of items or prompts like these, what percentage (0% to 100%) would the student perform correctly?"
10. Each judge records the estimated percentage of students who will correctly perform items like those noted in the cell.
11. Average judgments across all judges are computed and recorded, as shown in Table 6.3.
12. A weighted mean is computed for each row of the matrix, defined as the number of items in the cell multiplied by the mean rating for that cell, and then summed.
13. Adding the total for each row of the matrix gives the raw passing score as determined by the Ebel judges.

The Hofstee Method

The Hofstee method is sometimes referred to as the "relative-absolute compromise method," because it combines features of both relative and absolute standard setting (Hofstee, 1983, De Gruijter, 1985). Judges are asked to define minimum and maximum acceptable passing scores and failure rates. The standard is determined by the midpoint of the cumulative frequency curve of the exam scores as it passes through this bracketing rectangle (see Figure 6.2). Since it considers the assessment as a whole, it can be used conveniently for complex assessments composed of multiple disparate elements (for example, a clerkship grade composed of a written exam, faculty ratings, and an OSCE). Like the Ebel method, the Hofstee method requires analyzing and summarizing performance data prior to collecting judgments. Alternatively, performance data can be obtained from a subgroup of representative examinees or from a prior administration of the examination. If the judges do not take actual performance data under close consideration, the cumulative frequency distribution curve may not be included within the score boundaries they define. The graphical Hofstee (see procedure step 6/alternate) avoids this problem and ensures that the standard-setting exercise will result in judgments that are applicable to the specific group examined.

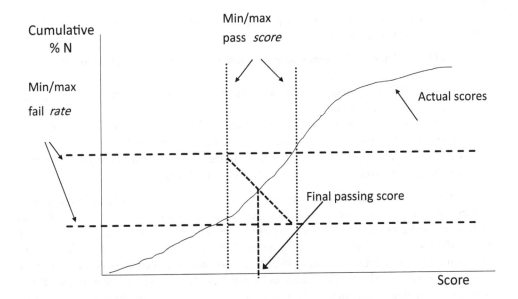

Figure 6.2 Hofstee method

Due to its normative considerations, the Hofstee method is not appropriate for use in mastery learning settings or in clinical contexts with patient safety concerns (Yudkowsky, Park, Lineberry, Knox, & Ritter, 2015). Some researchers discourage use of the Hofstee method for high-stakes examinations, perhaps feeling that it is less credible because the judgments are global rather than based on individual items (Norcini, 2003).

Hofstee Standard-Setting Procedures

A group of content-expert judges, who are familiar with the students and the performance examinations under consideration, are assembled and trained in the Hofstee method.

Before the Exercise

1. Based on actual performance data, compute the mean and standard deviation of the test and any other statistics (such as mean scores at quartile cutoffs) that would be helpful in describing the overall performance of students on the test.
2. Consider presenting graphical data showing the overall distribution of scores.
3. Optionally, calculate and present other examination data such as any historical data about student performance on the same or similar tests over time.
4. Calculate and graph the cumulative frequency distribution (as a cumulative percent) of the total performance test score for each case. (Statistical software such as SPSS can be used to plot the cumulative frequency percent.)

During the Exercise

1. Present and discuss the data discussed above with the standard-setting judges.
2. Review the cases and the items, the scoring methods, and other relevant details of the exam.
3. Discuss the borderline examinee with the group of judges, coming to a consensus agreement on the characteristics of the examinee who just barely passes or just barely fails.
4. Present and discuss the four Hofstee questions, ensuring that each judge fully understands each question (see #6 below) and its implications.
5. Consider doing a practice run to be certain that judges fully understand the Hofstee procedures.
6. Have each judge bracket the acceptable passing score and failure rate by answering each of the four questions, as noted here:

    a. The **LOWEST acceptable percentage** of students to **FAIL** the examination is: _____ percent (minimum fail rate).

    b. The **HIGHEST acceptable percentage** of students to **FAIL** the examination is: _____ percent (maximum fail rate).

    c. The **LOWEST acceptable percent-correct score** which allows a borderline student to pass the examination is: _____ percent (minimum passing score).

    d. The **HIGHEST acceptable percent-correct score** required for a borderline student to pass the examination is: _____ percent (minimum passing score).

7. Alternate: Graphical Hofstee. Alternatively, have judges draw lines designating the highest and lowest acceptable pass scores and fail rates *directly on the cumulative score graph*, with instructions to be sure to include the cumulative score line within the rectangle thus defined. Have judges specify and record the exact numerical value represented by their lines. Note: this method requires judges to wrestle with the consequences of their standards and to make judgments about the relative importance of high standards vs. acceptable failure rates. If you want to reserve that judgment for administrative decision makers, use the standard method.

Table 6.4 Sample Hofstee Ratings and Calculation of Passing Score

	Rater 1	Rater 2	Rater 3	Rater 4	Mean
Minimum passing *score*	65	70	60	60	64
Maximum passing *score*	75	75	65	70	71
Minimum fail *rate*	5	0	10	7	6
Maximum fail *rate*	20	25	30	30	26

Note: Use rater means to obtain passing score by graphing onto cumulative percent graph, see Figure 6.3.

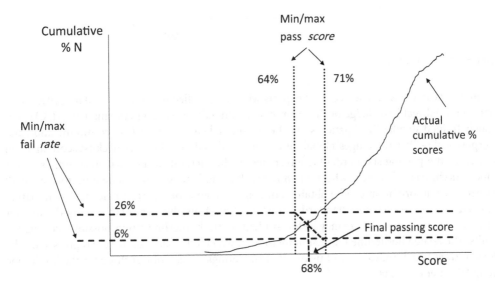

Figure 6.3 Hofstee example

After the Exercise

1. Compute the mean percentage for each of the four questions, across all judges.
2. Plot the mean of the four data points (minimum and maximum acceptable fail percent and pass score) on the cumulative frequency distribution. The four lines should define a rectangle containing the cumulative frequency line.
3. Draw a diagonal in the rectangle to intersect the frequency line. Drop a perpendicular from this intersection to the X-axis to find the passing score.

See Table 6.4 and Figure 6.3 for a worked example.

Using the traditional method, if the cumulative frequency distribution curve does not fall within the score boundaries defined by the judges and the judges cannot be recalled to run the exercise again, the standard can default to the minimum acceptable passing score or the maximum acceptable failure rate determined by the judges. Use of the graphical Hofstee method (#6/ alternate, above) will help prevent this problem, since judges can immediately see the results of their judgments and whether the cumulative score line falls within the defined boundaries.

Borderline Group Method

The borderline group method (Livingston & Zieky, 1982) is an examinee-centered rather than an item-centered method: judgments are made about individual test-takers, not test items or content.

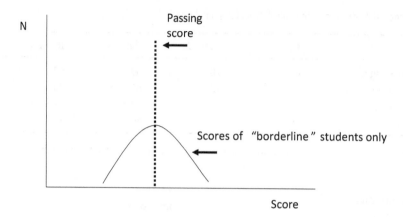

Figure 6.4 Borderline group

The method can be used when content experts who are qualified to serve as standard setters (e.g., faculty) have direct knowledge of the examinees or directly observe a performance test. (Appropriately trained standardized patients may be considered content experts in communication and interpersonal skills.) The judges' global ratings are used to determine the checklist score that will be used as the passing standard. One advantage of the method for performance tests is that it empowers clinician observers, who are familiar with the task of assessing student performance; all the necessary information can be obtained during the course of a performance test, eliminating the need to convene a separate standard-setting meeting. A disadvantage of this method is that for small-scale examinations, there may be few students in the borderline group, possibly skewing the results. The related borderline regression method in which (checklist) scores are regressed on the global ratings has the advantage of using all of the ratings instead of just those for the borderline group (Kramer et al., 2003).

Borderline Group Standard-Setting Procedures

1. Prepare judges by orienting them to the test, station, or case and to the checklist or other rating instruments.
2. Judges may have prior classroom or clinical-setting knowledge of the examinees, or alternatively they may directly observe the test performance of each examinee. Each judge should observe multiple examinees on the same station rather than following an examinee across several stations. The test performance observed may consist, with appropriate training, of performance products such as individual checklist item scores or post-encounter notes (in that case, this method is similar to the body of work method).
3. The judge provides a global rating of (the overall performance of) each examinee on a three-point scale: fail, borderline, pass.
4. The performance is also scored (by the judge or another rater) using a multiple-item checklist or rating scale.
5. The mean or median checklist score of those examinees rated "borderline" becomes the passing score for the test (see Figure 6.4). Alternatively, regress the checklist scores on the global ratings and use the resulting equation to obtain a cut score.

Contrasting Groups Method

The contrasting groups method (Livingston & Zieky, 1982; Burrows et al., 1999; Clauser & Clyman, 1994) is another examinee-centered standard-setting method, which requires using an external criterion or other method to divide examinees into two groups: experts vs. novices; passers vs.

failers; or competent vs. non-competent. The standard is the score that best discriminates between the two groups. One of the advantages of this method is that the standard can easily be adjusted to minimize errors in either direction. Thus, if the error of greatest concern is mistakenly categorizing an examinee as a "pass" when they should have failed (for example, in certifying examinations), the standard can be moved to the right (see Figures 6.5 and 6.6).

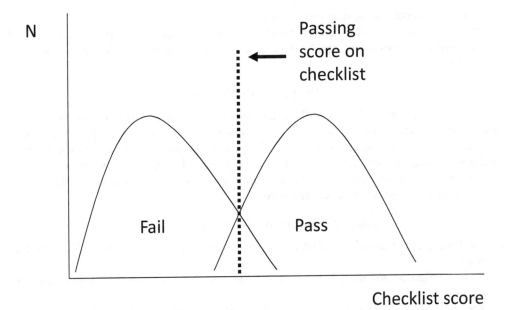

Figure 6.5 Contrasting groups

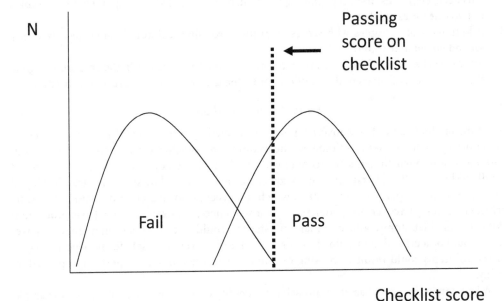

Figure 6.6 Contrasting groups: minimizing errors. The passing score has been moved up to avoid passing examinees who should have failed

Contrasting Groups Standard-Setting Procedures

1. Examinee performance is scored by judges or other raters using a multiple-item checklist or rating scale.
2. Examinees are divided into expert and non-expert groups, based on an external criterion or by having expert observers provide a global pass/fail rating of the student's overall performance.
3. Graph the checklist score distributions of the two groups.
4. The passing score is set at the intersection of the two distributions if false-positive and false-negative errors are of equal weight, or moved to the right or the left to minimize the error of greater concern.

Body of Work Method

Like the Hofstee, the body of work method (Kingston & Tiemann, 2012) can be used to set standards for an assessment that is composed of multiple disparate components. The general approach is similar to that of contrasting groups, but the judgments are made about samples of examinee's durable work (such as essays, chart notes, or portfolios) rather than about the examinees and their directly observed performance. Work samples are typically scored by judges or other persons before the standard-setting exercise takes place.

Body of Work Standard-Setting Procedures

1. Work samples are scored by judges or other raters using a multiple item checklist or rating scale.
2. Prepare judges by orienting them to the test, the examinees, and the definitions of any relevant categories.
3. Present judges with a large number of real, complete examinee work samples, spanning the range of obtained scores.
4. Judges assign each sample into one of the required categories (pass/fail, basic/proficient/advanced, etc.). This first *range-finding* round defines a "borderline region" where the scores of two categories overlap.
5. Additional work samples with scores from the borderline region only are categorized in a second *pinpointing* round.
6. The final cut score can be derived from the mean or median of scores in the borderline region, the intersection of adjacent distributions, or by the use of a logistic regression procedure.

Patient Safety Method

All of the methods described above, originally developed for written tests in K–12, take a compensatory approach to items on the test: the examinee must achieve a set percentage of items, without regard to which items are accomplished and which are not. The patient safety method (Yudkowsky et al., 2014; Barsuk, Cohen, Wayne, McGaghie, & Yudkowsky, 2018) was developed to set standards for performance tests in which incorrect performance or omission of specific critical items may have serious patient safety consequences. For example, for a basic procedural skill such as phlebotomy, failure to maintain sterility could lead to infection; maintaining sterility would be a critical item. Allowing non-critical items to compensate for non-performance of critical items could result in passing examinees who are not able to perform a procedure safely.

A key step in the patient safety approach is to identify criteria for critical items—for example, items that impact patient or provider safety, patient comfort, and/or the outcome of the procedure. Standards are then set separately and conjunctively for critical and non-critical items. Frequently a 100% pass score is expected for critical items, i.e., *all* must be accomplished in order to pass.

The patient safety method is especially appropriate for basic procedural skills and mastery learning settings (see Chapter 18). It can also be useful in other clinically oriented performance tests such as mannequin-based and standardized patient simulations (Chapters 9 and 14). While procedural skills checklists will often be composed entirely of critical items, more complex simulations or challenges may have a smaller proportion of truly critical actions. As in other mastery assessments, the target performance category for this method is typically the "well-prepared" learner rather than the "minimally competent" learner. Prior performance of first-time test-takers is generally not relevant since learners have the opportunity to retest until the mastery standard is achieved.

Patient Safety Standard-Setting Procedures

1. Judges or other stakeholders determine criteria for critical items.
2. Judges individually apply criteria to identify critical and non-critical items; may include iterative discussion. Average across judges to determine final categories.
3. Judges individually determine separate passing scores for critical and non-critical items. This can be done on an item-by-item basis ("Would a well-prepared learner accomplish this item?") or for the class of items ("What percent of critical items would a well-prepared learner accomplish? What percent of non-critical items?"). May include iterative discussion.
4. Average across judges to determine final cut scores for critical and non-critical items.
5. Apply standards conjunctively: examinees must accomplish x% of critical items AND y% of non-critical items in order to pass.

CONCLUSION

This chapter described the procedures for seven different methods of setting standards. Which method should you choose for your examination? The choice will depend on the purposes and practical realities of the test. See Table 6.5 for a comparison of the seven methods across several important dimensions.

Different standard-setting methods and different groups of judges will produce different passing scores; there is no "gold standard." The key to defensible standards lies in the choice of credible judges and in the use of a systematic approach to collecting their judgments. As such, it is important to document all information gathered as part of the standard-setting process. Ultimately, all standards are policy decisions, reflecting the collective, subjective opinions of experts in the field.

Table 6.5 Comparison of Standard-Setting Methods

	Judgment Focused On:	Judgments Require Exam Data?	Requires Expert Observers of Performance?	Timing of Judgments
Angoff	Test items	No	No	Before exam
Ebel	Test items	Yes	No	After exam
Hofstee	Whole test	Yes	No	After exam
Borderline Group	Examinee performance	No	Yes	During exam
Contrasting Groups	Examinee performance	No	Yes	During exam
Body of Work	Examinee products	No	Yes	After exam
Patient Safety	Test items	No	No	Before exam

ACKNOWLEDGEMENTS

This chapter is an updated and expanded version of a paper that appeared in *Teaching and Learning in Medicine* in 2006:

Downing, S., Tekian, A., & Yudkowsky, R. (2006). Procedures for Establishing Defensible Absolute Passing Scores on Performance Examinations in Health Professions Education. *Teaching and Learning in Medicine*, *18*(1), 50–57.

Reprinted by permission of Taylor & Francis Ltd, www.tandfonline.com.

Note: Additional material and resources may be available at the UIC AHPE website: https://go.uic.edu/AHPE

REFERENCES

Angoff, W.H. (1971). Scales, norms, and equivalent scores. In R.L. Thorndike (Ed.), *Educational measurement* (2nd ed., pp. 508–600). Washington, DC: American Council on Education.

Barsuk, J.H., Cohen, E.R., Wayne, D.B., McGaghie, W.C., & Yudkowsky, R. (2018). A comparison of approaches for mastery learning standard setting. *Academic Medicine*, *93*, 1079–1084.

Boulet, J.R., de Champlain, A.F., & McKinley, D.W. (2003). Setting defensible performance standards on OSCEs and standardized patient examinations. *Medical Teacher*, *25*(3),245–249.

Boursicot, K.A.M., Roberts, T.E., & Pell, G. (2006). Standard setting for clinical competence at graduation from medical school: A comparison of passing scores across five medical schools. *Advances in Health Sciences Education*, *11*, 173–183.

Burrows, P.J., Bingham, L., & Brailovsky, C.A. (1999). A modified contrasting groups method used for setting the passmark in a small scale standardized patient examination. *Advances in Health Sciences Education*, *4*(2), 145–154.

Chapman, B. (2014). Angovian methods for standard setting in medical education: Can they ever be criterion referenced? *International Journal of Learning, Teaching and Educational Research*, *4*(1), 1–26.

Cizek, G.J. (2006). Standard setting. In S.M. Downing & T.M. Haladyna (Eds.), *Handbook of test development* (pp. 225–258). Mahwah, NJ: Lawrence Erlbaum Associates.

Cizek, G.J. (2012). *Setting performance standards: Foundations, methods and innovations* (2nd edition). New York, NY: Routledge.

Cizek, G.J., Bunch, M.B., & Koons, H. (2004). Setting performance standards: Contemporary methods. *Educational Measurement: Issues and Practice*, Winter, 31–50.

Clauser, B.E., & Clyman, S.G. (1994). A contrasting-groups approach to standard setting for performance assessments of clinical skills. *Academic Medicine*, *69*(10), S42–S44.

Clauser, B.E., Margolis, M.J., & Case, S.M. (2006). Testing for licensure and certification in the professions. In R.L. Brennan (Ed.), *Educational measurement* (4th ed.). American Council on Education. Westport, CT: Praeger Publishers.

Cohen, A., Kane, M., & Crooks, T. (1999). A generalized examinee-centered method for setting standards on achievement tests. *Applied Measurement in Education*, *14*, 343–366.

De Gruijter, D.N. (1985). Compromise models for establishing examination standards. *Journal of Educational Measurement*, *22*, 263–269.

Downing, S., Tekian, A., & Yudkowsky, R. (2006). Procedures for establishing defensible absolute passing scores on performance examinations in health professions education. *Teaching and Learning in Medicine*, *18*(1), 50–57.

Dylan, W. (1996). Meaning and consequences in standard setting. *Assessment in Education: Principles, Policy and Practice*, *3*(3), 287–308.

Ebel, R.L. (1972). *Essentials of educational measurement* (2nd ed.). Englewood Cliffs, NJ: Prentice-Hall.

Friedman, M. (2000). AMEE Guide No. 18: Standard setting in student assessment. *Medical Teacher*, *22*(2), 120–130.

Hambleton, R.M., & Pitoniak, M.J. (2006). Setting performance standards. In R.L. Brennan (Ed.), *Educational measurement* (4th ed.). American Council on Education. Westport, CT: Praeger Publishers.

Hambleton, R.M., & Plake, B.S. (1995). Using an extended Angoff procedure to set standards on complex performance assessments. *Applied Measurement in Education*, *8*, 41–56.

Hofstee, W.K.B. (1983). The case for compromise in educational selection and grading. In S.B. Anderson & J.S. Helmick (Eds.), *On educational testing* (pp. 107–127). Washington, DC: Jossey-Bass.

Jaeger, R.M. (1991). Selection of judges for standard setting. *Educational Measurement: Issues and Practice, 10*(2), 3–10.

Kane, M. (1994). Validating the performance standards associated with passing scores. *Review of Educational Research, 64*, 425–461.

Karam, V.Y., Park, Y.S., Tekian, A., & Youssef, N. (2018). Evaluating the validity evidence of an OSCE: Results from a new medical school. *BMC Medical Education, 18*, 313.

Kingston, N.M., & Tiemann, G.C. (2012). Setting performance standards on complex assessments: The body of work method. In G.J. Cizek (Ed.), *Setting performance standards: Foundations, methods and innovations* (2nd ed., pp. 201–224). New York: Routledge.

Kramer, A., Muitjens, A., Jansen, K., Dusman, H., Tan, L., & van der Vleuten, C. (2003). Comparison of a rational and an empirical standard setting procedure for an OSCE. *Medical Education, 37*, 132–139.

Livingston, S.A., & Zieky, M.J. (1982). *Passing scores: A manual for setting standards of performance on educational and occupational tests.* Princeton, NJ: Educational Testing Service.

Meskauskas, J.A. (1986). Setting standards. *Evaluation & the Health Professions, 9*, 188–203.

Norcini, J., & Guille, R. (2002). Combining tests and setting standards. In G.R. Norman, C.P.M. van der Vleuten, & D.I. Newble (Eds.), *International handbook of research in medical education* (pp. 811–834). Dordrecht, The Netherlands: Kluwer Academic Publishers.

Norcini, J.J. (2003). Setting standards on educational tests. *Medical Education, 37*, 464–469.

Norcini, J.J., & Shea, J.A. (1997). The credibility and comparability of standards. *Applied Measurement in Education, 10*(1), 39–59.

Ross, L.P., Clauser, B.E., Margolis, M.J., Orr, N.A., & Klass, D.J. (1996). An expert-judgment approach to setting standards for a standardized-patient examination. *Academic Medicine, 71*, S4–S6.

Schindler, N., Corcoran, J., & DaRosa, D. (2007). Description and impact of using a standard-setting method for determining pass/fail scores in a surgery clerkship. *American Journal of Surgery, 193*, 252–257.

Stern, D.T., Friedman Ben-David, M., Norcini, J., Wojtczak, A., & Schwarz, M.R. (2006). Setting school-level outcome standards. *Medical Education, 40*, 166–172.

Wainer, H., & Thissen, D. (1996). How is reliability related to the quality of test scores? What is the effect of local dependence on reliability? *Educational Measurement: Issues and Practice, 15*(1), 22–29.

Ward, H., Chiavaroli, N., Fraser, J., Mansfield, K., Starmer, D., Surmon, L., Veysey, M., & O'Mara, D. (2018). Standard setting in Australian medical Schools. *BMC Medical Education, 18*(1), 80.

Wayne, D.B., Barsuk, J.H., Cohen, E., & McGaghie, W.C. (2007). Do baseline data influence standard setting for a clinical skills examination? *Academic Medicine, 82*(10 Supplement), S105–S108.

Yudkowsky, R., Downing, S.M., & Wirth, S. (2008). Simpler standards for local performance examinations: The yes/no Angoff and whole-test Ebel. *Teaching and Learning in Medicine, 20*(3), 212–217.

Yudkowsky, R., Park, Y.S., Lineberry, M., Knox, A., Ritter, E.M. (2015). Setting mastery learning standards. *Academic Medicine, 90*, 1495–1500.

Yudkowsky, R., Tumuluru, S., Casey, P., Herlich, N., & Ledonne, C. (2014). A patient safety approach to setting pass/fail standards for basic procedural skills checklists. *Simulation in Healthcare, 9*(5), 277–282.

PART II

ASSESSMENT METHODS

7

WRITTEN TESTS: WRITING HIGH-QUALITY CONSTRUCTED-RESPONSE AND SELECTED-RESPONSE ITEMS

Miguel Paniagua, Kimberly A. Swygert, and Steven M. Downing

INTRODUCTION

This chapter provides an overview of two commonly used written test item formats that are crucial to assessment in health professions education: the *constructed-response* (CR) format and the *selected-response* (SR) format, which most often takes the form of a one-best-answer multiple-choice question (MCQ). These two formats can be used to assess a wide variety of cognitive knowledge and skills within the framework of the foundational and clinical sciences. This chapter also highlights some key concepts, guidelines, and relevant research that support the development and use of these item formats. This chapter is not intended to be a complete item writing guide, nor is it intended to be a comprehensive review of the current literature on these formats. Instead, the overall aim of this chapter is to provide a practical summary of information about developing and effectively using CR and SR formats in the assessment of trainee performance in health professions education programs, along with suggestions for their appropriate use and discussion of areas for future research.

ASSESSMENT USING WRITTEN TESTS

One primary purpose of creating an assessment is to communicate what you, as the instructor and item writer, view as important. Tests are a powerful motivator, and your test-takers or learners will strive to learn the educational concepts they believe you (and your curriculum) value. This position is in alignment with recent shifts in the design of assessment programs in health professions education, which have in some ways moved away from assessment *of* learning and more toward assessment *for* learning (Chapter 17), with an emphasis on formative feedback and integrated assessments (Lockyer et al., 2017). The building block of any assessment, whether summative or formative, is the test item, so it is important to develop items and tests that align with educational and professional goals. In this chapter, we focus on written assessments for measurement of knowledge and skills (where "written," in the current century, encompasses computer-based assessments as well as traditional handwritten ones).

The primary guiding factors in determining the appropriateness of any item or testing format include the purpose and desired interpretations of scores, the construct hypothesized to be measured, and the ultimate consequences of the test. Often, these factors are summarized in the language of test validity as the *inferences* to be made from the test scores and whether these inferences are *generalizable* to the domain of interest (see Chapter 2, and the American Educational Research Association (AERA), American Psychological Association (APA), and National Council on Measurement in Education (NCME) Joint Committee for the Revision of the Standards for Educational, & Psychological Testing, 2014). Inferences are defined here as decisions, judgments, or conclusions that generalize or extend beyond a particular set of exam items into the larger domain from which the items were sampled. Performance of a set of items provides a basis for estimating achievement in the broader domain of interest. The characteristics of the item format should match the validity needs of the assessment.

Written test items are well suited for the assessment of cognitive knowledge acquired during courses of study in the health professions and can be used to great effect to assess knowledge acquisition, reasoning skills, and understanding of basic principles. While these types of skills tend to fall into the "knows" and "knows how" sections of Miller's pyramid (Figure 7.1), they arguably form a foundational set of skills for students to master prior to the gamut of oral exams, simulated patients, multi-source feedback, and direct observation assessments they will encounter along their educational journey (Miller, 1990; Nyquist, 2014). It can be challenging to expand into the assessment of higher-order skills performance with written test items. For example, if the goal is to test baseline cognitive knowledge—the "knows" and "knows how"—about the principles of effective patient communication, written test items may meet the required needs for these specific types of validity evidence to support score inferences. However, if the goal is to measure students' use of communication or physical examination skills with patients—the "does"—a performance test such as a simulation, a standardized oral exam, or a structured observation of student communication with patients in a real setting may be more appropriate (Swygert & Williamson, 2015). Some innovative written item types, such as situational judgment tests (SJTs), have been developed in order to bridge this gap and provide a more efficient and inexpensive measure of tasks such as interpreting social cues. In this chapter, we will focus solely on assessment of cognitive knowledge or performance that is best addressed with CR and SR items. The reader interested in learning more about SJTs and other performance items best suited for non-cognitive assessments are referred to Chapter 15 by Reiter and Roberts, or Kyllonen's chapter on the topic in the *Handbook of Test Development* (2015, 190–211). For a recent discussion of the potential of SJTs

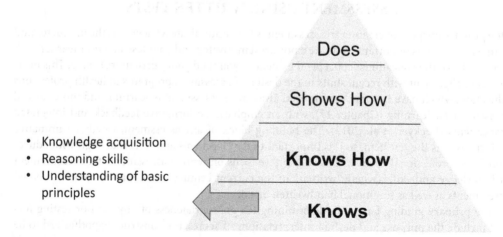

Figure 7.1 Miller's pyramid: cognitive abilities to assess with written examinations

for improving the quality of medical school admissions, see Fitzpatrick and Dunleavy (2016) as well as Chapter 15.

CR AND SR ITEM FORMATS: DEFINITION

Constructed-response (CR) items are defined here as non-cued, open-ended questions that require test-takers to provide written responses or answers. CR items are read and scored by judges with the necessary content expertise and training (almost always human judges, but increasingly supplemented by computer-based automated systems). The two main CR examples upon which this chapter will focus are written tasks such as *short-answer*, sometimes called open-ended items, and long-answer or *essay* questions. These CR formats allow for flexibility and creativity on the part of the item writer while retaining many assessment strengths. CR tasks require non-cued written answers from test-takers, so the effect of guessing is reduced and has little to no influence on the choice of answer. CR formats may be time efficient (for the instructor) when creating tests for small groups of learners, since less time is required to write a few short essay prompts than to create a large set of effective SR items. The CR item format may permit the rater to score specific steps the learner takes in working through a problem, or their demonstrated logic of each step used in reasoning or problem solving, and this facilitates partial credit scoring. Because learners are usually required to "show their work," the instructor will have a great deal of insight into not only the learner's cognitive knowledge, but also into their reasoning and logical abilities; the scoring rubrics can be designed to take advantage of this. CR items are not without their limitations, as will be discussed further in this chapter; these include the time needed to develop scoring rubrics and train raters, as well as the increased testing time required to adequately cover the domain of interest. It should be noted that the narrow definition of CR items used in this chapter is not intended to be dismissive of other types of CR items common in medical education performance assessments, such as the written communication sections (e.g., patient notes) on objective structured clinical examinations (OSCEs). We focus on short- and long-answer items solely for the sake of clarity and brevity in this chapter; for more information on constructed-response tasks for OSCEs, see Chapter 9.

On the other hand, SR items—especially in their most typical form of MCQs—have long been known to be the most efficient and cost-effective means of developing objectively scored tests for large classrooms of test-takers (Downing, 2002a; Downing & Haladyna, 1997; Haladyna, Downing, & Rodriguez, 2002). MCQs are useful for testing cognitive knowledge, not only for assessment of simple recall of information, but also for more advanced levels of reasoning. This item type is efficient for use with large groups of test-takers because these items can be easily and objectively scored even at the large volume required for broad testing of knowledge domains. This latter point is crucial in high-stakes and summative assessments; the broad domain ensures the test is a representative sample of the total content domain, thus increasing the content-related validity evidence and permitting better inferences or generalizations to the whole of the domain of interest. MCQs are more likely than CR item formats to be highly discriminating, allowing for a sharper distinction between those who demonstrate knowledge mastery overall and those who do not (for more discussion of item statistics such as difficulty and discrimination, see Chapter 5). Meaningful MCQ score reports—those providing feedback to learners on specific strengths and weaknesses—can be produced easily by computer and in a timely and cost-effective way, thus potentially improving the learning environment for learners. The most obvious drawback to SR items is inherent to the format: due to the cueing provided by the answer options, a learner who doesn't know the answer has a better chance to guess it correctly than with CR items. While SR items can be quickly and objectively scored, the time required to write many high-quality SR items is not insignificant; a flawless, relevant SR item can take between 30 and 60 minutes to compose (Rush, Rankin, & White, 2016). Some specific strengths and limitations of CR and SR items are noted in Table 7.1, and examples of typical CR and SR item formats are presented in Table 7.2.

Table 7.1 Strengths and Limitations of Constructed-Response and Selected-Response Item Formats

	Constructed-Response Format	Selected-Response Format
Strengths	• Demonstrates clearly the link between the item and the construct of interest • Avoids cueing responses • Allows for a more in-depth assessment of knowledge, such as assessing logic, reasoning, and steps in problem solving • Allows for partial credit scoring	• Allows for a broad and representative set of test content • Provides clear and defensible assessment • Allows for quick and straightforward computation of accurate, objective, and reproducible scores and feedback • Reduces the time and cost of assessment while increasing the potential scope of the domain to be measured • Provides more opportunity for item banking and re-use, due to lower memorability
Limitations	• Requires substantial testing time, which can lead to a limited breadth of content and negatively impact score generalizability • Requires substantial time to develop scoring rubrics, quality control measures, and score feedback • Allows for introduction of construct-irrelevant variance due to subjective human scoring and known rater biases	• Requires substantial time and training to write good items and to avoid known item flaws • Allows for introduction of construct-irrelevant variance because test-takers can answer correctly by guessing

Table 7.2 Examples of Constructed-Response and Selected-Response Items

Constructed-Response—Short Answer (Three sentences maximum)

Name and describe the function of each of the bones of the human inner ear.

Constructed-Response—Long Answer (Five pages maximum)

Discuss the human inner ear, describing in detail how the inner ear structures relate to hearing.

Selected-Response—Traditional Multiple-Choice Question (MCQ)

A 63-year-old woman comes to the physician because of a 2-week history of fatigue, malaise, nausea and vomiting, and decreased appetite; these symptoms have worsened during the past week. She was diagnosed with tuberculosis 3 months ago; a multidrug regimen was initiated at that time. Her temperature is 37.1 °C (98.8 °F). Physical examination shows scleral icterus and tenderness over the right upper quadrant of the abdomen; there is no hepatomegaly. Serum studies show a total bilirubin concentration of 6.5 mg/dL, AST activity of 580 U/L, and ALT activity of 650 U/L. Which of the following drugs is the most likely cause of these findings?

A. Ethambutol

B. Isoniazid

C. Levofloxacin

D. Streptomycin

E. Vitamin B$_6$ (pyridoxine)

Selected-Response— True/False (TF)

Which of the following is/are an X-linked recessive condition?

A. Cystic fibrosis

B. Duchenne's muscular dystrophy

C. Hemophilia A (classic hemophilia)

D. Tay-Sachs disease

Selected-Response—Testlets or Context-Dependent Item Sets

A 2-year-old girl is brought to the office by her mother for evaluation of fever. You have been the girl's physician since birth. While in the office, the girl stiffens and then has bilateral, symmetrical shaking of her upper and lower extremities; she becomes mildly cyanotic. The episode lasts for approximately 45 seconds, after which she becomes relaxed and appears to fall asleep. Vital signs at this time are temperature 40.0 °C (104.0 °F), pulse 120/min, and respirations 40/min. On physical examination she has a generally pink complexion and flushed cheeks. She is limp and somnolent and responds with a cry to noxious stimulus. Tympanic membranes are inflamed bilaterally; nose has a scant, clear discharge, and throat is mildly erythematous. Lungs are clear to auscultation except for transmitted upper airway sounds. Heart has rapid rate with a grade 1/6 systolic murmur at the left sternal border. Complete blood count, blood culture, lumbar puncture, and catheterized urine specimen are obtained and sent for stat analysis. Acetaminophen is administered by rectal suppository. Thirty minutes later the patient awakens and is smiling. She is afebrile. Additional history discloses that she was born at term, had an uneventful neonatal course, and has had normal growth and development, and vaccinations are up-to-date. She has never had an episode similar to this. Initial laboratory results are shown:

Blood

WBC 10,400/mm^3

Neutrophils, segmented 25%

Neutrophils, bands 5%

Lymphocytes 65%

Monocytes 5%

Cerebrospinal fluid 0 RBC/mm^3

Urinalysis normal

Other laboratory studies pending

1. In addition to ampicillin for otitis media and acetaminophen, this child also should receive which of the following?

A. Oral ethosuximide

B. Oral phenobarbital

C. Oral phenytoin

D. Rectal diazepam

E. No additional medications

2. Two weeks later the patient is brought to the office for a follow-up visit. Her mother says that she is doing well and has had no recurrence of her symptoms. Examination of the ears shows resolution of the otitis media. Which of the following is the most important diagnostic step at this time?

A. Audiology testing

B. Cognitive testing

C. CT scan of the head

D. EEG

E. No additional testing

CONSTRUCTED-RESPONSE ITEMS: SHORT-ANSWER VS. LONG-ANSWER FORMATS

The first step in composing a CR item is to identify the skill or cognitive performance of interest and determine what type of CR item can best assess such skills (Lane & Iwatani, 2015). This choice, known as format specification, is determined by the purpose of the assessment, the defined constructs and required content-related validity evidence, and the test platform (American Educational Research Association et al., 2014). As mentioned above, testing environments in which non-cued writing skills can be used to demonstrate mastery of knowledge and proficiency are ideal for CR item formats, and the first determination the item writer should make is whether to use short-answer or long-answer (typically essay) items. CR formats of either type typically require a substantial amount of testing time, meaning relatively few items can be administered within a reasonable testing time period. The extent to which the test content generalizes to the larger domain is therefore limited, and this implication should be used to guide the choice of format. Short-answer CR items permit a broader sampling of content because more questions can be asked and answered per hour of testing time, and the reliability of the test scores is thus improved. However, if the purpose of the test is to sample a narrow domain of knowledge in great depth, long-answer essays may be the most appropriate format. The essay format permits asking a test-taker to produce answers of great detail that probe the depths of knowledge about a single topic or content area. It is important to keep this trade-off in mind and to understand that even when long-answer essay items are well-written and accurately scored, the reduced number of items available during a testing time period can lead to a narrower sample of the construct, which in turn can have a substantial negative impact on score generalizability for broader educational domains.

CONSTRUCTED-RESPONSE ITEMS: SCORING

Scoring can be a major challenge for CR items, both in terms of operationalizing the scoring method and in developing and presenting final scores that provide necessary feedback while supporting the intended inferences. For CR prompts, whether essay length or short-answer, the scoring procedures require careful attention in order to reduce the common negative effects of subjective scoring by human raters. It is crucial that the choice of scoring procedure, training of raters, and scoring methods be suited to the particular CR task and the domain that the task represents (Chapter 2; Lane & Stone, 2006; Messick, 1994). Here, we discuss scoring procedures (aka *rubrics*) and common types of scoring scales, along with important aspects of training human CR task raters, as part of our recommendations to increase the scoring accuracy and validity of CR task score interpretations. We also briefly discuss the use of computer-based methods of scoring that may reduce the scoring time and need for ongoing rater work but are still heavily dependent on human expertise.

SCORING RUBRICS

A scoring rubric is a detailed guide showing raters how to assign numeric scores to CR task responses, in a way that aims to standardize the scoring and reduce some of the inherent subjectivity of human raters. Scoring rubrics can take many forms in the method of providing anchors and specific details for a particular scoring task, but the vast majority of rubrics for short-answer or essay tasks will be in the form of a *rating scale* (as opposed to checklists that are popular for true performance tasks). An appropriate rating scale for a written CR task will allow for a high differentiation of the quality of the written responses and will allow raters to use expert or trained judgment to provide a more nuanced rating as needed. The scale should leave open the possibility of single or multiple ratings to be generated from one CR task response (Kobrin & Kimmel, 2006; Welch, 2006). Rating scales may be used to generate a single *global* or *holistic* score that captures the overall performance of the item in a single score, or multiple scales might be used as a form of *analytic* scoring. Holistic ratings are useful when the goal is to capture a single, overall rating of the quality of a response to a CR task, where levels of the scale represent increasing or decreasing levels of quality. In contrast, with analytic methods, CR tasks are rated in several different categories or for several different characteristics. For example, an analytic scoring rubric could allow a rater to generate, from a single essay, separate ratings for the accuracy of the answer to the question, the specificity of the answer, the organization of the written answer, and other measures of writing quality such as spelling or grammar.

Two of the more common types of rating scales are Likert-type scales and behaviorally anchored rating scales (discussed in more detail in Chapter 9 on performance assessments). On a Likert-type scale, holistic impressions are captured for a single judgment on a task (e.g., the classic "Agree-Disagree" rating as applied to a measurement of competency). Behaviorally anchored rating scales, which are more likely to be employed for written CR tasks, also require a holistic judgment for each scale, but the rubric provides descriptive behavioral anchors for performance at multiple scale points. An additional consideration is to provide further quantitative guidance as to the relative meaning of scale terms (e.g., "most," "sometimes," "many," "few") to further guide judges. A simplified example of a behaviorally anchored rating scale that contains multiple elements for analytic scoring for an essay prompt is shown in Table 7.3.

What is the best scoring combination of score scale and scoring method to use? Holistic ratings representing an expert's global judgment about performance have a long history in health professions education work, including licensure and certification (Holmboe & Hawkins, 2008; Yudkowsky, Downing, & Sandlow, 2006). Ultimately, the intended use of the CR rating data should be a major factor in deciding on analytic or holistic methods. If a holistic judgment of performance is used, detailed feedback for examinees is unlikely to be generated. Analytic scoring methods may permit feedback to test-takers on more specific aspects of performance than do global methods; however, many of the separate characteristics rated in the analytic method may correlate highly with each other, thus reducing this presumed benefit of analytic scoring methods. Analytic methods usually require more scoring time than global methods, so feasibility and practicality are also factors in the choice of method. Analytic methods may permit the weighting or differential allocation of partial credit scores somewhat more easily or logically than global methods. For an essay item in which several different essay traits are rated, it is possible to allocate the total score for the essay differentially across the rating categories; for example, the content and structure of the essay answer may be weighted more highly than the writing quality or the organization.

Table 7.3 An Example of a Behaviorally Anchored Rating Scale for Analytic Scoring of an Essay Prompt on the Anatomy of the Inner Ear

Scale	Scale Point Description	Factual Accuracy	Structural Relationships	Writing
5	Excellent	All (100%) facts presented completely accurately	All structural relationships accurately described	Writing well organized, clear, grammatical
4	Good	Most (>75%) facts correct	Most structural relationships correct	Writing fairly well organized, good clarity, mostly grammatical
3	Satisfactory	Many (>50%) facts correct, some incorrect	Many structural relationships correct	Moderate organization and clarity, some grammatical errors
2	Marginal	Few (<50%) facts correct	Few structural relationships correct	Little organization or clarity of writing, many grammatical errors
1	Unsatisfactory	No facts correct	No structural relationships correct	No organization or clarity, many serious grammatical errors

Whatever scoring method is used, the test developer should begin by generating a model answer for each essay question rated, and the model answer should list all of the required components to the answer to serve as a starting point for the scoring rubric (Lane & Iwatani, 2015). Model answers are analogous to the scoring key for an SR test, so these should be reviewed for accuracy and completeness by content experts. Model answers should be constructed with a sufficient amount of objectivity and standardization in the scoring rubric to minimize the subjectivity of human raters. For example, if a behaviorally anchored rating scale is to be used, model answers can serve as useful examples at each point on the scale. The length of rating scales and the description of each point on the scale are also crucial for accurate measurement of performance. There should be a well-defined description to guide the raters, and the number of scale points should be enough to identify meaningful differences in performance without providing so many that the rater is making distinctions that are not meaningful (Lane & Stone, 2006; Shumate, Surles, Johnson, & Penny, 2007). The example responses for each scale point that illustrate the level of performance associated with each score should include both responses that are clearly assigned a particular score, as well as any on the borderline between two score points.

HUMAN RATERS OF CR TASKS

The quality of CR task scoring and the benefits of the information this item format provides depend greatly on the expertise and judgment that human raters bring to scoring. However, as noted previously, this same human input also has the potential to introduce subjectivity and "noise" to the scores that are unrelated to the construct of interest. The type of rating scale and the clarity of the rating guidelines play an important role in reducing this subjectivity, as does a careful recruiting and training of CR task raters. Best practices for training raters include ensuring that (1) raters are properly recruited based on their subject expertise, (2) rater qualifications are clearly linked to the CR tasks at hand, and (3) a clear training process is instituted (Educational Testing Service, 2009). The training process should involve introducing the raters to the exact tasks that test-takers will see, explaining the scoring methods fully, providing sufficient time for practice with the rating scale, providing feedback on rater accuracy via the use of quality control task responses, and discussion of unexpected genuine test-taker responses (especially those not captured by the rating scale). For a single classroom set of CR prompts to be scored by one educator, the full set of guidelines does not apply, but the rationale behind these should still be a consideration.

Regardless of whether there is one faculty member or a team of trained raters evaluating the responses to CR tasks, the potential for *rater bias* is always present, where bias is narrowly defined as the tendency on the part of the rater to rate in ways that vary systematically from the scoring rubric and construct of interest (Feldman, Lazzara, Vanderbilt, & DiazGranados, 2012). There are several well-known rater biases for all performance tasks that often remain despite careful training, and the education of raters should focus on awareness and correction of these biases. Formal written model answers seek to lessen the subjectivity of ratings, as do the use of written scoring rubrics, but instructors should keep in mind that rater bias can persist after training. The most common biases are the *halo effect*, the *leniency/severity bias*, the *central tendency/restriction of range bias*, and the *primacy effect* (Iramaneerat &Yudkowsky, 2007). The halo effect occurs when raters rate participants on characteristics other than the targeted ability or trait to be measured. For example, a rater may give a higher score to an essay where the test-taker has excellent handwriting or grammar, even when these are *not* explicitly part of the scoring rubric. Severity or leniency refers to the tendency of raters to be "hawks" or "doves," and raters should be trained to a shared idea of acceptable levels of severity (or leniency) in order to prevent extreme ratings. Restriction of range or central tendency refers to the likelihood of raters to rate all performances in the middle of the scale (e.g., every test-taker gets a "5"), regardless of the extreme options available. Finally, the primacy effect encourages raters to assume that the next examinee's performance will be similar to the performances they have just seen, causing them to compare an individual to their group and not the scoring rubric. This bias would be in effect if a rater sees several excellent essays and then assigns a moderately good essay a lower score than the scoring rubric demands, because the moderately competent essay writer is being scored relative to his or her peers rather than to the scoring rubric.

Because these biases are so common, it is recommended that rater performance be tracked and raters provided with frequent feedback on their performance relative to their rater peers, on both quality control task responses and genuine task responses, to help temper these effects. Another option is to use multiple independent raters per CR task prompt and average their ratings. If they have different biases, this may diminish some of the ill effects of rater bias. For example, if one rater tends to be a "hawk" or severe and the other rater tends to be a "dove" or lenient, their mean rating will offset both the severity and the leniency bias. Other recommendations include training raters to specific prompts, so that the raters read all the answers to one CR prompt for all test-takers, rather than reading all answers to all questions for a single test-taker. Having raters view and rate known samples is also useful in quality control, as long as raters are blinded to the known samples when rating. Raters should also be provided with adequate time and protection against fatigue when rating.

COMPUTER-BASED RATINGS OF CR TASKS

CR tasks are used in some large-scale tests, such as the Graduate Record Exam (GRE°) and Advanced Placement (AP°) exams, and computer-based CR task scoring models and software have been developed out of necessity to scale up the required score work. The first electronic rating system to be rolled out for large scale exams was Educational Testing Service's (ETS) e-rater°, which was met with a mixture of enthusiasm and skepticism (Powers, Burstein, Chodorow, Fowles, & Kukich, 2001), and research related to the accuracy and best use of e-rater continues to the current day. Haberman (2007) provides a handy overview of multiple electronic essay scoring systems and highlights specific findings that indicate some electronic grading methods produce results on par with human ratings, albeit much more quickly. Educators considering the use of electronic rating systems should keep several caveats in mind. First, there are multiple electronic scoring methods, and these methods vary in terms of the ease of explanation to learners, their suitability for different types of essays, and their expected contribution to increased efficiency. Second, there are multiple human interventions that may be as effective in improving score validity and reliability as the introduction of a computer-based scoring system, including improvement of rater training, more careful assignments of CR tasks to raters, and adjustments for rater effects. Last and perhaps most important to remember, an electronic CR task rating system is not a magic wand. The magic of computer scoring of essays does not remove the need for careful human effort in constructing CR task prompts and developing scoring rubrics, nor does it prevent the efforts of learners to try to game a system and artificially inflate their CR task scores. If anything, it underscores these needs, as the computer, unlike a human rater, will not be able to make adjustments after the fact to counteract any deficiencies in these areas.

CONSTRUCTED-RESPONSE ITEMS: THREATS TO SCORE VALIDITY

This chapter has already touched upon two major threats to the construct validity evidence of CR test score inferences. The first is the potential *construct underrepresentation* (CU) of the domain of interest from the reduced number of assessment points. Even a perfect set of essay items will have reduced construct validity evidence for the total score if the number of items is too limited to allow generalization to the full domain of interest. The second, the introduction of *construct-irrelevant variance* (CIV), is defined as the introduction of variability in the measurement or score that is systematic and unrelated to the construct of interest. The most obvious source of CIV for CR item formats is the lack of objective scoring; the subjectivity of rating scales and use of human raters (or computer-rating systems that rely on human judgments) has the potential to negatively impact the generalizability of scores (Downing, 2002b; Downing & Haladyna, 2004; Haladyna & Downing, 2004; Messick, 1989).

In addition to recommendations already listed, the CR task developer should evaluate the testing scenario and test-taker group for additional sources of CIV. These could include deliberate, test-wise behavior, such as bluffing, or inadvertent test-taker behavior related to response style. Test-taker bluffing can take the form of the test-taker restating the question to use up required space; restating the question in such a way as to answer a different question; writing correct answers to different questions (which were not posed in the prompt); writing answers to appeal to the biases of the essay reader, and so on (e.g., Linn & Miller, 2005). If bluffing attempts are successful for the test-taker, CIV is introduced and may artificially inflate test scores, because the scores are biased by assessment of traits not intended to be measured by the CR prompt. Test-taker style of responding includes aspects of handwriting, and writing skill in the use of grammar, spelling, and punctuation, when these are not intended to be related to the construct of interest but result in either a positive or negative bias on the part of the human raters.

Despite these concerns, the CR item format is one that continues to be useful and defensible in health professions education. You as the educator should be prepared to provide evidence to show that you are using the CR format to assess skills that are not readily measurable by SR items; that the CR prompts are clearly linked to relevant content; that the scoring rubrics are comprehensive and well-documented; and that there is appropriate attention being paid to the potential for rater bias.

SELECTED-RESPONSE ITEMS

The most classic example of an SR item is the multiple-choice question, or MCQ. The structure of the MCQ is deceptively simple: the most basic format consists of a stem or lead-in, which presents a stimulus containing all the necessary information required to answer a direct or implied question and is followed by a listing of possible answers or options. The most common format is the *single-best-answer*, where one option is the most correct or appropriate response to the item. From this simplicity comes a great deal of flexibility, as well as several traps in the form of item flaws for the unwary SR item writer. Other SR formats are often used in educational (formative assessment) settings, such as true/false (TF) items, simple recall, and matching items; these are now less common in high-stakes exams, such as admissions and licensure exams, than in years past, but can have value in lower-stakes and classroom settings. This chapter focuses primarily on the MCQ item type but will refer to other formats where applicable. In this section, we cover some basic principles for writing effective MCQs, methods to detect and remove known MCQ flaws, and factors impacting the reliability and validity evidence in SR item use.

SR ITEM FORMATS: GENERAL GUIDELINES FOR WRITING MCQS

Over many years of development, research, and widespread use, various sets of principles for creating effective and defensible SR item formats have emerged (Haladyna & Downing, 1989a, 1989b; Haladyna et al., 2002). Several user-friendly and detailed item writing guides exist, such as *Writing Test Items to Evaluate Higher Order Thinking* (Haladyna, 1997). Guides aimed specifically toward the health professions educator include the recently updated *Constructing Written Test*

Questions for the Basic and Clinical Sciences (Paniagua & Swygert, 2017). Selected guidelines from these sources are summarized as a set of best practices or principles for writing effective MCQs in Table 7.4.

The first and most important goal when writing any SR item is to ensure that the item content is relevant, important, and appropriate for the purpose of the assessment. There should be a good match between the cognitive level posed by the question and its instructional objective. In essence, examinees with mastery of a given content area may be able to recall an answer with little or no conscious thought, whereas others may need to reason out the answer from basic principles. The cognitive processes involved in responding to a question are learner-specific, making a taxonomic approach difficult to use. One suggested approach is to divide SR items into two categories: *application of knowledge* versus *recall* of a fact (see Table 7.5 for more information).

If an item requires an examinee to reach a conclusion, make a prediction, or select a course of action, it can be classified as an application of knowledge question, whereas an item that assesses only rote memory of a fact (without requiring its application) is classified as a recall question. In the health professions education programs, the use of *clinical vignettes* as part of SR item stems is highly recommended to assess application of knowledge (Paniagua & Swygert, 2017). Clinical vignettes are defined as a collection of information, usually about a fictitious patient, that the test-taker must evaluate. We recommend that vignettes be included where possible to allow for assessment of higher-order thinking skills, integration of facts with clinical reasoning, and other

Table 7.4 Guidelines for Writing High-Quality MCQs

General

Consider using clinical or experimentally based vignettes as appropriate to test higher-order thinking skills, as opposed to simple recall of isolated facts

Avoid including window dressing (extraneous information) in the item; ideally, all item content is necessary to answer the item

Avoid teaching statements (include the central idea in the stem, not the options)

Use parallel construction and language throughout the entire item

Use correct grammar, punctuation, capitalization, and spelling (carefully proofread each item)

Stems/Lead-Ins

Use positive lead-ins (use "Which one of the following is correct?" rather than "Which one of the following is not correct?") to avoid confusing test-takers

Avoid repeating words in either stem or option to avoid cueing the correct answer

Eliminate absolute statements in lead-ins (avoid using "Which one of the following is never the case?") to avoid misinterpretations

Use focused, closed lead-ins (create lead-ins that end with a question mark) to avoid grammatical cueing

Options

Develop as many plausible distractors (wrong answers) as possible; aim for three to five total options per MCQ

Make sure there is only a single correct answer (for one-best-answer items), that options don't overlap, and that the options are of similar length and grammatical style (all options are diagnoses, or all options are plural)

Make options as homogeneous in length, structure, and style as possible (avoid making the correct answer the longest or most complex option)

Replace "none of the above" or "all of the above" options with a specific action ("no intervention needed" or "reassurance only")

Use single options whenever possible to avoid confusing test-takers

Table 7.5 Comparison of Recall Items vs. Application Items in Formative vs. Summative Assessments

Item Type	Formative Assessment	Summative Assessment
Recall (short item with no vignette)	• May be useful for assessing efficacy of classroom instruction • Allows for "rapid fire" stimulation of learning • May help keep test-taker attention focused on learning facts	• Allows for increased quantity of items (quicker to write and to answer) • Suitable for single-step questions and single concepts/facts
Application (with use of clinical or experimental vignette)	• Teaches test-takers to become familiar with a patient scenario • Allows for better assessment of problem-based learning • Allows for better assessment of team-based learning • Allows for better link to clinical or experimental scenarios during instruction	• Allows for assessment of higher-order thinking skills • May be a better approximation of real-world practice • Allows for integration and differentiation • Amenable to multi-step question formats

advanced knowledge and skills. Vignettes are also useful for multi-step item formats (attaching multiple SR items to a single vignette) and are often perceived by the examinee and other score users as more genuine or representative of real-life health professions practice. Media objects, such as images, photos, radiographs, and other media can be included as part of the vignette and are a useful way to add authenticity and information without increasing the reading load.

Once the content of the MCQ has been addressed, the style and formatting of the item should be evaluated. A badly formatted MCQ will result in the introduction of CIV in the test score, even if the content of the item is relevant. The wording of the MCQ should extremely clear so that there are no ambiguities of language. No attempt should be made to deliberately trick knowledgeable test-takers into giving an incorrect answer. The stem should be clear and complete enough that a test-taker could figure out the right answer before seeing the option set. The set of options should be homogeneous, such that all possible answers are of the same general class and every option is a plausible correct answer, to avoid cueing test-takers to the correct answer. One and only one of the options should be the correct (or best) answer to the question posed in the stem. Ideally, the writer of an MCQ will be an expert in the content of the item who, in addition to vouching for the relevance of the item content, allows for sufficient time to review items and remove any technical flaws, which are covered in detail in the next section.

SR ITEM FORMATS: AVOIDING KNOWN MCQ FLAWS

Flawed test items also have the potential to bias test scores in more than one direction; some flaws make a test item easy to guess correctly even if the test-taker doesn't know the answer, while other flaws may confuse the test-taker to the extent that even those who have mastered the material select an incorrect option. As an educator, you cannot assume that your MCQs do not have flaws, and you cannot assume that any CIV introduced by flaws impacts scores in only one direction. The presence of flaws has the potential to greatly negatively impact the validity evidence for the score interpretations, and any careful quality process will include a close review of MCQs for potential flaws (Baranowski, 2006). The most common MCQ flaws can be divided into three general areas: flaws of content, flaws of style, and flaws of formatting.

The content flaw, as mentioned earlier, can be devastating; a poorly crafted or flawed MCQ that tests trivial content, at a low level of the cognitive domain, will have limited generalizability and may not provide the test developer with important information about test-taker performance. Item writers who have content expertise may have trouble placing themselves into the mindset of test-takers and may incorrectly estimate what test-takers are likely to know, rather than what they should know (or would know if they were at the expert level). One of the advantages of using MCQs is that many can be administered in a relatively short time period, allowing for a broader domain assessment, but each MCQ that is trivial or not focused on an important content area represents a missed assessment opportunity. Before any item writing begins, test developers should carefully review the test blueprint to ensure the MCQs accurately reflect the constructs of interest, in the desired numbers, and should list out the exact testing points to be assessed by each item.

Flaws of style and formatting may be relatively easy to spot and correct, but can be extremely problematic if not detected. Common style and formatting flaws include unfocused or open-ended stems (incomplete sentences), where the question is not clearly focused or is ambiguously written so that test-takers are confused about the question being posed. Stems containing negative words ("Which of the following is NOT correct?") are likely to be misread by test-takers, even when the negative words are emphasized. The stem may incorporate inadvertent cues to the correct answer, so that savvy test-takers (the "testwise" examinee) can get the item correct without knowing the content, or the item may be so ambiguous that test-takers who actually know the content get the item wrong. It is best to avoid writing MCQ options that are of differing style and length; a common result is that the keyed correct answer is longest (due to the item writer focusing the most on this option), and this can cue the testwise examinee into selecting the longest or most complex option. If an option set's distractors are implausible (unrealistic options based on the vignette), this will help the examinee rule out some of the options, thereby making it easier to guess the answer. For a more comprehensive description of known style and formatting flaws, see Downing (2002a, 2002b, 2005), Rodriguez (2015), and Paniagua and Swygert (2017).

Item flaws are more common than faculty and educators realize, and their impact can be problematic. In one study, flawed items were artificially more difficult for medical students and misclassified 14% of students as failing the test when they passed the same content when tested by non-flawed MCQs (Downing, 2005). A study of a year-end basic science exam with 33 MCQs showed that one-third of the items were flawed; passing rates increased by over 20% when item flaws were corrected (Downing, 2002b). Another study for a new medical school found that despite faculty awareness and concern about item flaws, a majority of the MCQs on various faculty-developed assessment tools tested only simple recall, and almost half of the MCQs contained other style or formatting flaws such as implausible distractors or unfocused stems (Baig, Ali, Ali, & Huda, 2014). These results were in agreement with other research showing that a general review of classroom item banks reveals flaws in anywhere from one-quarter to three-quarters of the MCQs (Ellsworth, Dunnel, & Duell, 1990; Tarrant, Knierim, Hayes, & Ware, 2006; Khan, Danish, Awan, & Anwar, 2013).

Luckily, there is research to show that corrective action to remove item flaws can have substantial positive effects. A study by Downing (2005) demonstrated that elimination of just five common flaws in MCQs—unfocused stems, negative stems, the "all of the above" and the "none of the above" options, and the so-called partial-K type item—could greatly reduce the ill effects of poorly crafted MCQs. One study based on item options for classroom MCQs showed that removal of distractors that were non-functioning (for any reason, though implausibility was the most common reason) produced items that were more difficult but also more discriminating, thus providing better measurement quality (Tarrant, Ware, & Mohammed, 2009). Another study that compiled item banks across multiple medical schools concluded that items written by faculty with specialized item writer training were far more likely to be free of flaws than item written by faculty without such training (Jozefowicz et al., 2002). While specialized training may seem expensive or overly time-consuming, there is evidence to suggest that only one day of item writer training can have a significant positive impact on item quality (AlFaris et al., 2015).

The literature on MCQs flaws suggests several notable conclusions. First, there are multiple types of flaws that can occur with MCQs, even if the content to be targeted is clear. Next, classroom achievement tests in the health professions, and sometime even high-stakes exams, may contain multiple flawed items, and these flaws can negatively impact learner achievement measurement and thereby bias pass-fail decisions. Finally, specialized item writer training, even if undertaken with limited time and resources, is likely to help prevent flaws and improve the quality of item production. The end result is that writing effective MCQs is both art and science, where the quality of the final product is affected by a multitude of variables such as effective item writer training, use of effective training materials, practice, feedback, motivation, and even writing ability. Content expertise is the single most essential characteristic of an effective item writer, but this alone is not sufficient, and a content expert with an excellent grasp of the material can still benefit from lessons on item writing or external support for reviewing and editing items to remove flaws. Item writing is a specialized skill and, like all skills, must be mastered through guided practice and feedback on performance.

SR ITEM FORMATS: NUMBER OF MCQ OPTIONS

Traditionally, MCQs will have four or five options, but given that plausible distractors can be challenging to create, the question of the optimal number of MCQs options, and whether the fourth or fifth option is really needed, remains an open research question. A meta-analysis of studies by Rodriguez (2005) on the optimal number of options suggested that use of three options plus a correct answer is best for most MCQs. Prior research indicated that four- or five-option MCQs tend to have only about three options that are functional defined as those distractors selected by 5% or more of the test-takers that also have negative discrimination indices (Haladyna & Downing, 1993). The general item writing recommendation is to "develop as many effective choices as you can, but research suggests three is adequate" (Haladyna, Downing, & Rodriguez, 2002, p. 312). Using more than three options may not do much harm to the test, but will add inefficiencies for item writers and test-takers and may increase reading time and item response time, which permits the use of fewer total MCQs per hour (Schneid, Armour, Park, Yudkowsky, & Bordage, 2014).

It is true that the fewer the options, the higher the probability of getting an MCQ correctly solely by uninformed guessing—this probability increases to .33 for a three-option item, as opposed to .20 for a five-option item. If item flaws provide the savvy test-taker with some educated methods in which to guess, the probability can increase substantially. In addition, reducing the number of options has the potential to slightly reduce the discrimination of a given item, which can in turn impact the generalizability of the test scores (Rodriguez, 2005). For a set of well-written MCQs, targeted in difficulty appropriately and in sufficient numbers, these shifts in guessing probability and item discrimination are unlikely to meaningfully impact scores, but this remains a fertile area for research. It will be interesting to see, on exams with fewer distractors (such as the revamped SAT, administered in March 2016, on which the number of response options on all MCQs was reduced from five to four), whether changes in reliability are observed. A reasonable guideline to convey to subject matter expert item writers is to ensure the plausibility of all distractors by ensuring some connection to vignette content.

SR ITEM FORMATS: MCQ SCORING METHODS

One of the major strengths of SR items, in particular MCQs, is the clarity and objectivity of the scoring method, which is easy to define and straightforward to explain and defend to test-takers. There are two basic methods used to score SR tests: summing up the number of correct items (aka *number-correct* scoring) or employing a formula to try to "correct" the number-correct score for presumed guessing (aka *formula* scoring). The simple count of the number of items marked correctly is usually the best score to use, especially in the classroom context. This type of raw scores can be converted to any number of other metrics if needed, such as percent-correct scores, derived scores, standard scores, and any other linear transformation of the number-correct score (see Chapter 5).

All correction-for-guessing formula scores attempt to eliminate or reduce the perceived ill effects of random guessing on SR items. These formulas work in one of two ways: by rewarding test-takers for resisting the temptation to guess or by actively penalizing the test-taker for guessing (Downing, 2003). However intuitively appealing these guessing corrections may be, the literature indicates that both methods rank order test-takers identically, although the absolute values of scores may differ. Further, no matter whether test-takers are directed to answer all questions or only those questions they know for certain (i.e., to guess or not to guess), the more savvy test-takers know that they will usually maximize their score by attempting to answer every question on the test, no matter what the general directions on the test state or what formulas are used to derive a score. Ultimately, corrections for guessing may bias scores (for an example, see Muijtjens, van Mameren, Hoogenboom, Evers, & van der Vleuten, 1999) and negatively impact the validity argument for score use by adding CIV to scores.

Another question of scoring for MCQs that often arises is the question of differential weighting based on content—whether assigning more than one point per MCQ, depending on the topic of the item, produces a more reliable or valid score. For MCQ-based tests, this is sometimes accompanied by "killer items"; i.e., items related to crucial content on which an incorrect answer can have a disproportionate impact on the final score or passing outcome. From a psychometric perspective, it is not recommended that this scoring method be used in the classroom. Each MCQ is only a single assessment point, and many of the strengths of MCQ-based exams come from systematically sampling content across the test blueprint. If one or two particular topic areas are more important than others within a given domain, the best way to capture this is to develop more MCQs for those topic areas, rather than keeping the number of MCQs the same and changing the weights. Since test-takers can guess a correct answer on an MCQ, or accidentally select the wrong answer, differential weighting can only inflate the contribution of that construct-irrelevant variance to the total test score. Some item response theory models (see Chapter 19) effectively weight MCQs differently in scoring, but the weights are not subjective and are directly related to each item's estimated discrimination rather than content. The advice to increase the number of MCQs on important content remains the same whether classical scoring methods or item response theory is being used to score the test. In effect, it is important for the educator to consider the overall content balance and blueprinting of the test and develop MCQs in numbers that fully represent the exam blueprint.

SR ITEM FORMATS: NON-MCQ FORMATS

While many educators default to one-best-answer MCQs that independently assess content, there are other types of MCQs that can be of use in the classroom. One of the most common variations of the SR is the *true-false* (TF) item format. This format appears similar to one-best-answer MCQs, with a stem and a list of options, but the test-taker has to evaluate each option and identify each as either true or false (e.g., Ebel & Frisbie, 1991). One difficulty in composing TF items follows from the fact that options cannot fall on a continuum, as they can on one-best-answer items; the TF format requires that each option can be absolutely defended as being more true than false or more false than true (Paniagua & Swygert, 2017). Because of this, many educators believe the TF item format is best suited to test only low-level cognitive knowledge such as recall of direct facts, or for use in formative assessment or the classroom setting. Measurement error due to random guessing on TF items is also a frequent criticism. However, if true-false items are well written and used in sufficient numbers on a test form (e.g., 50 or more items), measurement error due to blind guessing will be minimized. Like one-best-answer MCQs, TF items are best scored as "right or wrong," with no formula scoring used to attempt to correct for guessing.

Another variation that can be used with any format of SR item is the *testlet* or context-dependent item set (Wainer & Lewis, 1989; Haladyna, 1992). Testlets consist of stimulus materials that are used for two or more independent items, presented in sets, where the items could be any variation of one-best-answer, TF, and so on. For example, a testlet could consist of a paragraph or two giving a detailed clinical description of a patient, in sufficient detail to answer several different questions based on the same clinical information such as case-based assessments. One item in the testlet might ask for a most likely diagnosis, another question for laboratory investigations, another on therapies, another on complications, and a final question on expected or most likely outcomes. The main strength of testlets is that they are efficient; a single stimulus (stem, lead-in) serves multiple items, and a long vignette or reading passage can be used because it applies to multiple items. Some basic principles of testlet use must be noted. All items appearing on the same test with a common stem must be reasonably independent aside from the stimulus, such that getting one of the items incorrect does not necessarily mean getting another item incorrect. Ideally, one item should not cue the answer to another item in the set due to information provided in the item stem or options. For computer-based test administrations, it is possible to use testlets in such a way that later items in the testlet provide information that cues the answers to earlier items within the testlet, but this requires the administration method prevent test-takers from being able to go back to earlier items in the testlet and change their earlier answers. For paper and pencil testing, and some basic computer-based testing that does not place limits on test-taker navigation within forms, this is not feasible. Each item in the testlet can be scored as an independent MCQ, but the proper unit of analysis is the testlet score and not the item score, especially for reliability analysis (Thissen & Wainer, 2001; Wainer & Thissen, 1996). If all of these conditions are met, testlets can be an excellent way to test some types of cognitive knowledge, but some care must be taken not to oversample areas of the content domain; when several items are presented on the same topic, it can become more challenging to build balanced test forms that represent all the necessary content areas.

SUMMARY AND CONCLUSION

The constructed-response (CR) and selected-response (SR) item formats are used widely in health professions education for the assessment of cognitive knowledge and skills and are essential for classroom assessments. Each format has strengths and limits, as summarized in this chapter. Overall, the SR format—particularly in its prototypic form, the multiple-choice question—is most appropriate for the vast majority of achievement testing situations in health professions education. When properly constructed, this format is extremely versatile in testing higher levels of cognitive knowledge, has a deep research base to support its validity, is efficient, and permits sound quality control measures in both paper-based and computer-based assessments. On the other hand, CR items—particularly the short-answer essay form—are appropriate for testing uncued written responses, but the item author should be aware that the scoring for these item types is inherently subjective, and they should actively employ methods that can help control or reduce rater biases. The goal in choosing the assessment methodology is to carefully weigh both the advantages and disadvantages of each item type, and to thoughtfully develop the item format that is best suited for the cognitive knowledge and skills of interest.

Note: Additional material and resources may be available at the UIC AHPE website: https://go.uic.edu/AHPE

REFERENCES

AlFaris, E., Naeem, N., Irfan, F., Qureshi, R., Saad, H., Al Sadhan, R., Abdulghani, H.M., & van der Vleuten, C. (2015). A one-day dental faculty workshop in writing multiple-choice questions: An impact evaluation. *Journal of Dental Education, 79*(11), 1305–1313.

American Educational Research Association, American Psychological Association, National Council on Measurement in Education, Joint Committee for the Revision of the Standards for Educational, & Psychological Testing (US). (2014). *Standards for educational and psychological testing*. Washington, DC: American Educational Research Assn.

Baig, M., Ali, S.K., Ali, S., & Huda, N. (2014). Evaluation of multiple choice and short essay question items in basic medical sciences. *Pakistani Journal of Medical Sciences, 30*, 3–6.

Baranowski, R.A. (2006). Item editing and item review. In S.M. Downing & T.M. Haladyna (Eds.), *Handbook of test development* (pp. 349–357). Mahwah, NJ: Lawrence Erlbaum Associates.

Downing, S.M. (2002a). Assessment of knowledge with written test forms. In G.R. Norman, C.P.M. van der Vleuten, & D.I. Newble (Eds.), *International handbook for research in medical education* (pp. 647–672). Dordrecht, The Netherlands: Kluwer Academic Publishers.

Downing, S.M. (2002b). Construct-irrelevant variance and flawed test questions: Do multiple-choice item-writing principles make any difference? *Academic Medicine, 77*(10), s103–104.

Downing, S.M. (2003). Guessing on selected-response examinations. *Medical Education, 37*, 670–671.

Downing, S.M. (2005). The effects of violating standard item writing principles on tests and students: The consequences of using flawed test items on achievement examinations in medical education. *Advances in Health Sciences Education, 10*, 133–143.

Downing, S.M., & Haladyna, T.M. (1997). Test item development: Validity evidence from quality assurance procedures. *Applied Measurement in Education, 10*, 61–82.

Downing, S.M., & Haladyna, T.M. (2004). Validity threats: Overcoming interference with proposed interpretations of assessment data. *Medical Education, 38*, 327–333.

Educational Testing Service. (2009). *Guidelines for constructed-response and other performance assessments*. Princeton, NJ: ETS.

Ebel, R.L., & Frisbie, D.A. (1991). *Essentials of educational measurement*. Englewood Cliffs, NJ: Prentice Hall.

Ellsworth, R.A., Dunnel, P., & Duell, O.K. (1990). Multiple-choice test items: What are textbook authors telling teachers? *Journal of Educational Research, 83*(5), 289–293.

Feldman, M., Lazzara, E.H., Vanderbilt, A.A., & DiazGranados, D. (2012). Rater training to support high-stakes simulation-based assessments. *The Journal of Continuing Education in the Health Professions, 32*(4), 279–286.

Fitzpatrick, S., & Dunleavy, D. (2016). *Exploring a situational judgment test for use in medical school admissions*. Retrieved October 2017 from www.aamc.org/download/462754/data/sjtupdatefor2016pdc.pdf.

Haberman, S.J. (2007). Electronic essay grading. In C.R. Rao & S. Sinrahay (Eds.), *Handbook of statistics 26: Psychometrics* (pp. 205–233). New York: Elsevier.

Haladyna, T.M. (1992). Context-dependent item sets. *Educational Measurement: Issues and Practice, 11*, 21–25.

Haladyna, T.M. (1997). *Writing test items to evaluate higher-order thinking*. Needham Heights, MA: Allyn & Bacon.

Haladyna, T.M., & Downing, S.M. (1989a). A taxonomy of multiple-choice item-writing rules. *Applied Measurement in Education, 1*, 37–50.

Haladyna, T.M., & Downing, S.M. (1989b). Validity of a taxonomy of multiple-choice item-writing rules. *Applied Measurement in Education, 1*, 51–78.

Haladyna, T.M., & Downing, S.M. (1993). How many options is enough for a multiple-choice test item. *Educational and Psychological Measurement, 53*, 999–1010.

Haladyna, T.M., & Downing, S.M. (2004). Construct-irrelevant variance in high-stakes testing. *Educational Measurement: Issues and Practice, 23*(1), 17–27.

Haladyna, T.M., Downing, S.M., & Rodriguez, M.C. (2002). A review of multiple-choice item-writing guidelines for classroom assessment. *Applied Measurement in Education, 15*(3), 309–334.

Holmboe, E.S., & Hawkins, R.E. (2008). *Practical guide to the evaluation of clinical competence*. Philadelphia, PA: Mosby/Elsevier.

Iramaneerat, C., & Yudkowsky, R. (2007). Rater errors in a clinical skills assessment of medical students. *Evaluation in the Health Professions, 30*(3), 266–283.

Jozefowicz, R.F., Koeppen, B.M., Case, S., Galbraith, R., Swanson, D., & Glew, R.H. (2002). The quality of in-house medical school examinations. *Academic Medicine, 77*(2), 156–161.

Khan, H.F., Danish, K.F., Awan, A.S., & Anwar, M. (2013). Identification of technical item flaws leads to improvement of the quality of single best multiple choice questions. *Pakistani Journal of Medical Science, 29*(3), 715–718.

Kobrin, J.L., & Kimmel, E.W. (2006). Test development and technical information on the writing section of the SAT Reasoning Test™. *College Board Research Notes, 25*.

Kyllonen, P.C. (2015). Designing tests to measure personal attributes and noncognitive skills. In M. Raymond, S. Lane, & T. Haladyna (Eds.), *Handbook of test development* (2nd ed., pp. 190–211). New York: Routledge.

Lane, S., & Iwatani, E. (2015). Design of performance assessments in education. In M. Raymond, S. Lane, & T. Haladyna (Eds.), *Handbook of test development* (2nd ed., pp. 274–293). New York: Routledge.

Lane, S., & Stone, C.A. (2006). Performance assessment. In R.L. Brennan (Ed.), *Educational measurement* (4th ed., pp. 387–432). Westport, CT: Praeger Publishers.

Linn, R.L., & Miller, M.D. (2005). *Measurement and assessment in teaching* (9th ed.). Upper Saddle River, NJ: Pearson/Merrill Prentice Hall.

Lockyer, J., Carraccio, C., Chan, M., Hart, D., Smee, S., Touchie, C., . . . & ICBME Collaborators (2017). Core principles of assessment in competency-based medical education. *Medical Teacher, 38*(6), 609–616.

Messick, S. (1989). Validity. In R.L. Linn (Ed.), *Educational measurement* (3rd ed., pp. 13–104). New York: American Council on Education and Macmillan.

Messick, S. (1994). The interplay of evidence and consequences in the validation of performance assessments. *Educational Researcher, 23,* 13–23.

Miller, G.E. (1990). The assessment of clinical skills/competence/performance. *Academic Medicine, 65,* S63–67.

Muijtjens, A.M.M., van Mameren, H., Hoogenboom, R.J.I., Evers, J.L.H., & van der Vleuten, C.P.M. (1999). The effect of a 'don't know' option on test scores: Number-right and formula scoring compared. *Medical Education, 33,* 267–275.

Nyquist, J.G. (2014). *Techniques for assessment of learner performance in teaching and assessing the competencies* (10th ed.). Los Angeles: University of Southern California.

Paniagua, M., & Swygert, K.A. (Eds.). (2017). *Constructing written test questions for the basic and clinical sciences.* Philadelphia: National Board of Medical Examiners.

Powers, D.E., Burstein, J.C., Chodorow, M., Fowles, M.E., & Kukich, K. (2001). Stumping *e-rater*: Challenging the validity of automated essay scoring. *ETS Research Report 01–03*. Princeton, NJ: Educational Testing Service.

Rodriguez, M.C. (2005). Three options are optimal for multiple-choice items: A meta-analysis of 80 years of research. *Educational Measurement: Issues and Practice, 24*(2), 3–13.

Rodriguez, M.C. (2015). Selected-response item development. In S. Lane, M.R. Raymond, & T.M. Haladyna (Eds.), *Handbook of test development* (2nd ed., pp. 259–273). New York: Routledge.

Rush, B.R., Rankin, D.C., & White, B.J. (2016). The impact of item-writing flaws and item complexity on examination item difficulty and discrimination value. *BMC Medical Education, 16,* 250.

Schneid, S., Armour, C., Park, Y.S., Yudkowsky, R., & Bordage, G. (2014). Reducing the number of options on multiple-choice questions. *Medical Education, 48,* 1020–1027.

Shumate, S.R., Surles, J., Johnson, R.L., & Penny, J. (2007). The effects of the number of scale points and nonnormality on the generalizability coefficient: A Monte Carlo study. *Applied Measurement in Education, 20,* 357–376.

Swygert, K.A., & Williamson, D.M. (2015). Using performance tasks in credentialing tests. In M. Raymond, S. Lane, & T. Haladyna (Eds.), *Handbook of test development* (2nd ed., pp. 294–312). New York: Routledge.

Tarrant, M.M., Knierim, A., Hayes, S.K., & Ware, J. (2006). The frequency of item writing flaws in multiple-choice questions use in high stakes nursing assessments. *Nursing Education Today, 26*(8), 662–671.

Tarrant, M.M., Ware, J., & Mohammed, A.M. (2009). An assessment of functioning and non-functioning distractors in multiple-choice questions: A descriptive analysis. *BMC Medical Education, 9*(40).

Thissen, D., & Wainer, H. (Eds.). (2001). *Test scoring.* Mahwah, NJ: Lawrence Erlbaum Associates.

Wainer, H., & Lewis, C. (1989). *RR-89-29: Toward a psychometrics for testlets.* Princeton, NJ: Educational Testing Services.

Wainer, H., & Thissen, D. (1996). How is reliability related to the quality of test scores? What is the effect of local dependence on reliability? *Educational Measurement: Issues and Practice, 15*(1), 22–29.

Welch, C. (2006). Item and prompt development in performance testing. In S.M. Downing & T.M. Haladyna (Eds.), *Handbook of test development* (pp. 303–327). Mahwah, NJ: Lawrence Erlbaum Associates.

Yudkowsky, R., Downing, S.M., & Sandlow, L.J. (2006). Developing an institution-based assessment of resident communication and interpersonal skills. *Academic Medicine, 81,* 1115–1122.

8

ORAL EXAMINATIONS

Dorthea Juul, Rachel Yudkowsky, and Ara Tekian

The oral examination, sometimes known as a *viva voce*, is characterized by a face-to-face inter-action between an examinee and one or more examiners. Test questions may be linked to a patient case, clinic chart, or other clinical material; examination sessions can range from focused five-minute probes to comprehensive "long cases" of up to an hour in length.

The stated purpose of an oral examination is to explore an examinee's thinking in order to assess skills such as critical reasoning, problem solving, judgment, and ethics, as well as the ability to express ideas, synthesize material, and think on one's feet. The potential advantage of the oral examination compared to a constructed-response written examination lies in the examiner's abil-ity to follow up with additional probes that explore the examinee's response and thereby deepen or broaden the challenge in order to better define the limits of the examinee's abilities. Oral exam-inations should not be used primarily to assess knowledge, which is better assessed with a written examination, or to evaluate elements of the patient encounter, better assessed with simulations, performance examinations, or direct observational methods (see Figure 8.1).

Despite the long history and widespread use of oral examinations, there are many threats to their validity (and they are often comparatively costly), and this has led to controversy and concern about their usefulness as an assessment strategy (see, for example, Hutchinson, Aitken, & Hayes, 2002; Yudkowsky, 2002; Wass, Wakeford, Neighbour, & van der Vleuten, 2003; Davis & Karunathilake, 2005; Burch, Norman, Schmidt, & van der Vleuten, 2008; Memon, Joughin, & Memon, 2010). In this chapter, we review these threats and suggest some ways to address them, primarily by means of *structured* oral examinations; but first, we will look at some examples of how oral examinations are used around the world.

ORAL EXAMINATIONS AROUND THE WORLD

Oral examinations are used both at undergraduate and postgraduate levels, as well as in licensure and certification examinations. For example, Hamdy, Prasad, Williams, and Salih (2003) describe what they call a direct observation clinical encounter examination (DOCEE) that is used to assess medical students at the Arabian Gulf University. After direct observation of encounters with real patients, the examiners discuss the case with the examinee and rate them in four domains:

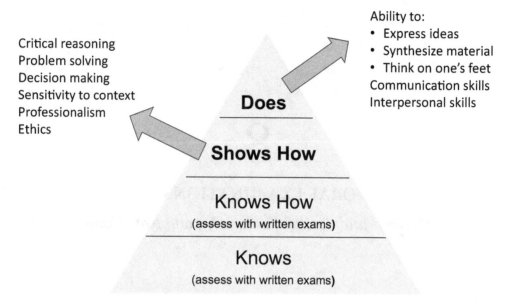

Figure 8.1 Miller's pyramid: competencies to assess with oral examinations

Source: Miller (1990)

data-gathering skills; reasoning and analytical skills; decision-making skills; and professional attitude. The examination has been shown to have good reliability and inter-rater agreement between the two examiners, and the information that it provides is not completely overlapped by other indicators of students' clinical competence.

The *CanMEDS Assessment Tools Handbook* includes the oral examination in the list of contemporary assessment tools and indicates that the format is well suited for assessing many of the key competencies of the medical expert role (Bandiera, Sherbino, & Frank, 2006). Chou, Lockyer, Cole, and McLaughlin (2009) surveyed Canadian residency program directors, and 86% reported that they used oral examinations to assess their trainees. Furthermore, it was the most utilized format other than the in-training evaluation report (ITER). Jefferies, Simmons, and Skidmore (2011) developed a structured oral examination to assess all seven CanMEDS roles in a subspecialty (neonatal/perinatal medicine) training program. They found that the test had reasonable psychometric properties for six of the seven roles and that it was feasible and economical to administer and very acceptable to trainees and faculty.

Chart-stimulated recall (CSR) is a format that, like a traditional oral examination, involves an interaction between an examiner and an examinee. The examiner's questions are based on the examinee's documented patient encounter and can address a wide range of competencies, including clinical reasoning, decision-making, documentation skills, communication with patients and families, and understanding of systems of care (Philibert, 2018). In effect, the examiner asks the examinee to "think aloud" and articulate the rationale for her actions. CSRs have been used to assess trainees as well as practicing physicians and to provide feedback (Al-Wassia, Al-Wassia, Shihata, Park, & Tekian, 2015; Goulet, Jacques, Gagnon, Racette, & Sieber, 2007; Reddy, Endo, Gupta, Tekian, & Park, 2015).

In the US, oral examinations were used as early as 1917 with the founding of the medical specialty boards (Mancall, 1995). As of 2018, about half of the 24 American Board of Medical Specialties member boards included some type of oral examination in their certification process, as did most specialties of the Royal College of Physicians and Surgeons of Canada, dentistry boards in the US and Canada, the Royal Colleges in Great Britain, and other certification bodies around the world.

Because of their use in US board certification, practice or "mock" oral examinations are conducted in many residency programs. In addition to assessing the residents' progress, a secondary goal is to provide exposure to the format and thereby enhance the odds of passing. There are examples in the literature for emergency medicine (Schwaab et al., 2011); ophthalmology (Wiggins, Harper, Landes, & O'Sullivan, 2008); physical medicine and rehabilitation (Engel, Pai, & Walker, 2014); radiology (Strickland, Jensen, & McArthur, 2017); and surgery (Fingeret et al., 2016).

In a study that directly addressed the "value added" of an oral examination to the certification process, researchers at the American Board of Anesthesiology demonstrated that the risk of disciplinary action against a physician's medical license was lower for those who passed both the MCQ and oral examination components of the certification process compared to those who only passed the MCQ test or who passed neither examination (Zhou et al., 2017). They concluded that these results supported the hypothesis that "an oral examination assesses domains important to anesthesiologist performance that are not fully assessed in a written examination" (Zhou et al., 2017, p. 1178).

THREATS TO THE VALIDITY OF ORAL EXAMINATIONS

Concerns about the validity of traditional unstructured oral examinations have led to their gradual replacement by written tests, performance tests using simulations and standardized patients, and structured oral examinations, especially for high-stakes assessments. To understand this shift we will look at the vulnerability of oral examinations to the two major threats to validity discussed in Chapter 2: construct underrepresentation (CU) and construct-irrelevant variance (CIV).

Construct underrepresentation or undersampling is a major challenge for oral examinations. Like any other assessment, an oral examination must provide multiple data points that systematically sample the domain to be assessed. As with other tests of clinical skills, content specificity (Elstein, Shulman, & Sprafka, 1978) limits the ability to generalize from competency in one topic to competency in another. An oral examination that consists of questions about two or three topics or clinical scenarios is not likely to provide a broad and systematic sampling of the content domain (Turnball, Danoff, & Norman, 1996; Norcini, 2002); an examination that assesses problem solving or clinical reasoning skills in only one or two scenarios is not sufficiently sampling that skill. Furthermore, if the oral examination is linked to encounters with real patients, the content that can be assessed may be limited by patient availability, the patient's ability to cooperate, and his/her ability to consent to the examination (Yudkowsky, 2002). If learners are tested on different patients, their tests may not be equivalent in either difficulty or content, compromising fairness and the ability to compare test scores across examinees.

Compounding the problem, early studies (Evans, Ingersoll, & Smith, 1966; McGuire, 1966) found that questions asked in oral examinations were not much different than questions in written examinations. Jayawickramarajah (1985) found that approximately two-thirds of the questions in an unstructured oral examination were simple recall. Regardless of the number of topics covered, these questions are not likely to elicit the higher-order thinking that is the appropriate focus of oral examinations.

Construct-irrelevant variance refers to score variance due to factors that are irrelevant to the competency being assessed; for example, when characteristics such as politeness, demeanor, and dress impact the rating of clinical reasoning (Williams, Klamen, & McGaghie, 2003). CIV is a substantial threat to traditional oral examinations that use a small number of examiners per learner, since there are likely to be too few raters to compensate for stringency (hawk/dove) and bias effects (Linn & Zeppa, 1976; Schwiebert & Davis, 1993; Weingarten, Polliack, Tabenkin, & Kahan, 2000; Wass et al., 2003; Houston & Myford, 2009).

Construct-irrelevant variables that can impact the scores in oral examinations include mannerism and behavior, language and fluency, appearance and attractiveness (e.g., dress code—professional or non-professional), physical abnormalities/peculiarities or oddness, anxiety/stress level, and emotional status (Pokorny & Frazier, 1966; Yaphe & Street, 2003; Lunz & Bashook, 2008). The level of confidence of candidates can have more influence on the score awarded by the examiners than what was actually said (Thomas et al., 1993).

In an interesting experiment on the effect of communication style, Rowland-Morin, Burchard, Garb, and Coe (1991) trained five actors and actresses to portray identical students with variations such as direct versus indirect eye contact and moderate versus slower response rate. Examiners rated ten categories of performance (knowledge of facts, understands concepts, identified problems, integrates relevant data, makes proper decisions, is motivated, communicates effectively, is resourceful, has integrity, and is attractive in appearance). The study found that examiners were strongly influenced by the students' communication skills. Conversely, an examiner's approving or disapproving facial expression can encourage or discourage an examinee's responses, introducing additional construct-irrelevant variance into the mix.

STRUCTURED ORAL EXAMINATIONS

The CU and CIV problems outlined above led many educators to replace oral examinations with more objective and controllable methods such as written examinations and performance tests using standardized patients and other simulations. Nonetheless, under controlled and standardized conditions as described below, oral examinations can provide added value within a comprehensive assessment approach.

A *structured* oral examination offers significant benefits in combating CU and CIV. In a structured oral examination, each examinee is exposed to the *same* or *equivalent tasks*, which are administered under the *same conditions*, in the *same amount of time*, and with *scoring as objective* as possible (Guerin, 1995). CU and CIV concerns can be addressed by assembling a series of oral examinations, with careful blueprinting of the examination stations, standardization of questions, and a rubric for scoring the answers; by utilizing multiple examiners with systematic training; by formal standard setting; and by systematic quality assurance efforts (Table 8.1).

Structured oral examinations share many of the characteristics of performance tests such as standardized patient examinations and objective structured clinical examinations (OSCEs) (see Chapter 9). As with performance tests, increasing the number of tests or stations can have a large impact on reliability/generalizability by increasing the sampling across content and raters, decreasing CU, and allowing CIV to cancel out across tests/examiners. Daelmans, Scherpbier, van der Vleuten, and Donker (2001) investigated the effect of multiple oral examinations in an internal medicine clerkship, aiming for two 30-minute patient-based orals a day for five days. They found it would take ten 30-minute examinations or about five hours of testing to reach a generalizability of 0.80, about comparable to the number of cases and time needed for a reliable OSCE

Table 8.1 Characteristics of a Structured Oral Examination

- Multiple examination "stations"
- Content blueprinting
- Standardization of initial questions
- Rubrics to assist in scoring answers
- Multiple examiners
- Examiner training
- Formal standard setting
- Quality assurance efforts

(van der Vleuten & Swanson, 1990). Just as in OSCEs, increasing the number of examinations with a single examiner at each "station" improves reliability more than doubling up examiners (Swanson, Norman, & Linn, 1995; Norman, 2000; Wass et al., 2003).

The multiple mini-interview or MMI described in Case Example 8.1 is an example of an OSCE-like series of short structured interviews, analogous to structured oral exams, replacing long unstructured interviews for the selection of medical students. Research has demonstrated the validity of the MMI for making admissions decisions (Eva et al., 2009; Eva et al., 2012; Knorr & Hissbach, 2014). Eva et al. (2012) reported that "compared with students who were rejected by an admission process that used MMI assessment, students who were accepted scored higher on Canadian national licensing examinations" (p. 2233).

An examination blueprint ensures that the domain of interest is systematically and representatively sampled (see Chapter 2; Haladyna, 2004; Lane, Raymond, & Haladyna, 2015). Use a specification table to identify the content area and skills to be assessed and provide examples of questions to elicit the skills to be assessed (see Table 8.2).

Depending on the purpose of the examination, a variety of trigger materials may be used to provide a clinical context for the examination questions. In addition to written/video cases, an oral examination can be based on a live or simulated patient encounter and can serve as the probe for an OSCE station. At times, the examiner may simulate a patient in order to assess a learner's data gathering or communication skills. The American Board of Emergency Medicine integrates computer-based graphics and images such as x-rays and ECGs into its oral examination (Kowalenko et al., 2017). The American Board of Anesthesiology recently began basing some of its oral examination stations on standardized patients, the first US medical specialty board to do so (American Board of Anesthesiology, 2018).

Case Example 8.1 An Oral Examination "OSCE"

Multiple Mini-Interview

The multiple mini-interview (MMI) is a creative example of a structured oral that was developed at the Michael G. DeGroote School of Medicine at McMaster University to provide a more valid assessment of noncognitive qualities of medical school applicants (Eva, Reiter et al., 2004, Eva, Rosenfeld 2004). The traditional interview for admission to a health professions program can easily be conceptualized as an "oral examination"—a high-stakes conversation between the interviewer and the applicant. The McMaster MMI was composed of a series of OSCE-like brief structured cases based on scenarios pertaining to ethical issues, communication skills, collaborative abilities, or some other noncognitive quality. In some stations, the examiner might discuss an issue with the candidate, and in others the examiner may observe the candidate interacting with a simulated "patient" or "colleague." The MMI method has been used for selection to dentistry, medicine, nursing, pharmacy, and veterinary schools, as well as for graduate-level medical and dentistry programs (Reiter & Eva, 2017).

Sample MMI-type question (8 minutes):

Your friendly neighbor plans to use only alternative medicine strategies to treat her stomach cancer. What do you tell her?

Would your answer be different if this were your sister?

Table 8.2 Blueprinting and Logistical Decisions

- Content domain and subdomains to be sampled
- Skills/competencies to be assessed
  - Decision-making
  - Patient management
  - Diagnostic interpretations
  - Sensitivity to contextual issues
  - Communication and interpersonal skills
  - Other
- Trigger materials (if any)
  - Real patients
  - Simulated patients
  - Written vignettes
  - Learner's own patient charts
  - Laboratory results
  - Examiner role play
- Desired breadth and depth of questions

Logistical Decisions:
- Number of oral examination stations
- Time/duration of each station
- Number of questions/cases per station
- Number of examiners per station

Another option is to use the examinee's own cases as trigger material in chart-stimulated recall (CSR), allowing the examiner to probe deeply into the learner's clinical reasoning and decision-making rationale in the context of care provided to his/her patients (Maatsch, 1981). The American Board of Obstetrics and Gynecology (2018) bases three of the six sections in its oral examinations on the case list submitted by the candidate. Case Example 8.2 provides examples of initial questions that might be pre-specified for a CSR-based assessment; follow-up questions would be at the discretion of the examiner.

SCORING AND STANDARD SETTING

Scoring issues for oral examinations are similar to those for performance tests (Chapter 9), including instrument design for capturing and rating a performance and procedures for combining marks. Checklists and rating scales can encourage examiners to focus on the critical components of the examination, and behaviorally anchored scoring rubrics can help standardize ratings. As in performance tests, including global ratings helps to tap the unique judgment and experience of expert examiners.

Standard setting is a particular challenge for oral examinations. If left to the sole judgment of the individual examiner, pass/fail decisions could be legitimately attacked as both arbitrary and capricious. Pooling the judgments of several experts through a formal standard-setting exercise will ensure that the cut scores are defensible and fair.

Any of the standard-setting methods used for performance tests such as OSCEs can be adapted for structured oral examinations with multiple stations and examiners. Examinee-based methods such as the borderline group method may be especially appropriate for oral examinations in which different learners are questioned by different examiners. In this method, the examiner scores or rates the examinee on several relevant items per the scoring rubric and also provides a global rating ranging from definite pass to marginal pass to definite fail. The final pass/fail cut score is determined by the mean item score of all examinees with a "marginal pass" rating.

Case Example 8.2 Chart-Stimulated Recall (CSR)

Philibert (2018) provides a worksheet that can be used to develop a CSR session. She estimates about 5 minutes for case selection and chart audit, and 10 to 15 minutes for discussion and feedback. There are sections for conducting a chart review, conducting a case discussion, giving verbal feedback, and probing understanding of the feedback. For the case discussion section, she lays out initial questions that can be used to probe thinking about the care of the patient. For example:

- What features of the patient's presentation led you to your top two diagnoses? Was there was ambiguity or uncertainty? If yes, how did you deal with it?
- What was your rationale for the labs or tests you ordered? Were there other tests that you thought of but decided against? Why?
- Did you inquire about the patient's experience of his/her illness and care (feelings, ideas, effect on function and expectations)? What did you learn?

Reddy et al. (2018) developed a CSR rating scale mapped to ACGME milestones, and also provides sample questions that can be used to develop a structured CSR session. For example:

- How did you decide the patient was ready for discharge?
- What did you learn from taking care of this patient?
- Knowing what you know now, what, if anything, could you do better to improve your own practice?

Here is an example of the Milestones-Based Rating Scale for Chart-Stimulated Recall:

Please Indicate the Resident's Ability to Accomplish This Task:
Item 3: Appropriately Use Consultants

Level 1 Critically deficient	Level 2	Level 3	Level 4 Ready for unsupervised practice	Level 5 Aspirational
Does not use consultant services when needed for patient care	Unable to justify reason(s) for consultation	Asks meaningful clinical questions that guide the input of consultants	Weighs recommendations from consultants in order to effectively manage patients	Manages discordant recommendations from multiple consultants

Source: Reddy, S.T., Tekian, A., Durning, S.J., Gupta, S., Endo, J., Affinati, B., & Park, Y.S. (2018). Preliminary Validity Evidence for a Milestones-Based Rating Scale for Chart-Stimulated Recall. *Journal of Graduate Medical Education, 10*(3), 269–275

In an Angoff-type method, standards can be set either at the individual oral examination station level or at the test level. A panel of carefully selected judges reviews each item or examination station, and each judge indicates the probability of the item or examination being successfully accomplished by a borderline examinee—an examinee just on the cusp of failure. The final cut score for the station or the test is the sum of the probabilities across items or stations.

See Chapter 6 for a more complete discussion of standard-setting issues and Chapter 9 for discussion of scoring and standard setting in the context of performance tests.

PREPARATION OF THE EXAMINEE

Examinees should be oriented to the objectives, setting, duration, number of examiners, and the overall procedures in advance and informed about the type of questions they will be asked and the criteria for passing. If possible, opportunities to practice (particularly for high-stakes examinations) should be provided. Testing organizations often provide this information on their websites. For example, in addition to detailed written information, the American Board of Emergency Medicine (2018) has an "Oral Examination Candidate Orientation" video, and the American Board of Surgery (2018) provides one titled "Your Guide to a Successful Oral Examination."

SELECTION, TRAINING, AND EVALUATION OF THE EXAMINERS

Wakeford, Southgate, and Wass (1995) suggested that selection criteria for examiners include appropriate knowledge and skills in the subject matter, "an approach to the practice of medicine and the delivery of health care that is within the limits of that acceptable to the examiners as a whole," effective interpersonal skills, demonstrated ability of a good team player, and being active in general practice.

While selection of appropriate examiners is a critical step for any oral examination, one of the advantages of a structured oral examination is the opportunity to institute systematic training as well. In addition to reviewing the cases they will administer, examiners can be trained to ask open-ended questions at higher taxonomic levels to provide better assessment of the candidates' problem-solving skills (Des Marchais & Jean, 1993). Frame-of-reference training, in which examiners practice rating exemplars of different levels of responses, is an especially effective method for calibrating examiners to the rating scale (Bernardin & Buckley, 1981, and Chapter 9).

Newble, Hoare, and Sheldrake (1980) demonstrated that training tends to be ineffective for less-consistent examiners and suggested that inconsistent examiners and extremely severe or lenient raters be removed from the examiner pool. Jones (2016) describes the type of feedback on their rating behavior that the American Board of Surgery provides their examiners.

Systematic severity and leniency (but not inconsistency) can also be corrected by statistical adjustment of scores. Raymond, Webb, and Houston (1991) and Raymond, Harik, and Clauser (2011) used a relatively simple statistical procedure based on ordinary least squares (OLS) regression to identify and correct errors in leniency and stringency, resulting in a 6% change in the pass rate. In high-stakes examinations, more complex statistical methods such as many-facet Rasch measurement can help identify and correct for rater errors (Myford & Wolfe, 2003; Jones, 2012; see Chapter 19, Item Response Theory).

In addition to tracking examiners' scoring behavior, more senior examiners are often assigned to mentor and evaluate their colleagues. Chiodo (2016) and Harman (2016) provide examples of the forms that their boards use to monitor examiners.

See Case Example 8.3 for a description of examiner training for The American Board of Emergency Medicine (ABEM) Oral Certification Examination, and Table 8.3 for a summary of examiner training steps.

Case Example 8.3 Training and Assessing Examiners

The American Board of Emergency Medicine (ABEM) Oral Certification Examination

The ABEM oral certification examination (as of 2018) consists of seven structured oral simulations based on actual cases: five single-patient scenarios and two scenarios in which the candidate has to manage multiple patients concurrently. A single examiner scores each simulation, rating candidates on eight performance criteria based on critical actions relevant to that case. The examination blueprint (content specification) and pass/fail criteria can be found on the ABEM website (www.abem.org).

The ABEM expects their examiners to undergo six hours of training on case administration and scoring, achieving a high degree of inter-examiner agreement. Their examiners are monitored and evaluated on 17 criteria at each examination. Some of these are listed below.

- Established a comfortable tone of interaction with candidates
- Started cases on time
- Maintained control of case timing
- Finished cases on time
- Introduced cases according to guidelines
- Managed case material appropriately
- Administered cases according to agreed upon standards
- Played roles appropriately
- Cued appropriately
- Took comprehensive and readable notes

Examiners are assessed by senior examiners who rotate between rooms. Examiners who repeatedly deviate from training guidelines are not invited to return.

Note: For more about the American Board of Emergency Medicine Examination, see Reinhart (1995) and Bianchi (2003).

Table 8.3 Steps in Examiner Training for a Structured Oral Examination

1. Select examiners who are knowledgeable in the domain to be tested, familiar with the level of learners to be tested (e.g., second-year nursing students), and have good communication skills.
2. Orient examiners to the examination purpose, procedure, and consequences (stakes).
3. Explain the competencies to be assessed, types of questions to be asked, and how to use any trigger material. Have examiners practice asking higher-order questions.
4. Review and rehearse rating and documentation procedures.
5. If possible, provide frame-of-reference training to calibrate examiners to scoring of different levels of responses.
6. Have new examiners observe an experienced examiner and/or practice via participation in a simulated oral examination.
7. Observe new examiners and provide feedback, after which an examiner is either invited or rejected. Examiners who are inconsistent or have clearly deviant patterns of grading (very lenient or very severe) should not be allowed to serve as examiners.
8. Continue ongoing calibration/fine-tuning of examiners, particularly in high-stakes examinations.

QUALITY ASSURANCE

Quality assurance (QA) efforts can focus on preventing and checking for and remedying threats to the validity of the examination (Table 8.4) and on obtaining the five types of validity evidence described in Chapter 2. These might include activities such as reviewing the blueprint for content validity; ensuring that examiners adhered to implementation guidelines for questions, scoring, and managing the examination; obtaining reliability indicators such as inter-rater reliability or generalizability estimates; investigating the relationship between scores on the oral examination and other assessments; and assessing the consequences of the cut score standards set for the examination.

AFTER THE EXAMINATION

Planning for an oral examination includes consideration of post-examination issues common to all assessment methods. These include questions such as mechanisms for disseminating the results to examinees and other stakeholders, dealing with failing or marginal candidates, and developing an adjudication process to review disputed scores.

Table 8.4 Threats to Validity*: Oral Examinations

	Problem	Remedy
Construct Underrepresentation (CU)	Too few questions to sample domain adequately	Use multiple cases/stations
	Unrepresentative sampling of domain	Blueprint to be sure examinations systematically sample the domain
	Lower order questions (mismatch of questions to competencies)	Train examiners to use higher order questions Standardize the questions
	Too few independent examiners	Use multiple examiners Use one examiner per station
Construct-Irrelevant Variance (CIV)	Flawed or inappropriate questions	Train examiners Standardize questions
	Flawed or inappropriate case scenarios or other prompts	Pilot test cases and prompts
	Examiner bias	Provide scoring rubric Train examiners to use rubric
	Systematic rater error: halo, severity, leniency, central tendency	Frame-of-reference training for examiners
	Question difficulty inappropriate (too easy/too hard)	Train examiners Standardize questions
	Bluffing by examinees	Train examiners
	Language/cultural bias	Train examiners Review and revise questions
	Indefensible passing score methods	Use formal standard-setting procedures
Reliability Indicators	Generalizability	
	Inter-rater reliability	
	Rater consistency	

* For more about CU and CIV threats to validity, see Chapter 2.

COST

There are many expenses involved in an oral examination: examination preparation and production (including item/case generation and scoring); examiners' training and travel; other reimbursements particularly if standardized or real patients are utilized; and venue/site expenses. The logistics of a structured oral examination are particularly complex but are worth the extra cost and effort to be able to respond affirmatively to questions such as "Are we measuring what we intended to measure?", "Are the results reliable?" and "Is the examination worth the investment in time and money?"

SUMMARY

Oral examinations remain the subject of debate and dispute, but when properly implemented, orals can be credible components of the assessment toolbox. In the context of a low-stakes, formative assessment, an unstructured oral examination can provide an invaluable opportunity for faculty to engage in a conversation with learners, understand their thinking, and provide immediate feedback based on the encounter. In high-stakes settings, a structured, OSCE-like oral examination can provide a unique opportunity for in-depth probing of decision-making, ethical reasoning, and other "hidden" skills.

When planning a structured oral examination, follow these evidence-based recommendations:

- Use multiple cases/stations with multiple examiners.
- Use a blueprint to guide question development.
- Use a structured scoring system.
- Select consistent, well-trained examiners.
- Monitor the preparation, production, training, implementation, evaluation, and feedback phases of the examination process.
- Use oral examinations as one component of a comprehensive assessment system.

Note: Additional material and resources may be available at the UIC AHPE website: https://go.uic.edu/AHPE

REFERENCES

Al-Wassia, H., Al-Wassia, R., Shihata, S., Park, Y.S., & Tekian, A. (2015). Using patients' charts to assess medical trainees in the workplace: a systematic review. *Medical Teacher, 37*, S82–S87.

American Board of Anesthesiology. (2018). Staged examinations policy book. Retrieved from www.theaba.org/PDFs/BOI/StagedExaminations-BOI. Accessed 23 January 2018.

American Board of Emergency Medicine. (2018). Oral examination candidate orientation. Available at www.abem.org/public/emergency-medicine-(em)-initial-certification/oral-examnation/familiarize-yourself-with-the-oral-examination/candidate-video-and-sample-cases. Accessed January 24, 2018.

American Board of Obstetrics and Gynecology. (2018). 2018 bulletin for the certifying examination for basic certification in obstetrics and gynecology. Retrieved from www.abog.org/Bulletins/2018%20Basic%20Certifying%20Bulletin.pdf. Accessed August 31, 2018.

American Board of Surgery. (2018). General surgery certifying exam. Retrieved from www.absurgery.org/default.jsp?certcehomewebsite. Accessed January 23, 2018.

Bandiera, G., Sherbino, J., & Frank, J.R. (2006). *The CanMEDS assessment tools handbook: An introductory guide to assessment methods for the CanMEDS competencies.* Ottawa, ON: The Royal College of Physicians and Surgeons of Canada.

Bernardin, H.J., & Buckley, M.R. (1981). Strategies in rater training. *Academy of Management Review, 6*(2), 205–212.

Bianchi, L., Gallagher, E.J., Korte, R., & Ham, H.P. (2003). Interexaminer agreement on the American Board of Emergency Medicine oral certification examination. *Annals of Emergency Medicine, 41*, 859–864.

Burch, V.C., Norman, G.R., Schmidt, H.G., & van der Vleuten, C.P.M. (2008). Are specialist certification examinations a reliable measure of physician competence? *Advances in Health Sciences Education, 13*, 521–533.

Chiodo, A. ABPMR Part II examiner training. (2016). Retrieved from www.abms.org/media/119998/tues_2_chiodo_oralexams.pdf. Accessed January 23, 2018.

Chou, S., Lockyer, J., Cole, G., & McLaughlin, K. (2009). Assessing postgraduate trainees in Canada: Are we achieving diversity in methods. *Medical Teacher, 31*(2), e58–63.

Daelmans, H.E.M., Scherpbier, A.J.J.A., van der Vleuten, C.P.M., & Donker, A.J.M. (2001). Reliability of clinical oral examinations re-examined. *Medical Teacher, 23*, 422–424.

Davis, M.H., & Karunathilake, I. (2005). The place of the oral examination in today's assessment systems. *Medical Teacher, 27*(4), 294–297.

Des Marchais, J.E., & Jean, P. (1993). Effects of examiner training on open-ended, higher taxonomic level questioning in oral certification examinations. *Teaching and Learning in Medicine, 5*, 24–28.

Elstein, A.S., Shulman, L.S., & Sprafka, S.A. (1978). *Medical problem solving: An analysis of clinical reasoning.* Cambridge, MA: Harvard University Press.

Engel, J., Pai, A.B., & Walker, W.C. (2014). Can American Board of Physical Medicine and Rehabilitation Part 2 board examination scores be predicted from rotation evaluations or mock oral examinations? *American Journal of Physical Medicine and Rehabilitation, 93*, 1051–1056.

Eva, K.W., Reiter, H.I., Rosenfeld, J., & Norman, G.R. (2004). The ability of the multiple mini-interview to predict preclerkship performance in medical school. *Academic Medicine, 79*(10 Suppl), S40–42.

Eva, K.W, Rosenfeld, J., Reiter, H.I., & Norman, G.R. (2004). An admissions OSCE: The multiple mini-interview. *Medical Education, 38*(3), 314–326.

Eva, K.W., Reiter, H.I., Rosenfeld, J., Trinh, K., Wood, T.J., & Norman, G.R. (2012). Association between a medical school admission process using the multiple mini-interview and national medical licensing examination scores. *JAMA, 308*, 2233–2240.

Eva, K.W., Reiter, H.I., Trinh, K., Wasi, P., Rosenfeld, J., & Norman, G.R. (2009). Predictive validity of the multiple mini-interview for selecting medical trainees. *Medical Education, 43*, 767–775.

Evans, L.R., Ingersoll, R.W., & Smith, E.J. (1966). The reliability, validity, and taxonomic structure of the oral examination. *Journal of Medical Education, 41*, 651–657.

Fingeret, A.L., Arnell, T., McNelis, J., Statter, M., Dresner, L., & Widmann, W. (2016). Sequential participation in a multi-institutional mock oral examination is associated with improved American Board of Surgery certifying examination first-time pass rate. *Journal of Surgical Education, 73*, e95–e103.

Goulet, F., Jacques, A., Gagnon, R., Racette, P., & Sieber, W. (2007). Assessment of family physicians' performance using patient charts: Interrater reliability and concordance with chart-stimulated recall interview. *Evaluation in the Health Professions, 30*(4), 376–392.

Guerin, R.O. (1995). Disadvantages to using the oral examination. In E.L. Mancall & P.G. Bashook (Eds.), *Assessing clinical reasoning: The oral examination and alternative methods* (pp. 41–48). Evanston, IL: American Board of Medical Specialties.

Haladyna, T. (2004). *Developing and validating multiple-choice test items* (3rd ed.). Mahwah, NJ: Lawrence Erlbaum Associates.

Hamdy, H., Prasad, K., Williams, R., & Salih, F.A. (2003). Reliability and validity of the direct observation clinical encounter examination (DOCEE). *Medical Education, 37*, 205–212.

Harman, A.E. (2016). American Board of Anesthesiology oral examiner management. Retrieved from www.abms.org/media/120002/tues_2_harman_oralexams.pdf. Accessed January 23, 2018.

Houston, J.E., & Myford, C.M. (2009). Judges' perception of candidates' organization and communication, in relation to oral certification examination ratings. *Academic Medicine, 84*, 1603–1609.

Hutchinson, L., Aitken, P., & Hayes, T. (2002). Are medical postgraduate certification processes valid? A systematic review of the published evidence. *Medical Education, 36*, 73–91.

Jayawickramarajah, P.T. (1985). Oral examinations in medical education. *Medical Education, 19*, 290–293.

Jefferies, A., Simmons, B., Ng, E., & Skidmore, M. (2011). Assessment of multiple physician competencies in postgraduate training: Utility of the structured oral examination. *Advances in Health Sciences Education, 16*, 569–577.

Jones, A. (2016). Examiner management. Retrieved from www.abms.org/media/120005/tues_2_jones_oralexams.pdf. Accessed January 23, 2018.

Jones, A.T. (April 2012). Leveling the field in performance assessment: A deviation model for adjusting rater leniency. Paper presented at the annual meeting of the American education Research Association, Vancouver, BC, Canada.

Knorr, M., & Hissbach, J. (2014). Multiple mini-interviews: Same concept, different approaches. *Medical Education, 48*(12), 1157–1175.

Kowalenko, T., Heller, B.N., Strauss, R.W., Counselman, F.L., Mallory, M.N.S., Joldersma, K.B., et al. (2017). Initial validity analysis of the American Board of Emergency Medicine enhanced oral examination. *Academic Emergency Medicine, 24*(1), 125–129.

Lane, S., Raymond, M.R., & Haladyna, T.M. (2015). *Handbook of test development* (2nd ed.). New York: Routledge.

Linn, B.S., & Zeppa, R. (1976). Team testing: One component in evaluating surgical clerks. *Journal of Medical Education, 51*, 672–674.

Lunz, J.E., & Bashook, P.G. (2008). Relationship between candidate communication ability and oral certification examination scores. *Medical Education, 42*, 1227–1233.

Maatsch, JL. (1981). Assessment of clinical competence on the Emergency Medicine Specialty Certification Examination: The validity of examiner ratings of simulated clinical encounters. *Annals of Emergency Medicine, 10*, 504–507.

Mancall, E.L. (1995). The oral examination: An historic perspective. In E.L. Mancall & P.G. Bashook (Eds.), *Assessing clinical reasoning: The oral examination and alternative methods* (pp. 3–7). Evanston, IL: American Board of Medical Specialties.

McGuire, C.H. (1966). The oral examination as a measure of professional competence. *Journal of Medical Education, 41*, 267–274.

Memon, M.A., Joughin, G.R., & Memon, B. (2010). Oral assessment and postgraduate medical examinations: Establishing conditions for validity, reliability and fairness. *Advances in Health Sciences Education, 15*, 277–289.

Miller, G.E. (1990). The assessment of clinical skills/competence/performance. *Academic Medicine, 65*, S63–S67.

Myford, C.M., & Wolfe, E.W. (2003). Detecting and measuring rater effects using many-facet Rasch measurement: Part I. *Journal of Applied Measurement, 4*(4), 386–422.

Newble, D.I., Hoare, J., & Sheldrake, P.F. (1980). The selection and training of examiners for clinical examinations. *Medical Education, 14*, 345–349.

Norcini, J.J. (2002). The death of the long case? *British Medical Journal, 324*, 408–409.

Norman, G. (2000). Examining the examination: Canadian versus US certification exam. *Canadian Association of Radiologists Journal, 51*, 208–209.

Philibert, I. (2018). Using chart review and chart-stimulated recall for resident assessment. *Journal of Graduate Medical Education, 10*(1), 95–96.

Pokorny, A.D., & Frazier, S.H. (1966). An evaluation of oral examinations. *Journal of Medical Education, 41*, 28–40.

Raymond, M.R., Harik, P., & Clauser, B.E. (2011). The impact of statistically adjusting for rater effects on conditional standard errors of performance ratings. *Applied Psychological Measurement, 35*, 235–246.

Raymond, M.R., Webb, L.C., & Houston, W.M. (1991). Correcting performance-rating errors in oral examinations. *Evaluation and the Health Professions, 14*, 100–122.

Reddy, S.T., Endo, J., Gupta, S., Tekian, A., & Park, Y.S. (2015). A case for caution: Chart-stimulated recall. *Journal of Graduate Medical Education, 7*(4), 531–535.

Reddy, S.T., Tekian, A., Durning, S.J., Gupta, S., Endo, J., Affinati, B., & Park, Y.S. (2018). Preliminary validity evidence for a milestones-based rating scale for chart-stimulated recall. *Journal of Graduate Medical Education, 10*(3), 269–275.

Reinhart, M.A. (1995). Advantages to using the oral examination. In E.L. Mancall & P.G. Bashook (Eds.), *Assessing clinical reasoning: The oral examination and alternative methods* (pp. 31–39). Evanston, IL: American Board of Medical Specialties.

Reiter, H., & Eva, K. (2017). Vive la difference: The freedom and inherent responsibilities when designing and implementing multiple mini-interviews. *Academic Medicine, 93*(7), 969–971.

Rowland-Morin, P.A., Burchard, K.W., Garb, J.L., & Coe, N.P. (1991). Influence of effective communication by surgery students on their oral examination scores. *Academic Medicine, 66*, 169–171.

Schwaab, J., Kman, N., Nagel, R., Bahner, D., Martin, D.R., Khandelwal, S., et al. (2011). Using second life virtual simulation environment for mock oral emergency medicine examination. *Academic Emergency Medicine, 18*, 559–562.

Schwiebert, P., & Davis, A. (1993). Increasing inter-rater agreement on a family medicine clerkship oral examination—A pilot study. *Family Medicine, 25*, 182–185.

Strickland, C., Jensen, A., & McArthur, T. (2017). Does the oral "mock board" examination still have a role as a training tool? *Academic Radiology, 24*, 1463–1467.

Swanson, D.B., Norman, G.R., & Linn, R.L. (1995). Performance-based assessment: Lessons from the health professions. *Educational Researcher, 24*, 5–11.

Thomas, C.S., Mellsop, G., Callender, K., Crawshaw, J., Ellis, P.M., Hall, A., et al. (1993). The oral examination: A study of academic and non-academic factors. *Medical Education, 27*, 433–439.

Turnball, J., Danoff, D., & Norman, G. (1996). Content specificity and oral certification exams. *Medical Education, 30*, 56–59.

van der Vleuten, C.P.M., & Swanson, D.B. (1990). Assessment of clinical skills with standardized patients: State of the art. *Teaching and Learning in Medicine, 2*, 58–76.

Wakeford, R., Southgate, L., & Wass, V. (1995). Improving oral examinations: selecting, training, and monitoring examiners for the MRCGP. *British Medical Journal, 311*, 931–935.

Wass, V., Wakeford, R., Neighbour, R., & van der Vleuten, C. (2003). Achieving acceptable reliability in oral examinations: An analysis of the Royal College of General Practitioners membership examination's oral component. *Medical Education, 37*, 126–131.

Weingarten, M.A., Polliack, M.R., Tabenkin, H., & Kahan, E. (2000). Variations among examiners in family medicine residency board oral examinations. *Medical Education, 34*, 13–17.

Wiggins, M.N., Harper, R.A., Landes, R.D., & O'Sullivan, P.S. (2008). Effects of repeated oral examinations on ophthalmology residents. *British Journal of Ophthalmology, 92*, 530–533.

Williams, R.G., Klamen, D.A., & McGaghie, W.C. (2003). Cognitive, social and environmental sources of bias in clinical performance ratings. *Teaching and Learning in Medicine, 15*, 270–292.

Yaphe, J., & Street, S. (2003). How do examiners decide? A qualitative study of the process of decision making in the oral examination component of the MRCGP examination. *Medical Education, 37*, 764–771.

Yudkowsky, R. (2002). Should we use standardized patients instead of real patients for high-stakes exams in psychiatry? *Academic Psychiatry, 26*(3), 187–192.

Zhou, Y., Sun, H., Culley, D.J., Young, A., Harman, A.E., & Warner, D.O. (2017). Effectiveness of written and oral specialty certification examinations to predict actions against the medical licenses of anesthesiologists. *Anesthesiology, 126*, 1171–1179.

9

PERFORMANCE TESTS

Rachel Yudkowsky

A performance test is an examination designed to elicit performance on an actual or simulated real-life task. In contrast to observation of naturally occurring behavior "in vivo," the task is contrived for the purpose of the examination and explicitly invites the examinee to demonstrate the behavior to be assessed. Thus, a performance test is an "in vitro" assessment, at Miller's "shows how" level (Miller, 1990); see Figure 9.1. Since the examinees know they are being assessed, their performance likely represents their personal best or maximum performance, rather than a typical performance. Examples of performance tests include a road test to obtain a driver's license, an undersea diving test, and the Unites States Medical Licensing Exam (USMLE) Step 2 Clinical Skills Assessment. In this chapter, we review some of the purposes, advantages and limitations of performance tests, and provide practical guidelines for the use of standardized patients (SPs), a simulation modality commonly used in health professions education. Focusing on the use of SPs for assessment rather than instruction, we discuss scoring options, multiple-station objective structured clinical exams, standard setting, and threats to validity in the context of SP exams; the same principles apply to performance tests using other modalities. There are several other types of simulations currently in use, such as bench models, virtual (computer-based) models, and mannequins. Many of the assessment issues addressed here also apply to these forms of simulation, which are discussed in greater detail in Chapter 14.

STRENGTHS OF PERFORMANCE TESTS

Performance tests provide the opportunity to observe learners in action as they respond to complex challenges, while controlling when, where, how, and what will be tested. Performance tests are not limited to patients and problems that chance to present in clinical settings in a specific span of time. The simulation option provides a high degree of control over the examination setting, allowing standardization across examinees, advance training of examiners, and a systematic sampling of the domain to be assessed. When used formatively, performance tests provide unique opportunities for feedback, coaching, and debriefing, thus facilitating deliberate practice (Ericsson, Krampe, & Tesch-Römer, 1993; Ericsson, 2004) and the development of skills and expertise. From a patient safety perspective, performance tests allow educators to ensure that learners have reached a minimal level of competency and skill before they are allowed to work with real

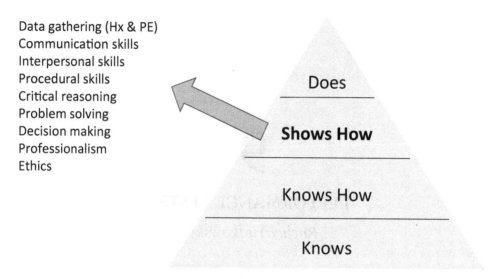

Data gathering (Hx & PE)
Communication skills
Interpersonal skills
Procedural skills
Critical reasoning
Problem solving
Decision making
Professionalism
Ethics

Does

Shows How

Knows How

Knows

Figure 9.1 Miller's pyramid: competencies to assess with performance tests

patients. Disadvantages of performance tests are related to the complex logistics and difficulty of realistically modeling clinical tasks; simulations can be expensive, and the need for multiple stations or cases (see "Multiple-Station Performance Tests" later in this chapter) increases the resource cost in terms of both money and time.

DEFINING THE PURPOSE OF THE TEST

As with all assessments, faculty must be clear about the purpose of the test. What are the underlying constructs (competencies or skills) to be assessed?

Since performance tests are time consuming and expensive, they are best reserved for the assessment of skills that cannot be observed or assessed effectively elsewhere or by other means. Skills that involve interactions with patients are particularly amenable to performance tests. Communication and interpersonal skills with patients, family, staff, and colleagues; data gathering by means of a history and physical exam; clinical reasoning and decision-making; documentation in the patient chart; ethical and professional behavior; and procedural skills all can be elicited and assessed effectively in simulated settings.

The choice of whether to assess individual skills or a complete clinical encounter depends in part on the level of the learner (Petrusa, 2002). Students early in training often learn discrete skills such as "examining the shoulder" or "taking a sexual history." These skills can be assessed by means of brief, 5–7 minute stations in which they are instructed to demonstrate the particular skill: "please examine the shoulder of this patient." Intermediate learners must select salient history and physical exam items on their own when encountering a patient and must construct a differential diagnosis and management plan. These learners are more appropriately tested in a longer, integrated patient encounter that elicits these competencies in the context of a given complaint. For more advanced learners, the ability to handle complex critical situations can be tested in an "error prone" environment that features staff blunders, non-functioning equipment, and distracting family members.

An observation of an actual (not simulated) clinical encounter can be part of a performance test if the encounter is taking place for the purpose of an assessment: for example a mini-CEX (Chapter 10), the live interview in the US Psychiatry Board exam, or the first part of a traditional "viva," in which a preceptor rates the performance of a history and physical exam on an unknown patient. Note that a performance test does not require the subsequent oral examination or discussion of the patient—the encounter itself is the object of the rating. All of the principles discussed in this chapter, such as blueprinting, scoring the encounter, and standard setting, apply equally to performance tests based on real patients and to simulations.

STANDARDIZED PATIENTS

Standardized patients (SPs) are persons who are trained to portray a given patient presentation in a consistent and believable manner, allowing the realistic simulation of patient encounters (Barrows & Abrahamson, 1964; Barrows, 1993). SPs can come from a range of backgrounds including professional actors, retired teachers, community volunteers, patients with stable physical findings, nurses, medical residents, and students. "Hybrid" or multimodal simulations use SPs in conjunction with bench models and/or mannequins to encourage a patient-centered approach to procedural skills and to enhance the realism and challenge of critical care and team scenarios (Kneebone et al., 2005; Black et al., 2006; Nestel, Mobley, Hunt, & Eppich, 2014). Unannounced SPs can be sent incognito into clinician offices and clinics to assess performance in actual practice (Rethans, Drop, Sturmans, & van der Vleuten, 1991; Rethans, Gorter, Bokken, & Morrison, 2007; Weiner et al., 2010; Schwartz, Weiner, & Binns-Calvey, 2013). The SP methodology also has been extended to the portrayal of standardized students for faculty development (Gelula & Yudkowsky, 2003) and standardized family members, colleagues (Gangopadhyaya, Kamin, Kiser, Shadrake, & Yudkowsky, 2013), and staff. Standardized patients are deployed across the health professions, in medicine, nursing, pharmacy, dentistry, physiotherapy, occupational therapy, dietetics, veterinary medicine, and others.

"Simulated patient" is a generic term that includes portrayals that do not need to be highly consistent across encounters, for example patient simulation for the purpose of small group instruction. In contrast, the "standardized" aspect of the SP is crucial to the use of SPs for assessment. In a high-stakes assessment setting, SPs must be able to keep the portrayal consistent across a large number of examinees, each bringing his or her own idiosyncratic questions and behaviors to the encounter. Consistent portrayal requires two elements: a highly specified script and rigorous training of the SP.

The *SP script* contains the details of the portrayal. The script stipulates the age, gender, and other salient characteristics of the patient and describes the patient's medical history and physical exam findings, their "backstory" (family, job, and life circumstances), and their personality and affect. The script specifies information to be provided in response to open-ended questions, information to be provided only if specifically elicited by the examinee, SP prompts for the examinee (e.g., questions such as, "Can I go home now?"), and the desired SP responses to different examinee behaviors. The extent and richness of the script depends in part on the length and nature of the expected interaction. A five-minute encounter in which a student examines the shoulder of the SP without gathering any historical information may require only a description of physical exam findings to be simulated (if any). A 30-minute encounter in which an examinee is asked to develop a differential diagnosis and treatment plan for a depressed elderly woman demands a highly detailed and elaborated script.

SP scripts should be written by teams of experienced clinicians, preferably based on their own experiences with an actual patient, with modifications to maintain patient confidentiality. Basing the script on a real patient provides the foundation for a rich backstory, supporting details such as laboratory results, and the assurance that the script "hangs together" to present a plausible and realistic patient. Box 9.1 lists suggested elements of an effective script. SP scripts can also be found in published casebooks (e.g., Macy Initiative, 2003) and in online resource banks such as MedEd Portal (www.aamc.org/mededportal) and the Association of Standardized Patient Educators (www.aspeducators.org).

Box 9.1 Sample Elements of a Standardized Patient Case

General Case Information

- ☐ Presenting complaint
- ☐ Diagnosis
- ☐ Case author contact information
- ☐ Learning objectives, competencies addressed in case
- ☐ Target learner group (e.g., medical students, residents, nursing students, nurse practitioner students, other)
- ☐ Level of learner (year of training, advanced clinician, etc.)
- ☐ Duration of patient encounter

Case Summary and SP Training Notes

- ☐ SP demographics: name, gender, age range, ethnicity
- ☐ Setting (clinic, ER, etc.)
- ☐ History of present illness
- ☐ Past medical history
- ☐ Family medical history
- ☐ Social history and backstory
- ☐ Review of systems
- ☐ Physical examination findings (if indicated)
- ☐ Special instructions for the SP:
  - ☐ Patient presentation (affect, appearance, position of patient at opening, etc.)
  - ☐ Opening statement
  - ☐ Embedded communication challenges
  - ☐ Responses to open-ended questions
  - ☐ Responses to specific interviewing techniques or errors
- ☐ Special case considerations/props:
  - ☐ Specific body type/physical requirements
  - ☐ Props (e.g., pregnancy pillow)
  - ☐ Makeup (please include application guidelines if available)

Additional Materials

- ☐ Door chart information
- ☐ Laboratory results, radiology images (if indicated)
- ☐ Student instructions
- ☐ Student pre- or post-encounter challenge
- ☐ SP checklist or rating scale for scoring the encounter
- ☐ Observer checklist or rating scale
- ☐ SP feedback guidelines
- ☐ Other supporting documents (faculty instructions, etc.)

Source: Adapted with permission from the Association of Standardized Patient Educators (ASPE) Copyright 2008

SP training: Once the script is available, an SP can be trained to portray the patient accurately, consistently, and believably (van der Vleuten & Swanson, 1990; Tamblyn, Klass, Schnabl, & Kopelow, 1991; Colliver & Williams, 1993; Errichetti & Boulet, 2006; Wallace, 2007). Training includes review, clarification, and memorization of the case material, followed by rehearsal of the material in simulated encounters with the trainer and/or simulated examinees. The SP must be able to improvise appropriately and in character when confronted with unexpected questions from the examinee. If more than one SP will be portraying the same case, training them together will promote consistency across different SPs. Video recordings of previous SPs portraying the case help provide consistency across different administrations of the test (Schlegel, Bonvin, Rethans, & van der Vleuten, 2015). If the SPs will be providing verbal or written feedback to the examinee, they should be trained to do so effectively (e.g., Howley, 2007). If the SPs will be rating the examinees, this requires training as well (see rater training, later). The entire training process can range from 30 minutes to eight hours and more, depending on the complexity of the script, the responsibilities of the SP, and the extent of standardization needed. Once the SP is performing at the desired level, periodic assessment and feedback can help maintain the quality of the exam (Wind, Van Dalen, Muijtjens, & Rethans, 2004).

SCORING THE PERFORMANCE

Checklists and rating scales are used to convert the examinee's behavior during the SP encounter (or other observed performance) into a number that can be used for scoring. *Checklist* items are statements or questions that can be scored dichotomously as "done" or "not done"—for example, "The examinee auscultated the lungs." *Rating scales* employ a range of response options to indicate the quality of what was done—for example, "How respectful was the examinee?" might be rated on a four-point scale ranging from "extremely respectful" to "not at all respectful."

Case-specific checklists identify actions essential to a given clinical case, and are usually developed by panels of content experts or local faculty (Gorter et al., 2000). Checklist items can also be derived by observing the actions of experienced clinicians as they encounter the SP (Nendaz et al., 2004). Ideally, items should be evidence-based and reflect best-practice guidelines. Since checklists are intended simply to record what took place in the encounter, completing the checklist does not necessarily require expert judgment. Nonetheless, to minimize disagreements between raters, the checklist items must be very well specified, and raters must be trained to recognize the parameters of examinee behaviors that merit a score of "done" for a particular action. For example, the checklist item cited above "the examinee auscultated the lungs" might be more fully specified as "the examinee auscultated the lungs on skin, posteriorly, bilaterally, at three levels, while asking the patient to breathe deeply through the mouth." If any one of these conditions is not met, the item is scored as "not done" or as "done incorrectly." The item could be split into individual items for each of the essential conditions (on skin, bilateral, three levels, etc.) if more detailed feedback is desired. Checklists may be completed by observers during the encounter or by the SP immediately after the encounter. Checklists of 12–15 items can be completed quite accurately by well-trained SPs (Vu et al., 1992). Some extensively trained SPs can complete much longer checklists, such as those required for a full head-to-toe screening physical exam (Yudkowsky et al., 2004). Trained non-experts such as SPs, non-SP lay persons, and medical students are as reliable as expert observers (e.g., physicians) when using checklists and checklist-calibrated rating scales (Swanson & van der Vleuten, 2013).

While checklists can be used effectively with beginning learners to confirm that they followed all steps of a medical procedure or elicited a thorough medical history, comprehensive checklists are not always appropriate for more advanced examinees (Hodges, Regehr, McNaughton, Tiberius, & Hanson, 1999; Swanson & van der Vleuten, 2013). Expert clinicians often receive relatively low scores on history and physical exam (H&P) checklists that reward thoroughness; they tend to reach a diagnosis based on non-analytic processes such as pattern matching and thus perform a highly abbreviated H&P. Checklists that focus on clinically discriminating items (items that discriminate between competing diagnoses) (Yudkowsky, Park, Riddle, Palladino, & Bordage, 2014) and key feature items (see Chapter 13) may better identify advanced learners. Weighting check-list items is not generally useful (Sandilands, Gotzmann, Roy, Zumbo, & de Champlain, 2014). When assessing more complex performance and/or advanced clinicians, rating scales completed by experts may be a more appropriate tool (Swanson & van der Vleuten, 2013).

Rating scales provide the opportunity for observers to exercise expert judgment and rate the quality of an action. *Global* scale items rate the performance as an integrated whole; for example, "Overall, this performance was: excellent | very good | good | marginal | unsatisfactory." *Analytic* scale items allow polytomous (multiple-level) rating of a detailed list (similar to a check-list) of specific behaviors salient to a task. One item, for example, might be rated as "Student followed up on patient non-verbal cues: frequently | sometimes | rarely | never." *Primary trait* scale items are used to assess a small number of salient features or characteristics of the over-all performance; thus when assessing communication skills, one might be asked to rate verbal communication, non-verbal communication, and English language skills. While checklists are usually case-specific, rating scales can be used to score behaviors or skills that are demonstrated across different cases, such as data gathering, communication skills, or professionalism. A variety of instruments for rating communication and interpersonal skills have been published; see, for example, Stillman, Brown, Redfield, and Sabers (1977); Makoul (2001a, 2001b); Kurtz, Silverman, Benson, and Draper (2003); Iurameneerat, Myford, Yudkowsky, and Lowenstein (2009). Excellent guidelines for developing rating scales and survey items can be found in Artino, La Rochelle, Dezee, and Gehlbach (2014).

Because rating scales require the exercise of judgment, they are inherently more subjective than checklists. Providing anchors for the different rating options can improve agreement between raters (inter-rater reliability), especially if these anchors are behaviorally anchored (Bernardin & Smith, 1981a). The Accreditation Council for Graduate Medical Education (ACGME) Milestones (Holmboe, Edgar, & Hamstra, 2016) are examples of developmentally oriented behaviorally anchored rating scales (BARS). See Box 9.2 for examples of different types of rating scale anchors. *Rubrics* can be used to rate written products such as chart notes completed after an SP encounter. The rubric is, in effect, a behaviorally anchored rating scale providing detailed information about the performance expected at each score level (see Chapter 7 for more about rubrics in the context of written tests). A sample rubric for scoring a chart note is shown in Box 9.3.

Box 9.2 Rating Scale Anchors

A. Likert Scale Item*

The student provided a clear explanation of my condition and the treatment plan.

1	2	3	4
Strongly disagree	Disagree	Agree	Strongly agree

* May include a middle anchor "neither agree nor disagree."

B. Linear Scale ("Likert-type") Item

How clear were the student's explanations?

1	2	3	4	5
Not at all clear	Somewhat clear	Clear	Very clear	Extremely clear

C. Behaviorally Anchored Rating Scale (BARS) Item

Did the student provide a clear explanation of your condition?

1	2	3	4
Provided little or no explanation of my condition	Provided brief or unclear explanations of my condition	Provided a full and understandable explanation of my condition	Provided a full and understandable explanation of my condition, and probed my understanding by asking me to summarize pertinent information

Box 9.3 Sample Post-Encounter Patient Note Scoring Rubric

Task	Scoring Levels
Documentation: Documentation of findings from the history (Hx) and physical examination (PE) 30 points total	1. Most key Hx and PE findings are missing or incorrect (7 points) 2. About half of the key positive and negative findings present; OR most findings are present but poorly documented or disorganized (15 points) 3. Most key positive and negative findings present, well documented and organized, may miss a few pertinent positive or negative findings (23 points) 4. All key information present, concise and well organized with little irrelevant information (30 points)
DDX: Differential diagnosis 30 points total	1. [0–1 of 3] or [0 of 2] of the correct diagnoses listed (7 points) 2. [2 of 3] or [1 of 2] of the correct diagnoses listed, in any order (15 points) 3. All diagnoses listed, incorrect rank order (23 points) 4. All diagnoses listed and correctly rank ordered (30 points)
Justification: Justification of the differential diagnosis 30 points total	1. No justification provided OR many missing or incorrect links between findings and Dx (7 points) 2. About half of the key links between findings and Dx are missing or incorrect (15 points) 3. Only a few missing or incorrect links to diagnoses (23 points) 4. Links to diagnoses are correct and complete (30 points)
Workup: Plans for immediate diagnostic workup 10 points total	1. Diagnostic workup ordered or omitted places patient in unnecessary risk or danger (2 points) 2. Ineffective plan with most essential tests missed, and/or inefficient plan with many irrelevant tests included (5 points) 3. Reasonable plan for diagnostic workup; may have some unnecessary tests or missing a few essential tests (8 points) 4. Plan for diagnostic workup is effective and efficient; includes all essential tests and few or no unnecessary tests (10 points)

Source: Reprinted with permission from Park, Y.S., Hyderi, A., Heine, N., May, W., Nevins, A., Lee, M., Bordage, G., & Yudkowsky, R. (2017): Validity Evidence and Scoring Guidelines for Standardized Patient Encounters and Patient Notes From a Multisite Study of Clinical Performance Examinations in Seven Medical Schools. *Academic Medicine, 92,* S12–S20.

Academic Medicine is the journal of the Association of American Medical Colleges, https://journals.lww.com/academicmedicine

TRAINING RATERS

Raters must be trained to use checklists and rating scales accurately and consistently. Training is best done with all raters in one group to facilitate consensus and cross-calibration. After reviewing the purpose of the exam and each of the items, frame of reference training (Bernardin & Buckley, 1981b; Newman et al., 2016) can help ensure that all raters are calibrated and using the scale in the same way. The raters observe and individually score a live or recorded performance such as an SP encounter or chart note, then together discuss their ratings and reach a consensus on the observed behaviors corresponding to the checklist items and rating anchors. Ideally, raters should observe performances at high, middle, and low levels of proficiency and identify behaviors that are characteristic of each level.

Many of the challenges facing developers and raters of performance tests are similar to those for written constructed-response items. See Chapter 7 for additional insights into item development and rater selection and training.

PILOT TESTING THE CASE

Before deploying the case in an assessment, the station and rating instruments should be piloted with a few representative raters and examinees to ensure that the test will function as intended. Pilot tests frequently result in changes to the examinee instructions, specification of SP responses to previously unanticipated queries, and clarification of checklist items and rating anchors.

MULTIPLE-STATION PERFORMANCE TESTS: THE OBJECTIVE STRUCTURED CLINICAL EXAM (OSCE)

Performance on one clinical case or challenge is not a good predictor of performance on another case; this phenomenon is known as "case specificity" (Elstein, Shuman, & Sprafka, 1978). The ability to manage a patient with an acute appendicitis does not predict the ability to diagnose depression; demonstrating an appropriate history and physical exam (H&P) for a patient with chronic diabetes does not predict the ability to conduct an appropriate H&P for a patient with acute chest pain. Just as one would not assess a student's knowledge based on a single multiple-choice question, one cannot assess competency based on a single observation. One solution is the objective structured clinical examination or OSCE (Harden, Stevenson, Downie, & Wilson, 1975), an exam format that consists of a series or circuit of performance tests. Within an OSCE, each test is called a "station"; students start at different points in the circuit and encounter one station after another until the OSCE is complete. A given OSCE can include stations of the same type (e.g., only SP encounters) or of different types: SP-based patient encounters, procedures such as IV insertion, written challenges such as writing prescriptions or chart notes, interpretation of lab results, EKGs or radiology images, and oral presentations to an examiner (Figure 9.2). A larger number of stations allows for better sampling of the domain to be assessed, thus improving the reliability and validity of the exam—see the threats to validity discussion later.

The duration of an OSCE station can range from five minutes to 30 minutes or longer, depending on the purpose of the exam (Petrusa, 2002). Shorter stations allow the testing of discrete skills such as eliciting reflexes; longer stations allow the assessment of complex tasks in a realistic context—for example, counseling a patient reluctant to undergo colorectal screening. Ten to 20 minutes are usually sufficient for a focused history and physical exam (Petrusa, 2002). For logistic convenience, all stations in a given OSCE should be of equal duration. "Couplet" stations consist of two linked challenges—for example, writing a chart note about the patient just seen in the previous station. The duration of the couplet station—the SP encounter plus note—will be equal to the combined time of two stations.

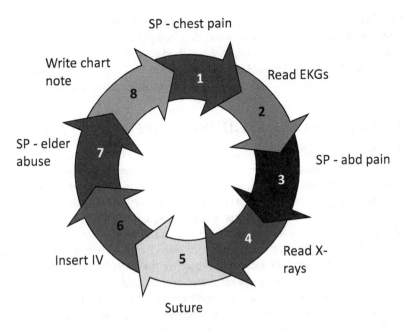

SP - chest pain

Write chart note

Read EKGs

SP - elder abuse

SP - abd pain

Insert IV

Read X-rays

Suture

1 2 3 4 5 6 7 8

Figure 9.2 An eight-station OSCE for an internal medicine clerkship

---

Box 9.4 OSCE Case Example: The United States Medical Licensing Examination (USMLE) Step 2 Clinical Skills Exam

Exam purpose	To ensure that new residents have the knowledge and skills needed to provide patient care under supervision
Content domain	Patients and problems normally encountered during medical practice in the United States
Level of skill assessed (discrete skills vs full encounter)	Full encounter: Ability to gather information from patients, perform physical examinations, and communicate findings to patients and colleagues
Format	(1) Standardized patient (SP) encounters (15 minutes each) (2) Patient note written after each encounter (10 minutes)
Number of stations (encounters)	Twelve
Skill section scores reported	(1) Integrated clinical encounter (ICE): Data gathering and data interpretation (from physical exam checklist and patient note) (2) Communication and interpersonal skills (CIS) (3) Spoken English proficiency (SEP)
Rating instruments	• Checklists for physical exam and CIS • Global rating scales for patient note and SEP
Raters	• SPs for physical exam checklist, CIS, and SEP • Trained physicians for patient note
Combining scores across cases, cut scores	Compensatory *within* skill section (ICE, CIS, SEP) Conjunctive *across* skills—must past each section separately

Source: www.usmle.org/step-2-cs/

High-stakes licensure OSCEs are conducted around the world. Boulet, Smee, Dillon, and Gimpbel (2009) provide a description of the use of standardized patient assessments in licensure examinations in the US and Canada. As an example of a high-stakes OSCE, Box 9.4 provides a summary description of the United States Medical Licensing Exam Step 2 Clinical Skills Assessment (USMLE Step 2CS). Additional information about this program is available at the USMLE website.

SCORING AN OSCE: COMBINING SCORES ACROSS STATIONS

The unit of analysis in an OSCE is the station or case, not the checklist item, since items within a case are mutually dependent: whether a resident examines the heart depends on whether she elicited a history of chest pain. Similarly, a couplet station is a single unit of analysis. Checklist or scale items should be aggregated to create a station score. Subsets of checklist items can give information about performance on different aspects of the task, for example history taking vs physical exam, but these subscales rarely have enough items to stand on their own as reliable measures. However, skills subscales or primary-trait ratings of skills that are common to several cases can be averaged across cases to obtain an exam-level score for that skill. For example, communication and interpersonal skills (CIS) scores show moderate correlations across cases, so it is reasonable to average CIS rating scale scores across cases to obtain an exam-level score.

Compensatory vs non-compensatory or conjunctive scoring issues were discussed in Chapter 6. Should good performance on one case or task compensate for poor performance on another? This is a policy-level decision. A skills-based compensatory approach would mean that good communication skills in one case could reasonably compensate for poor communication skills in another. On the other hand, decision makers may feel that examinees should demonstrate competency in an absolute number of critical clinical situations such as chest pain, abdominal pain, or shortness of breath—good performance on one would not compensate for poor performance on another. The ability to perform different clinical procedures is generally conjunctive—good performance inserting an IV does not compensate for poor performance obtaining an EKG.

STANDARD SETTING

Many of the standard-setting methods described in Chapter 6, originally developed for written tests, have been adapted for use with performance tests (Downing, Tekian, & Yudkowsky, 2006). Item-based methods such as Angoff are commonly and easily employed to set cut scores for checklists; however, the use of item-based methods for performance tests has been challenged, since items on a checklist are not mutually independent (Ross, Clauser, Margolis, Orr, & Klass, 1996; Boulet, de Champlain, & McKinley, 2003). Moreover, not all checklist items have equal clinical valence—the omission of one item may endanger a patient's life, while the omission of another may be of little import to the outcome of the clinical case. Standard-setting methods based on the direct observation of examinees' performance, such as borderline group (BG) and contrasting groups (CG), avoid these problems. Programs that use expert examiners (faculty) to observe and score SP encounters can easily use these examinee-based methods by having the examiners assign a global rating of fail, marginal pass, or pass in addition to completing the checklist for each examinee. The mean or median checklist score of examinees with a marginal pass rating is set as the cut score in the borderline group method, while the intersection of the passing and failing groups provides the basis for the cut score in the contrasting groups method (see Chapter 6 for details). Programs that use non-clinicians such as SPs to complete the checklists can have faculty experts rate the SP-scored checklists as proxies for examinee performance, use a whole-test method such as Hofstee, or opt to fall back on item-based methods such as Angoff or Ebel while acknowledging their limitations. Case-level cut scores can be aggregated across cases to provide a compensatory-type standard for the whole test. Conjunctive standards will require that a specific number of cases be passed, or that two or more subscales be passed (for example, both data gathering and communication skills). Conjunctive standards will always result in a higher failure rate than compensatory standards, since each hurdle adds its own probability of failure. See Chapter 6 for a more extended discussion of standard setting and the methods cited above.

Procedural skills testing brings a different set of challenges to standard setting. A mastery approach is especially appropriate in situations where the checklist is public and incorrect performance comprises a threat to patient safety or to the successful outcome of the procedure. See Chapter 18 (mastery learning) and Chapter 6 (standard setting) for details.

LOGISTICS

Conducting an OSCE can be daunting. Many schools have full-time SP trainers, paid professional actors or others who serve as SPs, and a dedicated facility that includes several clinic-type rooms with audiovisual recording capability, affording remote observation and scoring of SP encounters. Online data-management systems facilitate checklist data capture and reporting and allow both learners and faculty to view and comment upon digital recordings of encounters from remote locations. On the other hand, OSCEs also can be conducted on a more limited budget by using faculty as trainers and raters, recruiting students, residents, or community volunteers as SPs, and exploiting existing clinic space in the evening or weekend. Video recording the encounters is helpful but by no means essential.

THREATS TO THE VALIDITY OF PERFORMANCE TESTS

Threats to the validity of performance tests are summarized in Table 9.1. Our discussion will focus on the two main threats discussed in Chapter 2: undersampling (construct underrepresentation) and noise (construct-irrelevant variance).

Construct underrepresentation, or undersampling, can be a particular threat to the validity of performance tests since performance varies from station to station ("case specificity"), but only a small number of stations or performances can be observed. A multiple-station performance test (OSCE) thus falls between the written test with hundreds of multiple-choice questions and the traditional viva or oral exam that may include only a single observation or questions about a single patient case.

The validity of an OSCE depends primarily on its ability to sufficiently and systematically sample the domain to be assessed (Figure 9.3). Systematic sampling is supported by blueprinting and creating a table of test specifications (see Chapter 2). In the case of an SP-based OSCE, the blueprint should specify three Cs: *content* subdomains, *competencies* to be assessed, and patient *characteristics*; the OSCE should include cases that comprise a systematic sampling of these elements. Box 9.5 provides an example of blueprint elements for an SP-based assessment of occupational therapists on an inpatient rehabilitation rotation. A conceptual framework can assist in identifying salient elements to be sampled and assessed; examples of such frameworks are the Interprofessional Collaborative Practice Competency Domains (Interprofessional Education Collaborative Expert Panel, 2011), the American College of Clinical Pharmacy Clinical Pharmacist Competencies (Saseen et al., 2017), the ACGME competencies and milestones for residents in the US (Batalden, Leach, Swing, Dreyfus, & Dreyfus, 2002; Holmboe et al., 2016), and the Kalamazoo consensus statement on patient-centered communication (Makoul, 2001a); see Box 9.6. The multiple mini-interview (MMI) described in Chapter 8 (see Case Example 8.1, Eva, Rosenfeld, Reiter, & Norman, 2004, and many subsequent papers) applies the principles of blueprinting and

Table 9.1 Threats to the Validity of Performance Tests

Threat	Problem	Remedy
Construct Underrepresentation (CU) "Undersampling"	Not enough cases or stations to sample domain adequately	Use multiple stations (at least 8–10)
	Not enough items to reflect the performance in a given case	Use several checklist or rating scale items to capture the performance in each case
	Unrepresentative sampling of domain	Blueprint to be sure exams systematically sample the domain
Construct-Irrelevant Variance (CIV) "Noise"	Unclear or poorly worded items	Pilot stations and rating instruments Train raters on items
	Station or item difficulty inappropriate (too easy/too hard)	Pilot stations and rating instruments with learners of the appropriate level
	Checklist items don't capture expert reasoning (mismatch of items to competencies)	Careful design of checklist and rating scale items to match level of examinee Use content-expert raters who can rate the quality of the response (vs done/not done)
	Rater bias	Provide behaviorally anchored scoring rubric Train raters to use rubric Use multiple raters across stations
	Systematic rater error: halo, severity, leniency, central tendency	Frame of reference training for raters
	Inconsistent ratings	Remove rater
	Language/cultural bias	Train raters Pilot and revise stations
	Indefensible passing score methods	Formal standard-setting exercises
Reliability Indicators	Generalizability	
	Inter-rater reliability	
	Rater consistency	
	Internal consistency reliability of rating scale	

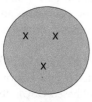

Construct under-representation or under-sampling: Not enough data points

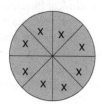

Construct under-representation or under-sampling: Data points do not systematically sample the entire domain

Data points systematically sample the domain to be assessed

Figure 9.3 Construct underrepresentation

Box 9.5 Creating Blueprint Specifications for an OSCE—Occupational Therapist Inpatient Rehabilitation Rotation

Content: *Identify the content subdomains to be assessed. For an inpatient rehabilitation OT rotation, these might include, for example:*

- Stroke, brain injury, spinal cord injury
- Other neurological conditions (Parkinson's, multiple sclerosis, etc.)
- Amputations and other orthopedic conditions
- Multiple trauma
- Cancer

Competencies: *Identify tasks, competencies, and skills to be assessed. For example, ability to:*

- Conduct chart review
- Obtain history and occupational profile
- Assess upper extremities (range of motion, sensation, tone)
- Assess cognitive and communication skills
- Assess vision and visual perceptual skills
- Assess balance skills
- Assess activities of daily living (ADLs) and instrumental activities of daily living (IADLs)
- Document all in chart

Characteristics: *Identify patient demographics and other salient dimensions to be sampled. For example:*

- Age, gender, ethnicity
- Chronic vs acute complaint
- Home environment, social support
- Previous level of functioning

Compile a set of cases or challenges that samples across the listed content, competencies, and characteristics. *Sample stations for an OT inpatient rehabilitation OSCE:*

- Complete an occupational profile for a previously independent 40-year-old woman with a new onset stroke.
- Counsel a spouse/caregiver who is having difficulty coping with their loved one's behavioral changes after a brain injury due to a car accident.
- Discuss implementation of a bowel program for a 20-year-old man with a complete C8 spinal cord injury with the patient, his primary nurse, and his mother; document in the chart.

---

sampling in the context of admission interviews, conceiving the interview as, in effect, a performance test.

To yield valid inferences, OSCE stations must be long enough to allow the observation of the behavior of interest. If the behavior of interest is the ability to conduct a focused history and physical exam and generate a differential diagnosis and treatment plan based on that H&P, the OSCE will need to utilize longer (10–20 minute) stations and extend the testing time to allow for

---

Box 9.6 Sample Frameworks to Assist in Blueprinting OSCEs

Interprofessional Collaborative Practice Competency Domains

- Values/Ethics for Interprofessional Practice
- Roles/Responsibilities
- Interprofessional Communication
- Teams and Teamwork

Source: Interprofessional Education Collaborative Expert Panel (2011). *Core Competencies for Interprofessional Collaborative Practice: Report of an Expert Panel.* Washington, DC: Interprofessional Education Collaborative.

American College of Clinical Pharmacy Clinical Pharmacist Competencies

- Direct patient care
- Pharmacotherapy knowledge
- Systems-based care and population health
- Communication
- Professionalism
- Continuing professional development

Source: Saseen, J.J. et al. (2017). ACCP Clinical Pharmacist Competencies. *Pharmacotherapy, 37*(5), 630–636, doi: 10.1002/phar.1923

The Kalamazoo consensus statement

Essential elements of communication in medical encounters:
- Build the doctor-patient relationship
- Open the discussion
- Gather information
- Understand the patient's perspective
- Share information
- Reach agreement on problems and plans
- Provide closure

Source: Makoul, G. (2001). Essential Elements of Communication in Medical Encounters: The Kalamazoo Consensus Statement. *Academic Medicine, 76*(4), 390–393.

---

a sufficient number of encounters. Generally about 4–8 hours of testing time are needed to obtain minimally reliable scores (van der Vleuten & Swanson, 1990).

The frequent disjunction between the exam and the clinical curriculum comprises an additional challenge to the content validity of the exam and may contribute to case specificity (Williams et al., 2014). An OSCE blueprint systematically maps the exam stations to the curriculum content and objectives. However, the clinical experiences of trainees are often opportunistic—the particular set of patient problems seen by a given student will depend on the patients who happen to be admitted to the hospital or seen in the clinic during the weeks of their clerkship. Comments from students that they have not encountered the clinical challenges included in the OSCE, or unusually low mean scores on a specific station, may provide valuable information regarding curricular gaps.

Another type of threat to validity is *construct-irrelevant variance*, in which the spread of scores across students (score variance) reflects something other than differences in student ability. Any source of variance other than that due to actual differences of ability between students is considered error variance ("noise"). In SP-based performance tests, the items, cases, SPs, raters, and occasion are all potential sources of measurement error. The generalizability coefficient G is a measure of the reliability of the exam as a whole (see Chapter 4); generalizability analyses can help identify the major sources of error for a given OSCE. Complementing the generalizability analysis, item response theory and many-facet Rasch measurement (MFRM) analyses (Chapter 19) can identify any individual items, cases, and raters that are problematic and the specific types of errors involved (Iramaneerat & Yudkowsky, 2007; Iramaneerat, Yudkowsky, Myford, & Downing, 2008; Pell, Fuller, Homer, & Roberts, 2010). Case specificity, the variance due to cases and the interaction between cases and persons, is usually the greatest source of variance in performance tests, and is a much greater source of error than differences between raters. Thus it is much more effective to use one rater per station and increase the number of stations than to have two or more raters per station with a smaller number of stations (van der Vleuten & Swanson, 1990; Swanson, Clauser, & Case, 1999). With proper training, SPs contribute little error variance; repeated studies have shown that SPs can be trained to portray cases and complete checklists with a high degree of accuracy and consistency (van der Vleuten & Swanson, 1990; Colliver & Williams, 1993). In general, if there is sufficient sampling of content via a sufficient sampling of cases or stations, and different raters and SPs are used across stations, then sampling across raters and SPs will also be sufficient to provide reproducible results.

Table 9.2 describes the sources of variance in a typical OSCE, along with typical errors and possible remedies.

Table 9.2 Sources of Error in an OSCE

Source of Variance	Reason	Result	Remedy
Person	Persons differ in their ability to do the behavior to be assessed	Differences in scores due to true differences in ability between persons	No remedy needed—this (and only this) is the desired score information
Item	Checklist or rating scale items or anchors not clear	Different raters will have different understandings of the item so will rate the same performance differently	Carefully word items Pilot the items Train raters
	Item-specific variance	Individual students find some items in a case more difficult than others (performance is variable across items within a case)	Use several items per case
Case	Case-specific variance	Individual students find some cases more challenging than others (performance is variable across cases within an exam)	Use many cases per exam
	Case situation or task is unclear or ambiguous	Students respond differently depending on their interpretation of the case	Pilot the case to be sure that it is clear and unambiguous
SP	SP portrays the case incorrectly	Students respond to a different case than authors intended	Train SP, quality assurance
	Different SPs vary in how they portray the case	Students respond differently to different SPs	

(Continued)

Table 9.2 (continued)

Source of Variance	Reason	Result	Remedy
Raters	Systematic rater error: halo, severity, leniency, central tendency	Systematically biased ratings—e.g., an individual rater gives consistently high or low ratings	Provide behaviorally anchored scoring rubric Frame of reference training for raters Use different raters across stations Statistical corrections for systematic errors
	Rater bias	Ratings depend on irrelevant characteristics such as gender or race	Rater training Remove rater
	Inconsistent ratings	A given rater gives randomly inconsistent ratings—adds to the random noise in the system	Rater training Remove rater
Occasion	Occasion-specific factors: environmental factors such as noise and temperature; individual factors such as illness or lack of sleep	Performance is affected by the occasion-specific factor	Control environmental factors Test on several different occasions

CONSEQUENTIAL VALIDITY: EDUCATIONAL IMPACT

One important aspect of an assessment is its impact on learning (van der Vleuten & Schuwirth, 2005; Swanson & van der Vleuten, 2013; see also Chapter 17). Adding an SP-based OSCE to the usual battery of MCQ written tests has been found to increase students' attention to clinical experiences and their requests for direct observation and feedback (Newble & Jaeger, 1983; Newble, 1988); testing procedural skills similarly leads students to seek opportunities for practicing these skills, a desirable result. However, the use of checklists in SP-based assessments can sometimes have unintended consequences. For example, if checklists require students to elicit a list of historical items and SPs are trained not to disclose the information unless specifically asked, students will learn to ask closed-ended questions in shotgun fashion instead of taking a patient-centered approach. Training SPs to give more elaborated and informative responses to open-ended questions can reduce this effect. Similarly, assessing the physical exam by means of a head-to-toe screening exam (Yudkowsky et al., 2004) ensures that students acquire a repertoire of PE maneuvers, but encourages students to learn these maneuvers by rote with no consideration of diagnostic hypotheses or potential physical findings. Using a hypothesis-driven PE approach to assessment (Yudkowsky et al., 2009; Nishigori et al., 2011) can promote the development of clinical reasoning instead of rote learning. Educators should be alert to the potential for both positive and negative consequences of any assessment method and ensure that the assessment experience encourages good habits of learning and practice.

CONCLUSION

Performance tests provide opportunities for examinees to demonstrate a particular competency or skill under controlled conditions. Performance tests utilizing standardized patients and other simulations can control or manage many elements that are not predictable in live patient settings. Systematic sampling across cases, items, and raters in performance tests is essential to minimizing sources of error and maximizing generalizability and validity of the score. The combination of systematic sampling, control, and standardization afforded by performance tests allows for a valid, fair, and defensible assessment of clinical skills.

Recommended Readings and Resources

- For summaries of research on standardized patients, see the reviews by van der Vleuten & Swanson, 1990; Colliver & Williams, 1993; and Petrusa, 2002. Swanson & van der Vleuten, 2013, provides an excellent discussion of more recent issues.
- For a fascinating narrative of the history of standardized patients, see Wallace, 1997.
- MedEdPortal, www.mededportal.org, includes a collection of peer-reviewed SP cases, indexed in PubMed. Consider publishing your own SP cases there!
- For additional resources and to network with health professions educators working with standardized patients and simulations around the world, go to the websites of the Association of Standardized Patient Educators at www.aspeducators.org/ and the Society for Simulation in Healthcare at www.ssih.org/.

Note: Additional material and resources may be available at the UIC AHPE website: https://go.uic.edu/AHPE

REFERENCES

Artino, A.R., La Rochelle, J.S., Dezee, K.J., & Gehlbach, H. (2014). Developing questionnaires for educational research: AMEE Guide No. 87. *Medical Teacher, 36*, 463–474.

Barrows, H.S. (1993). An overview of the uses of standardized patients for teaching and evaluating clinical skills. *Academic Medicine, 68*, 443–451.

Barrows, H.S., & Abrahamson, S. (1964). The programmed patient: A technique for appraising student performance in clinical neurology. *Journal of Medical Education, 39*, 802–805.

Batalden, P., Leach, D., Swing, S., Dreyfus, H., & Dreyfus, S. (2002). General competencies and accreditation in graduate medical education. An antidote to over specification in the education of medical specialists. *Health Affairs, 21*, 103–111.

Bernardin, H.J., & Smith, P.C. (1981a). A clarification of some issues regarding the development and use of behaviorally anchored rating scales (BARS). *Journal of Applied Psychology, 66*, 458–463.

Bernardin, H.J., & Buckley, M.R. (1981b). Strategies in rater training. *The Academy of Management Review, 6*(2), 205–212.

Black, S., Nestel, D., Horrocks, E., Harrison, R., Jones, N., Wetzel, C., Wolfe, J., et al. (2006). Evaluation of a framework for case development and simulated patient training for complex procedures. *Simulation in Healthcare, 1*(2), 66–71.

Boulet, J.R., de Champlain, A.F., & McKinley, D.W. (2003). Setting defensible performance standards on OSCEs and standardized patient examinations. *Medical Teacher, 25*(3), 245–249.

Boulet, J.R., Smee, S.M., Dillon, G.F., & Gimpel, J.R. (2009). The use of standardized patient assessments for certification and licensure decisions. *Sim Healthcare, 4*, 35–42.

Colliver, J.A., & Williams, R.G. (1993). Technical issues: Test application. *Academic Medicine, 68*, 454–460.

Downing, S., Tekian, A., & Yudkowsky, R. (2006). Procedures for establishing defensible absolute passing scores on performance examinations in health professions education. *Teaching and Learning in Medicine, 18*(1), 50–57.

Elstein, A.S., Shuman, L.S., & Sprafka, S.A. (1978). *Medical problem solving: An analysis of clinical reasoning.* Cambridge, MA: Harvard University Press.

Ericsson, K.A. (2004). Deliberate practice and the acquisition and maintenance of expert performance in medicine and related domains. *Academic Medicine, 79*(10 Suppl), S70–S81.

Ericsson, K.A., Krampe, R.T., & Tesch-Römer, C. (1993). The role of deliberate practice in the acquisition of expert performance. *Psychological Review, 100*, 363–406.

Errichetti, A., & Boulet, J.R. (2006). Comparing traditional and computer-based training methods for standardized patients. *Academic Medicine, 81*(10 Suppl), S91–S94.

Eva, K.W., Rosenfeld, J., Reiter, H.I., & Norman, G.R. (2004). An admissions OSCE: The multiple mini-interview. *Medical Education, 38*, 314–326.

Gangopadhyaya, A., Kamin, C., Kiser, R., Shadrake, L., & Yudkowsky, R. (2013). Assessing residents' interprofessional conflict negotiations skills. *Medical Education, 47*, 1139–1140.

Gelula, M., & Yudkowsky, R. (2003). Using standardized students in faculty development workshops to improve clinical teaching skills. *Medical Education, 37*, 621–629.

Gorter, S., Rethans, J.J., Scherpbier, A., van der Heijde, D., van der Vleuten, C., & van der Linden, S. (2000). Developing case-specific checklists for standardized-patient-based assessments internal medicine: A review of the literature. *Academic Medicine, 75*(11), 1130–1137.

Harden, R., Stevenson, M., Downie, W., & Wilson, M. (1975). Assessment of clinical competence using objective structured examinations. *British Medical Journal, 1*, 447–451.

Hodges, B., Regehr, G., McNaughton, N., Tiberius, R., & Hanson, M. (1999). OSCE checklists do not capture increasing levels of expertise. *Academic Medicine, 74*, 1129–1134.

Holmboe, E.S., Edgar, L., Hamstra, S. (2016). *The milestones guidebook*. Chicago, IL: Accreditation Council for Graduate Medical Education. Retrieved from www.acgme.org/What-We-Do/Accreditation/Milestones/Resources. Accessed July 2, 2019.

Howley, L. (2007). Focusing feedback on interpersonal skills: A workshop for standardized patients. MedEdPORTAL. Retrieved from www.mededportal.org/publication/339/

Interprofessional Education Collaborative Expert Panel. (2011). *Core competencies for interprofessional collaborative practice: Report of an expert panel*. Washington, DC: Interprofessional Education Collaborative.

Irameneerat, C., Myford, C.M., Yudkowsky, R., & Lowenstein, T. (2009). Evaluating the effectiveness of rating instruments for a communication skills assessment of medical residents. *Advances in Health Sciences Education, 14*, 575–594.

Iramaneerat, C., & Yudkowsky, R. (2007). Rater errors in a clinical skills assessment of medical students. *Evaluation & the Health Professions, 30*(3), 266–283.

Iramaneerat, C., Yudkowsky, R., Myford, C.M., & Downing, S. (2008). Quality control of an OSCE using generalizability theory and many-faceted Rasch measurement. *Advances in Health Sciences Education, 13*(4), 479–493.

Kneebone, R.L., Kidd, J., Nestel, D., Barnet, A., Lo, B., King, R., Yang, G.Z., & Brown, R. (2005). Blurring the boundaries: Scenario-based simulation in a clinical setting. *Medical Education, 39*, 580–587.

Kurtz, S.M., Silverman, J.D., Benson, J., & Draper, J. (2003). Marrying content and process in clinical method teaching: Enhancing the Calgary-Cambridge guides. *Academic Medicine, 78*(8), 802–809.

The Macy Initiative in Health Communication Casebook, 2003. Referenced in and available from the authors: Yedidia, M.J., Gillespie, C.C., Kachur, E., Schwartz, M.D., Ockene, J., Chepaitis, A.E., Snyder, C.W., Lazare, A., & Lipkin, M. (2003). Effect of communications training on medical student performance. *The Journal of the American Medical Association, 290*, 1157–1165.

Makoul, G. (2001a). Essential elements of communication in medical encounters: The Kalamazoo consensus statement. *Academic Medicine, 76*(4), 390–393.

Makoul, G. (2001b). The SEGUE Framework for teaching and assessing communication skills. *Patient Education and Counseling, 45*, 23–34.

Miller, G. (1990). The assessment of clinical skills/competence/performance. *Academic Medicine* (65 supplement), S63–67.

Nendaz, M.R., Gut, A.M., Perrier, A., Reuille, O., Louis-Simonet, M., Junod, A.F., & Vu, N.V. (2004). Degree of concurrency among experts in data collection and diagnostic hypothesis generation during clinical encounters. *Medical Education, 38*(1), 25–31.

Nestel, D., Mobley, B.L., Hunt, W.A., & Eppich, W.J. (2014). Confederates in health care simulations: Not as simple as it seems. *Clinical Simulation in Nursing, 10*(12),611–616.

Newble, D.I. (1988). Eight years' experience with a structured clinical examination. *Medical Education, 22*, 200–204.

Newble, D., & Jaeger, K. (1983). The effects of assessments and examinations on the learning of medical students. *Medical Education, 17*, 165–171.

Newman, L.R., Brodsky, D., Jones, R.N., Schwartzstein, R.M., Atkins, K.M., & Roberts, D.H. (2016). Frame-of-reference training: Establishing reliable assessment of teaching effectiveness. *The Journal of Continuing Education in the Health Professions, 36*(3), 206–210.

Nishigori, H., Masuda, K., Kikukawa, M., Kawashima, A., Yudkowsky, R., Bordage, G., & Otaki, J. (2011). A model teaching session for the hypothesis-driven physical examination. *Medical Teacher, 33*(5), 410–417.

Park, Y.S., Hyderi, A., Heine, N., May, W., Nevins, A., Lee, M., Bordage, G., Yudkowsky, R. (2017). Validity evidence and scoring guidelines for standardized patient encounters and patient notes from a multisite study of clinical performance examinations in seven medical schools. *Academic Medicine, 92*, S12–S20.

Pell, G., Fuller, F., Homer, M., & Roberts, T. (2010). How to measure the quality of the OSCE: A review of metrics—AMEE guide no. 49. *Medical Teacher, 32*, 802–811.

Petrusa, E. (2002). Clinical performance assessments. In G.R. Norman, C.P.M. van der Vleuten, & D.I. Newble (Eds.), *International handbook of research in medical education* (pp. 647–672). Dordrecht, The Netherlands: Kluwer Academic Publishers.

Rethans, J.J., Drop, R., Sturmans, F., & van der Vleuten, C. (1991). A method for introducing standardized (simulated) patients into general practice consultations. *British Journal of General Practice, 41*, 94–96.

Rethans, J.J., Gorter, S., Bokken, L., & Morrison, L. (2007). Unannounced standardized patients in real practice: A systematic literature review. *Medical Education, 41*(6), 537–549.

Ross, L.P., Clauser, B.E., Margolis, M.J., Orr, N.A., & Klass, D.J. (1996). An expert-judgment approach to setting standards for a standardized-patient examination. *Academic Medicine, 71*, S4–S6.

Sandilands, D.D., Gotzmann, A., Roy, M., Zumbo, B.D., de Champlain, A. (2014). Weighting checklist items and station components on a large-scale OSCE: Is it worth the effort? *Medical Teacher, 36*, 585–590.

Saseen, J.J., Ripley, T.L., Bondi, D., Burke, J.M., Cohen, L.J., McBane, S., McConnell, K.J., et al. (2017). ACCP clinical pharmacist competencies. *Pharmacotherapy, 37*(5), 630–636).

Schlegel, C., Bonvin, R., Rethans, J.J., & van der Vleuten, C. (2015). The use of video in standardized patient training to improve portrayal accuracy: A randomized post-test control group study. *Medical Teacher, 37*(8), 730–737.

Schwartz, A., Weiner, S.J., Binns-Calvey, A. (2013). Comparing announced with unannounced standardized patients in performance assessment. *Joint Commission Journal on Quality and Patient Safety, 39*, 83–88.

Stillman, P., Brown, D., Redfield, D., & Sabers, D. (1977). Construct validation of the Arizona clinical interview rating scale. *Educational and Psychological Measurement, 77*, 1031–1038.

Swanson, D.B., Clauser, B.E., & Case, S.M. (1999). Clinical skills assessment with standardized patients in high-stakes tests: A framework for thinking about score precision, equating, and security. *Advances in Health Sciences Education, 4*, 67–106.

Swanson, D.B., & van der Vleuten, C.P.M. (2013): Assessment of clinical skills with standardized patients: State of the art revisited. *Teaching and Learning in Medicine, 25*(sup1), S17–S25.

Tamblyn, R.M., Klass, D.J., Schnabl, G.K., & Kopelow, M.L. (1991). The accuracy of standardized patient presentation. *Medical Education, 25*, 100–109.

van der Vleuten, C.P., & Schuwirth, L.W. (2005). Assessing professional competence: From methods to programmes. *Medical Education, 39*, 309–317.

van der Vleuten, C.P., & Swanson, D.B. (1990). Assessment of clinical skills with standardized patients: state of the art. *Teaching and Learning in Medicine, 2*, 58–76.

Vu, N.V., Marcy, M.M., Colliver, J.A., Verhulst, S.J., Travis, T.A., & Barrows, H.S. (1992). Standardized (simulated) patients' accuracy in recording clinical performance check-list items. *Medical Education, 26*, 99–104.

Wallace, P. (1997). Following the threads of an innovation: the history of standardized patients in medical education. *CADUCEUS, 13*(2), 5–28.

Wallace, P. (2007). Coaching standardized patients: For use in the assessment of clinical competence. New York City, NY: Springer Publishing Company.

Weiner, S.J., Schwartz, A., Weaver, F., Goldberg, J., Yudkowsky, R., Sharma, G., Binns-Calvey, A., Preyss, G., Schapira, M.M., Persell, S.D., Jacobs, E., & Abrams, R.I. (2010). Contextual errors and failures in individualizing patient care: A multicenter study. *Annals of Internal Medicine, 153*, 69–75.

Williams, R.G., Klamen, D.L., Markwell, S.J., Cianciolo, A.T., Colliver, J.A., & Verhuls, S.J. (2014). Variations in senior medical student diagnostic justification ability. *Academic Medicine, 89*(5), 790–798.

Wind, L.A., Van Dalen, J., Muijtjens, A.M., & Rethans, J.J. (2004). Assessing simulated patients in an educational setting: the MaSP (Maastricht assessment of simulated patients). *Medical Education, 38*(1), 39–44.

Yudkowsky, R., Downing, S., Klamen, D., Valaski, M., Eulenberg, B., & Popa, M. (2004). Assessing the head-to-toe physical examination skills of medical students. *Medical Teacher, 26*, 415–419.

Yudkowsky, R., Otaki, J., Lowenstein, T., Riddle, J., Nishigori, H., & Bordage, G. (2009). A hypothesis-driven physical exam for medical students: Initial validity evidence. *Medical Education, 43*, 729–740.

Yudkowsky, R., Park, Y.S., Riddle, J., Palladino, C., & Bordage, G. (2014). Clinically discriminating checklists versus thoroughness checklists: Improving the validity of performance test scores. *Academic Medicine, 89*(7), 1057–1062.

10

WORKPLACE-BASED ASSESSMENT

Mary E. McBride, Mark D. Adler, and William C. McGaghie

This chapter has seven sections. We begin, in the first section, by introducing the concept of workplace-based assessment (WBA). The second section places WBA in the larger context of competency-based medical education (CBME). The third section discusses the importance of blueprinting or mapping competencies against curriculum objectives. The fourth section discusses WBA in more detail and reviews existing WBA tools. The fifth section addresses assessment administration and the tactics that must be followed for WBA programs to succeed. The sixth section discusses how we make sense of and use data from two perspectives: psychometric and socio-cultural. We conclude with a summary and a look ahead.

WORKPLACE-BASED ASSESSMENT

Singh and Norcini (2013) assert that workplace-based assessment involves direct observation of learners in a workplace for formative feedback or summative assessment within a competency-based medical education model. Knowledge, behavior, conduct, skills, and self-reflection are all assessment targets (Govaerts & van der Vleuten, 2013). WBA efforts are not the sole source of learner evaluation. WBAs are intended to be part of a well-considered, broadly sampled *program of assessment* including written evaluations, standardized tests, objective structured clinical exams (OSCEs), and simulation-based assessment, among others (van der Vleuten, 2016; van der Vleuten & Schuwirth, 2005). The purpose of WBA is to observe improvement, consistent with a learner's development, in skills, attitudes, and behaviors via direct observation using well-considered assessments in the hands of well-trained raters. The goal of a WBA process, in the terms of Miller's taxonomy, is to assess what the learner *can do or does* (Figure 10.1) as a proxy for what they *will do* in practice (Govaerts, 2015; Miller, 1990). The final measure of education quality is not just the learner but the patient and society who stand to benefit from high-quality care (Kogan & Holmboe, 2013).

The conceptual model for WBA within a competence framework has evolved over time. Data-driven outcomes derived from a variety of rating instruments, patient logs, portfolios, and other observational measures contribute to a system that favors an assessment-of-learning model. The learner is assessed by a rater and discrete data are passed up an evaluation chain to create a larger data compilation. Learner feedback is often a key feature of the process. However, learners often

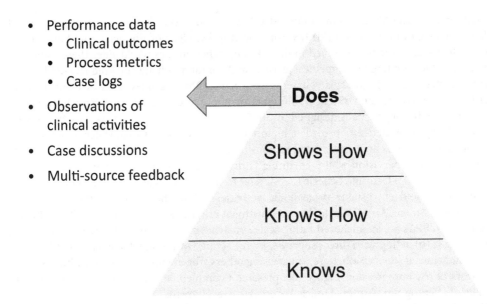

- Performance data
  - Clinical outcomes
  - Process metrics
  - Case logs
- Observations of clinical activities
- Case discussions
- Multi-source feedback

Does

Shows How

Knows How

Knows

Figure 10.1 Miller's pyramid: data sources for workplace-based assessments

do not experience observational assessment as primarily a learning experience. Responding to this sense that WBA is more summative than formative, learners quickly discern how to "game the system" via a variety of impression management strategies (McGaghie, 2018).

WBA programs assume there is an ideal clinical performance that can be achieved by a learner and assessed by raters without error who share the same mental model about a performance standard (Govaerts, 2015). Much of the published work over several decades focuses on describing and reporting validity evidence for WBA tools for a variety of uses and learner groups (Kogan, Holmboe, & Hauer, 2009). Existing assessment tools, however, do not produce strong validity evidence without a broad sample of ratings across time, settings, and raters to achieve adequate reproducibility (Crossley & Jolly, 2012).

WBA is seen in socio-cultural terms as the cornerstone of an assessment program that is learner-centric and seeks to provide a context for learning toward the goal of developing excellent healthcare providers. WBA, in a socio-cultural view, is primarily focused on an assessment-of-learning model that favors narrative feedback over numerical scores. In this view, there is no single "true" score that captures clinical fitness. When trained faculty raters see things differently, this variability should not be viewed as rater error but different views about performance standards (Govaerts & van der Vleuten, 2013). This simply reflects the understanding that most clinical problems have more than one correct answer and that faculty experts may disagree about the best course of action. Barriers in the path of this recognition are the realities of clinical demands on learners and faculty, financial drivers of healthcare education, and challenges of creating a learning culture to support more qualitative WBA.

COMPETENCY-BASED MEDICAL EDUCATION

McGaghie, Miller, Sajid, and Telder (1978) state that the intended output of a CBME program is a "health professional who can practice medicine at a defined level of proficiency, in accord with local conditions, to meet local needs." The proficiency or competency standards to which McGaghie et al. (1978) refer to are promulgated by national-level entities such as the Accreditation

Council for Graduate Medical Education (ACGME) and the Association of American Medical Colleges (AAMC) in the US; CanMEDS from the Royal College of Physician and Surgeons of Canada; the General Medical Council in the UK; and other entities worldwide. These standards form broad education targets for medical learners at the undergraduate and graduate levels.

This chapter addresses workplace-based assessments. Other sources of assessment data are described in the chapters on written, oral, and performance tests; narrative assessment; and portfolios. Together, the aggregate is designed to provide learner assessment across activity, assessor, and time. Such aggregated data provide a picture of learner readiness to advance to subsequent stages of education and clinical graduated responsibility. Educators assert we may *trust* the learner to work with less supervision while remaining faithful to goals of patient safety and providing high-quality care. Ten Cate and Scheele (2007) refer to these choices as *entrustment* decisions.

Entrustment and entrustable professional activities (EPAs) have entered the language of healthcare assessment. An EPA articulates entrustment criteria. Rather than a gestalt or a binary trust decision, EPAs are an anchored rating scale construct ranging from a learner (a) observing a clinical task; (b) acting with direct supervision; (c) acting with indirect supervision; (d) acting with distant clinical supervision; to (e) supervising others. The anchors may vary within a graded framework of trust progression. Figure 10.2 presents a complementary anchoring structure from the CanMEDS program (Gofton, Dudek, Wood, Balaa, & Hamstra, 2012).

The relationship between competencies, entrustment, WBA, and performance decisions is shown in Figure 10.3 (Gofton, Dudek, Barton, & Bhanji, 2017). Neither specific competencies nor EPAs were meant to be "in the moment" snapshots. More discrete evaluations, taken in the aggregate, fill that role (Holmboe, 2015). WBA provides an important data source for bidirectional feedback, with a data flow that allows for entrustment decisions and to chart progress toward developmental milestones.

BLUEPRINTING

Before probing WBA in greater depth, we touch on the process for linking broad education objectives to assessments. *Blueprinting* or content mapping is a mechanism that explicitly links assessment to learning objectives (Coderre, Woloschuk, & McLaughlin, 2009; Swanwick & Chana, 2009). The goal is to ensure alignment between assessment methods, including tools and settings

Level	Descriptor
1	**"I had to do"** i.e., requires complete hands on guidance, did not do, or was not given the opportunity to do
2	**"I had to talk them through"** i.e., able to perform tasks but requires constant direction
3	**"I had to prompt them from time to time"** i.e., demonstrates some independence, but requires intermittent direction
4	**"I needed to be in the room just in case"** i.e., independence but unaware of risks and still requires supervision for safe practice
5	**"I did not need to be there"** i.e., complete independence, understands risks and performs safely, practice ready

Figure 10.2 The O-SCORE entrustment scale

Source: Gofton, W.T., Dudek, N.L., Wood, T.J., Balaa, F., & Hamstra, S.J. (2012). The Ottawa Surgical Competency Operating Room Evaluation (O-SCORE): A Tool to Assess Surgical Competence. Academic Medicine, 87(10), 1401–1407. Academic Medicine is the journal of the Association of American Medical Colleges, http://journals.lww.com/academicmedicine

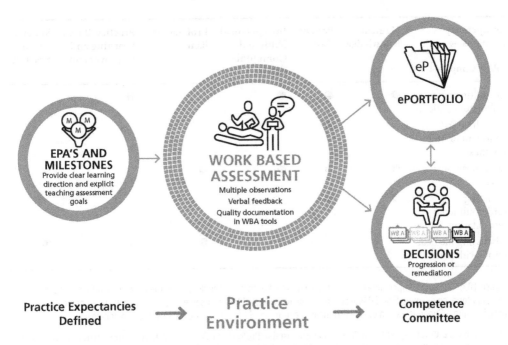

Figure 10.3 Situating WBA in a competency-based assessment framework

Source: Gofton, W., Dudek, N., Barton, G., and Bhanji, F. (2017). Workplace-Based Assessment Implementation Guide: Formative Tips for Medical Teaching Practice (1st ed.). (PDF) Ottawa: The Royal College of Physicians and Surgeons of Canada, pp. 1–12. Available at Royal College of Physicians and Surgeons, www.royalcollege.ca/rcsite/documents/cbd/work-based-assessment-practical-implications-implementation-guide-e.pdf. Reproduced with permission of the RCPSC.

and curriculum objectives. The intent is to evaluate learners across clinical domains in a balanced pattern without over- or underrepresenting specific content. Figure 10.4 illustrates how specific EPAs can be mapped to curriculum milestones to ensure adequate sampling across competency domains (ten Cate, 2014). Blueprinting has applicability at both the high-level curricular design stage and when creating individual WBA assessments. Blueprinting addresses concerns about purposeful content sampling in assessment programs that often emphasize ad hoc clinical encounters.

WORKPLACE-BASED ASSESSMENT

Direct clinical observation of learners with meaningful feedback and opportunities for incremental improvement is a key tenet of WBA. Watling and Ginsburg (2019) note that "to be effective, feedback should be timely, specific, actionable and task-oriented rather person-oriented." Provided over time, this adheres to the *deliberate practice* conceptual model where learners engage in sustained, purposeful practice with expert feedback. Deliberate practice has been shown to be effective in improving learner skills in healthcare education (Ericsson, 2004, 2015).

WBA programs seek to collect and use assessment data that focus, in part, on assessment *of* learning. Research in WBA, following this model, is marked by attempts to employ psychometric evidence to support the use of a variety of assessments. Schuwirth and van der Vleuten (2006) argue that a psychometrically driven approach does not align with the current WBA methods. They point out several assumptions made about using quantitative measures to evaluate WBAs outcomes: (a) that learning, measured by numerical scores, has meaning without regard to the context where the score was obtained; (b) competence, judged from a numerical score, is a stable trait; and (c) there is a "true" level of performance that could be scored if raters performed better.

Competency Domains → EPA Examples ↓	Medical Knowledge	Patient Care	Interpersonal Skills and Communi- cation	Professiona- lism	Practice-Based Learning and Improvement	Systems- Based Practice
Consulting new ambulatory patients	●	●	●		●	
Providing first treatment of mild traumas		●	●			
Leading an inpatient ward	●	●	●	●		●
Initiating cardiopulmonary resuscitation	●	●				
Discussing medical errors with patients		●		●	●	●

Figure 10.4 Multiple competencies are at stake with most activities. The dots show the most relevant competency domains for each example EPA. EPAs link competencies to work. EPAs can serve as the primary focus of competency-based training: Supervisors can observe trainees executing an EPA, but through a lens of competencies.

Source: ten Cate, O. (2014). AM Last Page: What Entrustable Professional Activities Add to a Competency-Based Curriculum, Academic Medicine, 89(4), 691. Academic Medicine is the journal of the Association of American Medical Colleges, https://journals.lww.com/academicmedicine.

These assumptions, they argue, cannot be justified (Govaerts & van der Vleuten, 2013). Context matters. A model of the interplay of key WBA factors is shown in Figure 10.5 (Durning et al., 2012).

While WBA programs do provide data for assessment, we clearly and explicitly use WBA events as opportunities for feedback. The one-on-one faculty-learner interaction is viewed as a primary driver of learning. There is tension in this model. There is, in today's model of CBME, a system-level need for data, and key portions of these data arise from workplace interactions between learner and faculty. The dual uses of WBA blur the lines between formative and summative assessment for both learner and assessor (Govaerts, 2015). Bok notes, "combining formative and summative assessment is very difficult, some would say almost impossible to achieve." Bok proceeds to describe how formative assessment was perceived as high stakes when data were also collected for grading (Bok et al., 2013). If there is confusion about an assessment purpose, then the default position does not favor learning. Learners should be oriented to the process and objectives of any WBA mechanism and how this process fits within an overall assessment program. Learners should be told what will be assessed, with what instruments, and under what conditions, such as observations with the medical team or with patients.

If WBA represents a cornerstone of an overall assessment program, then assessments must be done regularly and with purpose. This requires appropriate assessment tools, qualified raters, learners open to learning, and a conducive environment. We address these in order.

Assessment Tools

Published WBA tools range from checklists to anchored and global performance ratings, narrative feedback, and portfolio contributions. The assessment choice is sometimes informed by the skills or behavior that can be easily captured and the tools that are easiest to use. Crossley describes this as "measuring what is measurable rather than what is important" (Crossley & Jolly,

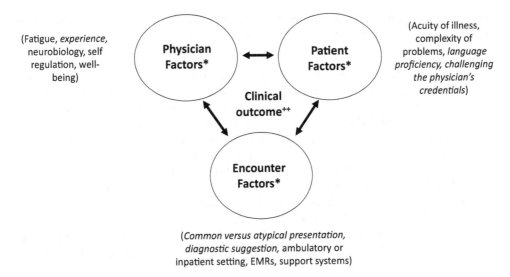

(Fatigue, *experience*, neurobiology, self regulation, well-being)

Physician Factors*

⟷

Patient Factors*

(Acuity of illness, complexity of problems, *language proficiency, challenging the physician's credentials*)

Clinical outcome++

Encounter Factors*

(*Common versus atypical presentation, diagnostic suggestion*, ambulatory or inpatient setting, EMRs, support systems)

Figure 10.5 Situated cognition and the context of the clinical encounter[+,^]

[+]Examples of each factor (physician, patient, and encounter) are shown next to each factor in parentheses (also known as factor elements). The factor elements that were specifically explored in this study are shown in italics. [^]Context refers to the three factors (patient, physician, and setting) and their interactions shown in this figure. *Factors that interact as shown by arrows; parentheses next to each factor are examples (factor elements). [++]Clinical outcome is dependent upon these three factors, their interactions, and possibly other inputs. Situated cognition takes the approach of the individual and the environment and all of the above interactions can and do influence the outcome (patient care) in such a model.

Source: Durning, S.J., Artino, A.R., Boulet, J.R., Dorrance, K., van der Vleuten, C., & Schuwirth, L. (2012). The Impact of Selected Contextual Factors on Experts' Clinical Reasoning Performance (Does Context Impact Clinical Reasoning Performance in Experts?). Advances in Health Sciences Education: Theory and Practice, 17, 65. Reprinted by permission from Springer Nature.

2012). Crossley summarizes this thought process succinctly: "[Assessment] works better if the right questions are asked, in the right way, about the right things, of the right people."

There is no shortage of published WBA tools. The Swanwick categorization of WBA tools is a useful structure (Swanwick & Chana, 2009).

1. *Analysis of performance data*: These data can be clinical outcomes (e.g., procedural success rates), process metrics (e.g., time to a specific intervention), and patient volume data (case logs, case data from an electronic health record). The original use of this data source was to provide learner feedback. One can also consider this data level as a means to provide evidence of value to patients in terms of safety and quality. Performance data can and has also been used to provide feedback and to investigate program outcomes. In two published works, patient outcome data were used to evaluate training programs. Smirnova et al. (2019) demonstrated a counterintuitive association within an obstetrical training program. Programs viewed by residents as having a better learning culture had *higher* perinatal complication rates. In another study, obstetricians' perinatal complication rates were linked to where they trained (Asch, Nicholson, Srinivas, Herrin, & Epstein, 2009). Smirnova and colleagues argue that clinical data use should target individual, training program, system, and GME collective levels with the goal of better aligning educational assessment and patient care outcomes (Smirnova et al., 2019).

2. *Observation of clinical activities*: Examples of the observation instruments discussed below can be found in Norcini and Burch (2007). This list is intended to be representative, not exhaustive.

   a. Mini-CEX (clinical evaluation exercise)—A learner is observed and assessed by a rater during direct patient care. The expectation is that each learner will be assessed by multiple raters across multiple cases (Norcini, 2003). Published work provides validity evidence for the mini-CEX (Durning, Cation, Markert, & Pangaro, 2002; Holmboe, Yepes, Williams, & Huot, 2004; Kogan, Bellini, & Shea, 2003). A 2013 meta-analysis demonstrated "small-to-large" effect sizes between trainee achievement and performance across 11 mini-CEX studies (Al Ansari, Ali, & Donnon, 2013). Much of this evidence is from internal medicine programs. Humphrey-Murto, Côté, Pugh, and Wood (2018) report validity evidence for a multidisciplinary mini-CEX that demonstrated a correlation between the mini-CEX and an OSCE but not with a written test.
   b. A MiniCard assessment tool has been shown to have validity evidence supporting its use for medical students in a single study (Donato, Park, George, Schwartz, & Yudkowsky, 2015).
   c. Direct observation of procedural skills (DOPS) is a variation on the mini-CEX. There is evidence supporting DOPS in surgical trainee assessment (Goff et al., 2002; Larson, Williams, Ketchum, Boehler, & Dunnington, 2005). System for Improving and Measuring Procedural Learning (SIMPL), a surgical WBA tool consistent with the DOPS model, uses smartphone-based data collection (Bohnen et al., 2016). Objective Structured Assessment of Technical Skills (OSATS) (Martin et al., 1997) and Non-Technical Skills (NOTECHS) (Flin, 2004) are additional examples of direct observational assessment of clinical skills. Both have been modified for a variety of uses.

3. *Discussion via cases*: Cased-based discussion (CbD), or chart-stimulated recall, is a focused discussion driven by an existing case the learner has addressed. The learning discussion is focused on what the learner did in the clinical case.

4. *Multi-source feedback*:

   a. The Mini-Peer Assessment Tool (Mini-PAT) is an anonymous feedback process from peer learners (Abdulla, 2008).
   b. Portfolios—Collection of learner-specific assessment from multiple sources (self, peer, supervisor) via different modalities and over time. There is evidence favoring portfolio use in the US (O'Brien, Sanguino, Thomas, & Green, 2016), Scotland (Davis et al., 2001), The Netherlands (Driessen, van Tartwijk, Vermunt, & van der Vleuten, 2003), Australia (O'Sullivan et al., 2012) and Canada (Hall, Byszewski, Sutherland, & Stodel, 2012). Portfolios draw upon a variety of evaluative sources to provide a broad, longitudinal picture of learner performance. Chapter 12 addresses portfolios in more detail.

Kogan and Holmboe (2013) note the abundance of existing assessment tools and state there is little need to create new assessments. They argue instead for a change in focus toward providing better training and preparing raters to provide feedback using existing tools (Kogan & Holmboe, 2013).

The Rater and Learner Dyad

Well-trained faculty raters interact with learners to create education opportunities that target identified gaps toward the goal of longitudinal improvement. The success of this endeavor is affected by each member of the dyad and their relationship. Factors to consider include:

- Learner-Centeredness—Learners come with expectations about the gaps they wish to address, from whom they wish to learn, in what place, and under what clinical conditions. The assessment expectation should be learner focused while following a sampling plan.
- Credibility of Assessors—Learners will accept feedback from raters they find credible. Credible feedback comes from a trusted source who *observed the behavior directly* and provides actionable recommendations for change. Criticism of intrinsic traits not amenable to change results in poor feedback reception (Watling & Ginsburg, 2019). Veloski, Boex, Grasberger, Evans, and Wolfson (2006) found, in a systematic review, that authoritative, longitudinal, clinical feedback was superior to shorter efforts.

  Feedback must be based on observed behavior to be credible. The end-of-rotation assessment, not surprisingly, is vulnerable to recall bias (Govaerts, 2015). Published evidence suggests that such tasks as taking patient histories and performing physical examinations are not often observed (Holmboe et al., 2004). Newer data from the Association of American Medical College's Annual Survey of students has shown a steady increase in student-reported clinical observation providing evidence of a gradual change. When asked, more than 80% of students said they were observed obtaining a history and performing a physical exam. Students on surgical clerkships reported history observation more than 70% of the time.

  Credibility also arises from the clinical competence of the assessor. There is evidence that graduates (and now assessors) may have gaps in their own skills and knowledge. Some deficiencies may be training-related and carried forward to practice and others are skill-related that fall into systems and professional competencies for which they may not have been trained (Holmboe et al., 2011).
- Clinicians today are under increasing time demands, have more documentation work, and have less time for learner observation. The success of any evaluative method relies on investing time and human resources. Evaluators need to be trained in assessment methods, including assessment tools. Continuity of learner-faculty dyads can only occur if sufficient time is permitted for its development.
- Learners and raters must have common expectations about the assessment purpose and the operative criteria and objectives. Learners and raters need a consensual understanding of the assessment purpose. Is the effort intended to provide learner feedback or are data also collected for summative purposes? Bok reported that students found it hard to separate formative from summative assessment (Bok et al., 2013). If assessment is viewed as summative, learner behavior may change to avoid observation except for "easier" cases or picking less judgmental assessors (Roberts, 2013). Haas and Shaffir (1982) refer to this as "impression management." McGaghie notes that in an effort to "look good," learners focus on how they are perceived. They seek to appear confident in all settings and avoid asking for help and thus avoid scrutiny (McGaghie, 2018). Patel investigated how surgical residents are focused on how they appear to supervisors (Patel et al., 2018). One trainee notes the motive for impression management as, "I know for a fact, in this program, if they brand you an idiot . . . you're done" (Patel et al., 2018).
- WBA requires trained, motivated, and available assessors. Years of experience, faculty rank, or clinical acumen do not automatically make an individual a "good" assessor (Herbers et al., 1989; Noel et al., 1992). Raters must be developed, and their skills maintained, if one hopes to acquire assessment data that are reliable. The aim is to reduce potential sources of bias so that WBA programs produce reliable data that lead to valid decisions and useful feedback.
- Rater background is a distinct factor in the data they provide. Physician raters vary, with increasing stringency as careers advance.

Holmboe et al. (2011) provide five key methods to improve faculty and program assessments:

1. Conduct frame-of-reference training—training raters in the area of performance standards typically with examples of different levels of performance, again, for example, through video-recorded vignettes. This training should be extended to program leadership.
2. Provide direct feedback to raters—in regard to their scoring range as it relates to other assessors. Programs should use these data to provide feedback to assessors.
3. Training in use of tools—both specific to a tool and general psychometric principles.
4. Common resources—national web-based resources to provide education and resources to local institutions.
5. Learner-centered—active involvement of learners in their assessments and taking on the task of self-directed improvement.

However, raters and the rating data produced via observation can never be fully free of bias. Tonesk and Buchanan (1987) interviewed clinical faculty members and clerkship coordinators, finding that many faculty members admitted to being unwilling to record negative evaluations. Yepes-Rio et al. (2016) reviewed the literature regarding what enabled and what served as a barrier to failing a trainee. They found barriers to be an assessor's professional considerations (taking more time and work to fail someone), the assessor's personal considerations (sense of failure of themselves), trainee-related considerations (impact on trainee's goals), and unsatisfactory evaluator development and evaluation tools (doubting their own judgement). Factors that enabled a negative or failing evaluation included the sense of duty to patients, society, and the profession; institutional support (e.g., backing a failing evaluation); support from colleagues; evaluator development; strong assessment systems; and opportunities for students after failing.

Environment

Specific considerations apply when using observation in a clinical context as a means of giving feedback for learning. Clinical settings allow for direct assessment of learners performing work tasks in an authentic environment. Distractions and competing care demands create a real-world milieu and interfere with assessment opportunities. However, time is the most common and pervasive barrier to WBA. Patient, assessor, and learner availabilities vary and often do not align.

ASSESSMENT ADMINISTRATION

Within the context of workplace assessment, we seek to balance consistency and fairness while recognizing the constraints the environment creates. Key features of high-quality implementation are consistency regarding how learners are rated, what instruments are used, what domains are evaluated, and how raters are trained. The more these conditions vary from standard conditions, the less meaningful the assessment will become. This requires effort that begins in the design phase and carries through when scheduling is done and assessment venues are set.

Data quality assurance requires equal attention. Data collection plans, whether on paper or using electronic media, must be tested rigorously. A simple text error may result in data loss that would not happen if pilot testing had been done. Pilot testing is also needed if data collection is designed to provide immediate feedback. How do learners feel about the assessment process and data display? Do the raters find the assessment process effective and consistent with formative feedback practice?

MAKING SENSE OF ASSESSMENT DATA

The end product of a WBA program is a pool of data that requires interpretation. There are two perspectives about how these data should be collected, used, and understood and what the primary purpose of WBA is.

Psychometric

In this view, we use mostly numeric score-based data as the primary basis for decisions. This viewpoint argues, as stated earlier, that there is a true, objective standard and the numeric data are a proximal measure of this construct. There is also an assumption that the constructs measured are stable over time and can be viewed independent from context (Govaerts & van der Vleuten, 2013). This assumption is needed if we are to "lump" data from various sources into a composite.

This view assumes that educators need evidence that assessment data are reliable and allow valid, accurate decisions about learners. Without such evidence, decision accuracy can and should be questioned. The meaning of data, in aggregate, depends on a number of factors:

- For the whole body of data, is there evidence that the assessment methods used have been employed successfully before in similar settings and for similar learners?
- Are there data about how instruments were used? What quality control measures were used to ensure that assessments were implemented as intended and data were captured consistently?
- What rater training efforts were implemented? Did the raters actually attend? If training was passive (e.g., web-based), is there evidence training was completed?
- How well do raters agree about scoring? Were there efforts to calibrate raters over time?
- Do the collected data measure the intended target construct?

Socio-Cultural

Social-culture theories assert that "learning outcomes emerge through active participation in activities of community and interaction with the complex and dynamic systems of the work environment" (Govaerts & van der Vleuten, 2013). In this framework, the view of WBA moves away from a score-driven approach towards understanding learners' progression. The departure from a psychometric view is stark. WBA data are considered to focus predominantly on process measures, which Crossley and Jolly (2012) argue are less discriminating than global assessments. We are less interested in process than performance. Raters are more consistent and can discriminate better for performance than process (Crossley & Jolly, 2012).

This viewpoint argues for narrative feedback over numeric scores (Govaerts & van der Vleuten, 2013; Hanson, Rosenberg, & Lane, 2013). Numbers (scores), it is argued, have no intrinsic meaning, whereas narratives provide a source of actionable feedback (Govaerts & van der Vleuten, 2013). "Performance can never be 'objective' but is always conceptualized and constructed according to the perspectives and values of an individual assessor, influenced by his or her unique experiences and social structures in the assessment task and its context" (Gipps, 1999; Govaerts & van der Vleuten, 2013).

Learner performance is not fixed or stable. Change over time is expected as an outcome of learning. However, there is also large intra-person variability between different performance domains (e.g., better at this task than another) and between occasions (e.g., better on same task on one day versus another).

A socio-cultural view calls into question the nature of assessment and assessment data. The purposeful sampling that we described earlier does not include all learning opportunities.

Purposeful sampling cannot cover "learning things 'that aren't there yet'" (Govaerts & van der Vleuten, 2013).

In the psychometric model, raters are a source of measurement *error* (Downing, 2005). In a socio-cultural approach, the same score variation across raters that one seeks to control in a psychometric approach is now viewed as having meaning. This variation is not "*error*" but a legitimate difference in rater's conceptions about what is acceptable performance (Govaerts & van der Vleuten, 2013).

Underlying this conception of WBA is a marked shift towards assessment *for* learning. Assessment should be a catalyst for learning as the endpoint. Assessment for learning is discussed in detail in Chapter 17 (Assessment Affecting Learning).

SUMMARY AND LOOK AHEAD

We provided one definition of WBA earlier in this chapter and provide a different version in closing. A 2010 systematic review of the previous literature provided this synthesis:

> Competency-based education (CBE) is an approach to preparing physicians for practice that is fundamentally oriented to graduate outcome abilities and organized around competencies derived from an analysis of societal and patient needs. It de-emphasizes time-based training and promises greater accountability, flexibility, and learner-centredness.
>
> (Frank et al., 2010)

This statement summarizes the contrast between our starting point and our closing thoughts. In one view, WBA is primarily a data-driven, psychometrically informed assessment-of-learning model. In the other view, it is a social experience that takes into account learner, assessor, and a broad concept of how WBA is situated within a learning culture. One view treats characteristics of the rater and learner as fixed over time and across context while the other questions such assumptions. Both concepts, in truth, are now in practice. Both models require sustained effort for implementation and maintenance, and both require strong rater support and institutional resources. WBA is firmly situated within a broader discussion about learning, developmental milestones, and how CBME impacts patients and society.

Note: Additional material and resources may be available at the UIC AHPE website: https://go.uic.edu/AHPE

REFERENCES

Abdulla, A. (2008). A critical analysis of mini peer assessment tool (mini-PAT). *Journal of the Royal Society of Medicine, 101,* 22–26.

Al Ansari, A., Ali, S.K., & Donnon, T. (2013). The construct and criterion validity of the mini-CEX: a meta-analysis of the published research. *Academic Medicine, 88,* 413–420.

Asch, D.A., Nicholson, S., Srinivas, S., Herrin, J., & Epstein, A.J. (2009). Evaluating obstetrical residency programs using patient outcomes. *The Journal of the American Medical Association, 302,* 1277–1283.

Bohnen, J.D., George, B.C., Williams, R.G., Schuller, M.C., DaRosa, D.A., Torbeck, L., . . . Procedural Learning and Safety Collaborative (PLSC). (2016). The feasibility of real-time intraoperative performance assessment with SIMPL (System for Improving and Measuring Procedural Learning): Early experience from a multi-institutional trial. *Journal of Surgical Education, 73,* e118–e130.

Bok, H.G.J., Teunissen, P.W., Favier, R.P., Rietbroek, N.J., Theyse, L.F.H., Brommer, H., . . . Jaarsma, D.A.D.C. (2013). Programmatic assessment of competency-based workplace learning: When theory meets practice. *BMC Medical Education, 13,* 123.

Coderre, S., Woloschuk, W., & McLaughlin, K. (2009). Twelve tips for blueprinting. *Medical Teacher, 31,* 322–324.

Crossley, J., & Jolly, B. (2012). Making sense of work-based assessment: Ask the right questions, in the right way, about the right things, of the right people. *Medical Education, 46,* 28–37.

Davis, M.H., Friedman Ben-David, M., Harden, R.M., Howie, P., Ker, J., McGhee, C., . . . Snadden, D. (2001). Portfolio assessment in medical students' final examinations. *Medical Teacher, 23,* 357–366.

Donato, A.A., Park, Y.S., George, D.L., Schwartz, A., & Yudkowsky, R. (2015). Validity and feasibility of the minicard direct observation tool in 1 training program. *The Journal of Graduate Medical Education, 7,* 225–229.

Downing, S.M. (2005). Threats to the validity of clinical teaching assessments: What about rater error? *Medical Education, 39,* 353–355.

Driessen, E., van Tartwijk, J., Vermunt, J.D., & van der Vleuten, C.P.M. (2003). Use of portfolios in early undergraduate medical training. *Medical Teacher, 25,* 18–23.

Durning, S.J., Artino, A.R., Boulet, J.R., Dorrance, K., van der Vleuten, C., & Schuwirth, L. (2012). The impact of selected contextual factors on experts' clinical reasoning performance (does context impact clinical reasoning performance in experts?). *Advances in Health Sciences Education : Theory and Practice, 17,* 65–79.

Durning, S.J., Cation, L.J., Markert, R.J., & Pangaro, L.N. (2002). Assessing the reliability and validity of the mini-clinical evaluation exercise for internal medicine residency training. *Academic Medicine, 77,* 900–904.

Ericsson, K.A. (2004). Deliberate practice and the acquisition and maintenance of expert performance in medicine and related domains. *Academic Medicine : Journal of the Association of American Medical Colleges, 79,* S70–81.

Ericsson, K.A. (2015). Acquisition and maintenance of medical expertise: A perspective from the expert-performance approach with deliberate practice. *Academic Medicine, 90,* 1471–1486.

Flin, R. (2004). Identifying and training non-technical skills for teams in acute medicine. *Quality and Safety in Health Care, 13,* i80–i84.

Frank, J.R., Mungroo, R., Ahmad, Y., Wang, M., De Rossi, S., & Horsley, T. (2010). Toward a definition of competency-based education in medicine: A systematic review of published definitions. *Medical Teacher, 32,* 631–637.

Gipps, C. (1999). Socio-cultural aspects of assessment. *Review of Research in Education, 24,* 355.

Goff, B.A., Nielsen, P.E., Lentz, G.M., Chow, G.E., Chalmers, R.W., Fenner, D., & Mandel, L.S. (2002). Surgical skills assessment: A blinded examination of obstetrics and gynecology residents. *American Journal of Obstetrics and Gynecology, 186,* 613–617.

Gofton, W., Dudek, N., Barton, G., & Bhanji, F. (2017). *Workplace-based assessment implementation guide: Formative tips for medical teaching practice* (1st ed.). Ottawa, ON: The Royal College of Physicians and Surgeons of Canada. Retrieved from www.royalcollege.ca/rcsite/documents/cbd/wba-implementation-guide-tips-medical-teaching-practice-e.pdf.

Gofton, W.T., Dudek, N.L., Wood, T.J., Balaa, F., & Hamstra, S.J. (2012). The Ottawa surgical Competency Operating Room Evaluation (O-SCORE): A tool to assess surgical competence. *Academic Medicine, 87,* 1401–1407.

Govaerts, M. (2015). Workplace-based assessment and assessment for learning: Threats to validity. *The Journal of Graduate Medical Education, 7,* 265–267.

Govaerts, M., & van der Vleuten, C.P.M. (2013). Validity in work-based assessment: Expanding our horizons. *Medical Education, 47,* 1164–1174.

Haas, J., & Shaffir, W. (1982). Ritual evaluation of competence: The hidden curriculum of professionalization in an innovative medical school program. *Work and Occupations, 9,* 131–154.

Hall, P., Byszewski, A., Sutherland, S., & Stodel, E.J. (2012). Developing a sustainable electronic portfolio (ePortfolio) program that fosters reflective practice and incorporates CanMEDS competencies into the undergraduate medical curriculum. *Academic Medicine, 87,* 744–751.

Hanson, J.L., Rosenberg, A.A., & Lane, J.L. (2013). Narrative descriptions should replace grades and numerical ratings for clinical performance in medical education in the United States. *Frontiers in Psychology, 4,* 668.

Herbers, J.E., Noel, G.L., Cooper, G.S., Harvey, J., Pangaro, L.N., & Weaver, M.J. (1989). How accurate are faculty evaluations of clinical competence? *Journal of General Internal Medicine, 4,* 202–208.

Holmboe, E.S. (2015). Realizing the promise of competency-based medical education. *Academic Medicine, 90,* 411–413.

Holmboe, E.S., Ward, D.S., Reznick, R.K., Katsufrakis, P.J., Leslie, K.M., Patel, V.L., . . . Nelson, E.A. (2011). Faculty development in assessment: The missing link in competency-based medical education. *Academic Medicine, 86,* 460–467.

Holmboe, E.S., Yepes, M., Williams, F., & Huot, S.J. (2004). Feedback and the mini clinical evaluation exercise. *Journal of General Internal Medicine, 19,* 558–561.

Humphrey-Murto, S., Côté, M., Pugh, D., & Wood, T.J. (2018). Assessing the validity of a multidisciplinary mini-clinical evaluation exercise. *Teaching and Learning in Medicine, 30,* 152–161.

Kogan, J.R., Bellini, L.M., & Shea, J.A. (2003). Feasibility, reliability, and validity of the mini-clinical evaluation exercise (mCEX) in a medicine core clerkship. *Academic Medicine, 78,* S33–S335.

Kogan, J.R., & Holmboe, E. (2013). Realizing the promise and importance of performance-based assessment. *Teaching and Learning in Medicine, 25*(Suppl 1), S68–74.

Kogan, J.R., Holmboe, E.S., & Hauer, K.E. (2009). Tools for direct observation and assessment of clinical skills of medical trainees: A systematic review. *The Journal of the American Medical Association, 302*, 1316–1326.

Larson, J.L., Williams, R.G., Ketchum, J., Boehler, M.L., & Dunnington, G.L. (2005). Feasibility, reliability and validity of an operative performance rating system for evaluating surgery residents. *Surgery, 138*, 640–647; discussion 647.

Martin, J.A., Regehr, G., Reznick, R., MacRae, H., Murnaghan, J., Hutchison, C., & Brown, M. (1997). Objective structured assessment of technical skill (OSATS) for surgical residents. *The British Journal of Surgery, 84*, 273–278.

McGaghie, William C. (2018). Evaluation apprehension and impression management in clinical medical education. *Academic Medicine, 93*, 685–686.

McGaghie, W.C., Miller, G.E., Sajid, A.W., & Telder, T.V. (1978). Competency-based curriculum development on medical education: an introduction. *Public Health Papers*, 11–91.

Miller, G.E. (1990). The assessment of clinical skills/competence/performance. *Academic Medicine: Journal of the Association of American Medical Colleges, 65*, S63–S67.

Noel, G.L., Herbers, J.E., Caplow, M.P., Cooper, G.S., Pangaro, L.N., & Harvey, J. (1992). How well do internal medicine faculty members evaluate the clinical skills of residents? *Annals of Internal Medicine, 117*, 757–765.

Norcini, J., & Burch, V. (2007). Workplace-based assessment as an educational tool: AMEE Guide No. 31. *Medical Teacher, 29*, 855–871.

Norcini, J.J. (2003). Work based assessment. *British Medical Journal (Clinical Research Ed.), 326*, 753–755.

O'Brien, C.L., Sanguino, S.M., Thomas, J.X., & Green, M.M. (2016). Feasibility and outcomes of implementing a portfolio assessment system alongside a traditional grading system. *Academic Medicine, 91*, 1554–1560.

O'Sullivan, A.J., Harris, P., Hughes, C.S., Toohey, S.M., Balasooriya, C., Velan, G., . . . McNeil, H.P. (2012). Linking assessment to undergraduate student capabilities through portfolio examination. *Assessment & Evaluation in Higher Education, 37*, 379–391.

Patel, P., Martimianakis, M.A., Zilbert, N.R., Mui, C., Hammond Mobilio, M., Kitto, S., & Moulton, C.-A. (2018). Fake it 'til you make it: pressures to measure up in surgical training. *Academic Medicine, 93*, 769–774.

Roberts, T.E. (2013). Assessment est mort, vive assessment. *Medical Teacher, 35*, 535–536.

Schuwirth, L.W.T., & van der Vleuten, C.P.M. (2006). A plea for new psychometric models in educational assessment. *Medical Education, 40*, 296–300.

Singh, T., & Norcini, J.J. (2013). Workplace-based assessment. In William C. McGaghie (Ed.), *International best practices for evaluation in the health professions* (pp. 257–279). London: Radcliffe Publishing.

Smirnova, A., Sebok-Syer, S.S., Chahine, S., Kalet, A.L., Tamblyn, R., Lombarts, K.M.J.M.H., . . . Schumacher, D.J. (2019). Defining and adopting clinical performance measures in graduate medical education: Where are we now and where are we going? *Academic Medicine, 94*, 671–677.

Swanwick, T., & Chana, N. (2009). Workplace-based assessment. *British Journal of Hospital Medicine, 70*, 290–293.

ten Cate, O. (2014). AM last page: What entrustable professional activities add to a competency-based curriculum. *Academic Medicine, 89*, 691.

ten Cate, O., & Scheele, F. (2007). Competency-based postgraduate training: Can we bridge the gap between theory and clinical practice? *Academic Medicine, 82*, 542–547.

Tonesk, X., & Buchanan, R.G. (1987). An AAMC pilot study by 10 medical schools of clinical evaluation of students. *Journal of Medical Education, 62*, 707–718.

van der Vleuten, C.P.M. (2016). Revisiting "Assessing professional competence: From methods to programmes." *Medical Education, 50*, 885–888.

van der Vleuten, C.P.M., & Schuwirth, L.W.T. (2005). Assessing professional competence: From methods to programmes. *Medical Education, 39*, 309–317.

Veloski, J., Boex, J.R., Grasberger, M.J., Evans, A., & Wolfson, D.B. (2006). Systematic review of the literature on assessment, feedback and physicians' clinical performance: BEME guide no. 7. *Medical Teacher, 28*, 117–128.

Watling, C.J., & Ginsburg, S. (2019). Assessment, feedback and the alchemy of learning. *Medical Education, 53*, 76–85.

Yepes-Rios, M., Dudek, N., Duboyce, R., Curtis, J., Allard, R.J., & Varpio, L. (2016). The failure to fail underperforming trainees in health professions education: A BEME systematic review: BEME Guide No. 42. *Medical Teacher, 38*, 1092–1099.

11

NARRATIVE ASSESSMENT

Nancy Dudek and David Cook

Educators and education researchers increasingly recognize that many aspects of trainee performance cannot be readily measured with numbers. For example, a numeric score might not explain the reasons for a trainee's low (or high) performance, or the predetermined items on a numeric scorecard might fail to capture important elements of overall performance. As such, there is growing recognition that performance can and often should be documented in the form of words in addition to—or sometimes instead of—only numbers (Hanson, Rosenberg, & Lane, 2013; Hodges, 2013; Holmboe, Sherbino, Long, Swing, & Frank, 2010; McConnell, Harms, & Saperson, 2016). Such narrative assessments can provide trainees with specific feedback to assist in their learning, fill in the gaps of a quantitative scale, and give competence committees the "why" information needed to make informed decisions about trainee achievement. As a result, narrative assessment is gaining popularity within the field of clinical performance assessment.

NARRATIVE ASSESSMENT INSTRUMENTS

Narrative assessment instruments come in a variety of forms and under many names. For example, some field notes and daily encounter cards are entirely narrative (i.e., they have no numeric or checklist ratings); these would be considered narrative reports. Other instruments, such as the typical in-training evaluation report (ITER) or end-of-rotation assessment, combine a numeric rating scale with narrative free-text comments. Learning portfolios typically contain a mix of narrative artifacts from trainees (e.g., essays, research reports, and clinical write-ups) and supervisors (e.g., the narrative portion of various assessment tools) and numeric items (e.g., test scores, supervisor ratings). For the purposes of this chapter, we will focus only on the narrative components of such mixed-methods sources. Although most narrative assessments are composed of words written by other people, sometimes the assessment involves words written by the trainees themselves, as when personal essays (e.g., reflecting upon a training experience) are used to make judgments about trainee achievements and level of performance.

Narrative assessment instruments may simply be a box labeled "Comments" or may have one or more prompts requesting specific information on, for example, positive aspects of the clinical performance, areas of deficiency, and specific recommendations for improvement.

STRENGTHS

There are several strengths of narrative assessment that are specific to the qualitative aspects of the assessment. A well-done narrative assessment provides rich descriptions of the performance. In doing so, it facilitates trainee learning (i.e., the formative aspect of clinical performance assessment) (Govaerts & van der Vleuten, 2013; McConnell et al., 2016). This is a necessary component of "assessment for learning," which is a cornerstone of competency-based education. It provides trainees with information regarding what they need to do to improve and work towards competent, independent practice. In addition to providing trainees with descriptions of their current performance, narrative assessment typically asks the observer to make recommendations for how the trainee can attain a higher level of performance (i.e., formative feedback). These directions provide much needed information to trainees about how to improve.

Narrative assessments provide more flexibility for the observer to decide on what aspects of performance to comment on. This can make these assessments more individualized and flexible. They also offer the opportunity to provide more detail to explain a complex situation. Providing this type of information about context affords a greater understanding of the decisions that may be made about a trainee's performance.

Although narrative assessments are commonly characterized as being more subjective than numeric assessments, evidence suggests that narrative assessments can support defensible (i.e., valid) decisions. Narrative assessments have been demonstrated to provide robust information about trainee performance (Bartels, Mooney, & Stone, 2017; Driessen, van der Vleuten, Schuwirth, van Tartwijk, & Vermunt, 2005; Ginsburg, van der Vleuten, & Eva, 2017). Narrative data can successfully identify students in difficulty, rank trainees, and predict trainee success versus failure (Cohen, Blumberg, Ryan, & Sullivan, 1993; Ginsburg, Eva, & Regehr, 2013; Guerrasio et al., 2012).

PRAGMATIC ISSUES IN USING NARRATIVE ASSESSMENT

In the next few sections, we outline several issues that must be addressed when using narrative assessments.

1. Define the Purpose of Narrative Assessment

The ultimate purpose of any assessment is to inform meaningful decisions about the person being assessed. Such decisions might be dichotomous (such as pass/fail or select/not select), granular (class rankings or grades), or qualitative (specific feedback). Narrative assessment can fulfill any or all of these purposes.

Some specific applications of narrative assessment include assessment of trainee portfolios, small group performance assessment, and workplace-based assessments. The latter may involve the direct observation of a performance in real time (e.g., watching a trainee perform a physical exam or procedural task) or appraisal of a piece of work that has been produced at an alternate time (e.g., a consult note or a suture placed in skin). Narrative assessments typically are used to support other quantitative assessments and for formative feedback. However, they may be used collectively to support a summative assessment of trainee performance (e.g., to provide supporting evidence to a competence committee) (Dudek et al., 2012; Hanson et al., 2013; Govaerts & van der Vleuten, 2013).

2. Document the Performance

High-quality assessments—and ultimately high-quality decisions—are grounded in high-quality raw data. For numeric assessment, the raw data are scores. For narrative assessment, the raw data are the narratives (e.g., written comments and other documents) that describe the trainee's performance. High-quality ("rich") narratives provide clear and detailed descriptions of strengths and weaknesses and specific recommendations for how the trainee could improve (Dudek, Marks, Lee, & Wood, 2008). Comments are further supported by specific examples of performance that illustrate the trainee's strengths and weaknesses. Descriptions and examples should contain sufficient detail that an independent analyst (e.g., competence committee member) can understand the performance without needing to contact the observer for clarification. Observers need to write their comments using a tone that is supportive of trainee learning by avoiding commenting on attitudinal issues without supporting those concerns with specific descriptions of the behavior in question. For example, rather than stating that a resident is "lazy" or that "he doesn't seem to care about surgery" (which represent high-level inferences), it is more useful to write descriptions of the observed behaviors that led to the inference, such as "the trainee was frequently late and did not complete assigned tasks." Finally, it is helpful to document the trainee's response to verbal feedback provided by the observer, as this can offer insight about this trainee's future learning needs (Dudek et al., 2008; Dudek & Dojeiji, 2014).

When narrative assessment is used in combination with numeric assessment, the narrative assessment should justify the assigned ratings. In other words, if the ratings suggest an excellent performance, then the comments should describe that in more detail. A mismatch between the numeric ratings and the narrative comments leads to confusion for trainees and those in charge of their learning plan (Dudek et al., 2008; Dudek & Dojeiji, 2014).

3. Train the Observers

Narrative assessment, like other forms of work-based assessment, ideally requires that the supervisor observe the trainee. This takes time on the part of the supervisor who often also has responsibilities for patient care. Excellent guidelines for directly observing trainees have been published (Kogan, Hatala, Hauer, & Holmboe, 2017). These guidelines should be used to train faculty on how to participate in direct observation.

Narrative assessments require rich, detailed descriptions in order to realize the potential strengths noted above, yet studies have shown that faculty comments on narrative reports are most often minimal and not specific (Dudek et al., 2012; Dudek, Marks, Bandiera, White, & Wood, 2013; Littlefield et al., 2005). When faced with poorly performing trainees, supervisors indicate that they often give a passing grade because they do not know what to write to support a failing grade (Dudek, Marks, & Regehr, 2005). Medical educators involved in trainee assessment are all too familiar with the common yet unhelpful comments of "good team player" and "needs to read more." Thus, there is a significant need for faculty development strategies aimed at encouraging observers to write more comments and higher quality comments (detailed, specific, behavioral) for their narrative assessments. There has been success with some such initiatives, but more work is required (Dudek et al., 2012; Dudek et al., 2013; Littlefield et al., 2005).

4. Manage the Collected Data

When done well, narrative assessment generates a lot of data. Using these data (e.g., for analysis, synthesis, and provision of feedback to trainees) requires a robust system for data storage, search, retrieval, and reporting. Paper archives can suffice, but educators are increasingly turning to electronic data systems that provide greater flexibility. Helpful features include the capacity to customize data collection forms for different trainees and rotations; remind people to submit incomplete forms; archive submitted data; search and retrieve data; contrast data across different completed forms (e.g., collate assessments across different supervisors or different rotations); annotate data (e.g., with comments from the competence committee); create synthesized reports and summaries; and provide feedback to trainees (e.g., both original and synthesized reports).

5. Combine Narratives Across Observers (Qualitative Synthesis)

Analyzing and pooling assessments from multiple observers is more difficult with narrative (qualitative) data than it is with numeric (quantitative) data. For the latter, psychometric approaches can be applied to large data sets, for example, to identify the average or median response and to estimate the reliability of scores. By contrast, narrative assessments require the use of qualitative research approaches such as thematic analysis to synthesize data across multiple observations and observers. While qualitative synthesis can require more time and a distinct skill set compared with quantitative synthesis, when done properly the results can be just as defensible—and insightful.

Combining narratives requires the analyst to look for common themes expressed by different observers in different contexts. For example, if communication skills are noted to be effective by multiple observers and in the context of both simple and challenging patient encounters, then this would support the theme of "effective communication skills." The analyst should also look for data that do not support these themes (i.e., contrasting perspectives). The quality (detail and specificity) and context of the data should be expressly considered during this synthesis, especially when data disagree (e.g., one detailed example of poor performance might have greater impact than several generic statements about "great team player").

The determination of themes should be reviewed by more than one person to ensure a consistent interpretation of the raw data. After individual consideration of the data, any differences in opinion regarding the themes should be resolved with group discussion. This is particularly important when narrative assessment is used to support higher-stakes decisions.

6. Provide Feedback to Trainees

Finally, consideration must be given to how the narrative assessment data will be provided to the trainee. When used for formative feedback, it may be useful to allow trainees to clarify their understanding of the information and then reflect upon how it can be incorporated into their future performance; this might be done in a one-on-one meeting with an advisor, via a confidential email, or through an interactive learning portfolio system. Trainees also may need guidance on how to interpret and use synthesized narrative data when used for summative purposes. Most trainees have an understanding of how numeric data are used to support a summative pass/fail decision (e.g., a pass threshold was set prior to the exam), but many are less familiar with how synthesized narrative data can be used to support a pass/fail decision (e.g., the deliberations of a competence committee). This could be particularly problematic when numeric and narrative data suggest different decisions, as when worrisome narrative comments accompany satisfactory numeric ratings. Providing trainees with access to both raw narratives and synthesized data, and explicitly explaining how numeric and narrative data are used in conjunction to make decisions, can be helpful.

EVALUATING THE VALIDITY OF NARRATIVE ASSESSMENT

Before we rely on any assessment (numeric or narrative) to make a decision, we must first establish that the proposed decision will be defensible. Such determinations are typically described in terms of validity, which is defined as "the degree to which evidence and theory support the interpretations of test scores for proposed uses of tests" (AERA, APA, & NCME, 2014). Although most often applied to numeric scores, this definition aptly applies to narrative assessment. One of us recently described how to apply contemporary models of assessment validation to narrative assessments (Cook, Kuper, Hatala, & Ginsburg, 2016). We will briefly review this approach below and refer readers to the more complete exposition for additional details.

Validation is a process in which evidence is collected to test (support or refute) the defensibility of the assessment interpretations, or more appropriately the decisions that are based on those interpretations. Such interpretations (and decisions) are grounded in raw scores or observations. People often speak casually of the validity or validation of instruments, but it is more accurate to speak of the validity or validation of scores, observations, interpretations, and decisions. Validation begins with a clear statement of the proposed interpretations (decisions). Evidence is then carefully planned, collected, appraised, and organized into an "argument" that renders judgment as to the defensibility of the proposed decisions. The statement of proposed interpretations together with the planned evidence is called the interpretation/use argument; the appraisal and judgment of collected evidence is called the validity argument (see Chapter 2).

Evidence to support these arguments can come from various sources. In planning, appraising, and organizing this evidence, it is helpful to use a comprehensive validation framework. There are currently two widely accepted frameworks, one proposed by Messick (1989) and currently endorsed by the American Educational Research Association, American Psychological Association, and National Council on Measurement in Education (2014) (the "five evidence sources" framework) and another proposed by Kane (2013) (see Chapter 2 for a discussion of these two frameworks). In this chapter, we will briefly review the former. Other sources offer readily accessible reviews of Kane's framework for medical education assessments broadly (Cook, Brydges, Ginsburg, & Hatala, 2015) and narrative assessments specifically (Cook & Lineberry et al., 2016).

The five evidence sources framework organizes evidence as representing *content, response process, internal structure, relationships with other variables*, or *consequences*. We emphasize that these are not different types of validity, but rather different types of evidence. Evidence is typically sought from several (but rarely, if ever, all) sources to support any given interpretation. We will briefly describe each evidence source as it relates to narrative assessment.

Content evidence examines the "relationship between the content of a test and the construct it is intended to measure" (AERA et al., 2014). Content evidence for a narrative assessment might include the method for selecting specific questions or prompts, the specific wording of prompts, and the selection of specific observation opportunities (i.e., sampling). Sampling is often purposeful or strategic, aiming to explore specific aspects of a trainee's performance by targeting specific situations or observers and to continue data collection until additional observations do not suggest new themes ("saturation"); content evidence would outline the strategy for such purposeful sampling.

Response process is defined as "the fit between the construct and the detailed nature of performance . . . actually engaged in" (AERA et al., 2014). Another way to think of this is what happens between the observation itself and the record (answer, numerical rating, or in this case narrative) that documents the observation. This might include the mental processes that influence the observer's interpretation of events, features of the context that influence observations (e.g., viewing angle or background noise), or the computer system used to document observer ratings and narratives. Response process *evidence* might show that observers follow instructions when completing reports, that narratives are based on observed performance rather than the trainee's reputation, or that the computer interface allows extended narratives.

Internal structure reflects the coherence among data elements from the same assessment and the appropriateness of the approach used to synthesize these elements into a meaningful message. In quantitative assessment, this typically involves reliability analyses and factor analyses. In qualitative assessment, this might involve triangulation among different data elements within a given assessment (e.g., different observers or time points), a detailed description of the analysis approach, including plans for iterative data collection and for the handling of outlier data points (e.g., were additional data sought to further explore discordant themes?), or a consideration of the analysts' background and training.

Whereas internal structure looks at associations among elements *within* an assessment, relationships with other variables examines the associations between the final synthesis and information sources *outside* this assessment. Key sources of evidence might include other concurrent, past, or future learning assessments, and consistency (or lack thereof) across assessments from different contexts (e.g., different clinical rotations), approaches (e.g., quantitative or narrative), or stages of training (i.e., with the assumption that more advanced trainees should perform better in most assessments). Having a predefined concept of the direction and magnitude of expected relationships (and articulating this in the interpretation-use argument) is particularly important when examining relationships with other variables, since without this it is possible to retrospectively interpret any relationship as favorable. For example, if a narrative assessment shows strong correlation with quantitative ratings, this could be interpreted as favorable validity evidence if both assessments are intended to measure the same trainee characteristic; or unfavorable, if they are intended to capture difference aspects of performance. Scientific integrity is preserved by committing to an expected relationship in advance. Note that some cross-assessment associations (such as quantitative scores and narrative comments on the same clinical rotation assessment form, or narrative comments from the surgery and medicine clerkships) could be considered either internal structure or relationships with other variables, depending on whether the assessments are viewed as "the same" or "different."

Finally, evidence of consequences looks at the impact of the assessment itself (and ensuing decisions) (Cook & Lineberry, 2016, and see Chapter 17). As noted above, the ultimate purpose of assessment is to inform meaningful decisions; consequences-type evidence seeks to determine whether this purpose has been achieved. Such evidence might explore objective evidence of intended and unintended consequences, agreement of others with the final interpretation and decision, or opinions about the assessment process. This evidence might be qualitative or quantitative, and might focus on the impact on or beliefs of trainees, instructors, institutions, or other stakeholders.

Table 11.1 summarizes the common threats to validity and potential remedies for narrative assessments.

SUMMARY

The use of narrative assessment in clinical training is increasing. Narrative assessment complements numeric scores by providing rich descriptions of current performance and identifying specific opportunities for improvement. Narrative assessment can support both formative feedback and summative decisions. Evidence suggests that narrative assessments can support defensible (i.e., valid) decisions. Table 11.2 summarizes best practices for narrative assessments.

Note: Additional material and resources may be available at the UIC AHPE website: https://go.uic.edu/AHPE

Table 11.1 Threats to Validity*: Narrative Assessment

	Problem	Remedy
Construct Underrepresentation (CU)	Too few observations (narratives)	Observer training (importance of observation and need for rich, detailed narrative) System that facilitates submission of incomplete assessments Prompts that encourage narrative comments in addition to numeric ratings
	Narratives come from limited diversity of contexts or observers	Blueprint to purposefully sample the domain (different contexts) Multiple, diverse observers
	Narratives lack detail	Prompts that encourage rich narrative comments
	Narratives focus on superficial aspects of performance	
Construct-Irrelevant Variance (CIV)	Narratives address irrelevant aspects of performance	Observer training (focus on relevant performances and relevant aspects; avoid euphemisms) Prompts that focus attention on relevant issues
	Observations based on irrelevant performances	System encourages observation of relevant performances (e.g., to "get in the room")
	Observer idiosyncrasies influence narratives	Multiple, diverse observers Rich narratives
	Idiosyncrasies of those performing analysis/synthesis Analysis/synthesis procedure introduces ideas not reflected in narratives	Defensible analysis/synthesis process Multiple, diverse, trained group of analysts Planned, defensible analysis/synthesis procedures Analysts trained to recognize euphemisms
	Narratives employ euphemisms and platitudes ("great team player")	

* For more about CU and CIV threats to validity, see Chapter 2.

Table 11.2 Narrative Assessment—Best Practices

- Define the purpose of the narrative assessment
- Document performance using detailed descriptions
- Train observers
- Develop systems to store and manage the data
- Follow robust procedures for narrative data analysis, using trained analysts
- Provide synthesized feedback to trainees, and support them in using this information to improve future performance

REFERENCES

American Educational Research Association, American Psychological Association, National Council on Measurement in Education. (2014). *Validity. Standards for educational and psychological testing* (pp. 11–31). Washington, DC: American Educational Research Association.

Bartels, J., Mooney, C.J., & Stone, R.T. (2017). Numerical versus narrative: A comparison between methods to measure medical student performance during clinical clerkships. *Medical Teacher, 39*(11), 1154–1158.

Cohen, G., Blumberg, P., Ryan, N., & Sullivan, P. (1993). Do final grades reflect written qualitative evaluations of student performance? *Teaching and Learning in Medicine, 5*(1), 10–15.

Cook, D.A., Brydges, R., Ginsburg, S., & Hatala, R. (2015). A contemporary approach to validity arguments: A practical guide to Kane's framework. *Medical Education, 49*, 560–575.

Cook, D.A., Kuper, A., Hatala, R., & Ginsburg, S. (2016). When assessment data are words: Validity evidence for qualitative educational assessments. *Academic Medicine 91*, 1359–1369.

Cook, D.A., & Lineberry, M. (2016). Consequences validity evidence: Evaluating the impact of educational assessments. *Academic Medicine, 91*, 785–795.

Driessen, E., van der Vleuten, C., Schuwirth, L., van Tartwijk, J., & Vermunt, J. (2005). The use of qualitative research criteria for portfolio assessment as an alternative to reliability evaluation: A case study. *Medical Education, 39*, 214–220.

Dudek, N.L., & Dojeiji, S. (2014). Twelve tips for completing quality in-training evaluation reports. *Medical Teacher, 36*(12), 1038–1042.

Dudek, N.L., Marks, M.B., Bandiera, G., White, J., & Wood, T.J. (2013). Quality in-training evaluation reports— Does feedback drive faculty performance? *Academic Medicine, 88*(8), 1129–1134.

Dudek, N., Marks, M., Lee, C., & Wood, T. (2008). Assessing the quality of supervisors' completed clinical evaluation reports. *Medical Education, 42*, 816–822.

Dudek, N.L., Marks, M.B., & Regehr, G. (2005). Failure to fail—The perspectives of clinical supervisors. *Academic Medicine, 80*(10), S84–S87.

Dudek, N.L., Marks, M.B., Wood, T.J., Dojeiji, S., Bandiera, G., Hatala, R., Cooke, L., & Sadownik, L. (2012). Quality evaluation reports: Can a faculty development program make a difference? *Medical Teacher, 34*(11), e725–e731.

Ginsburg, S., Eva, K.W., & Regehr, G. (2013). Do in-training evaluation reports deserve their bad reputations? A study of the reliability and predictive ability of ITER scores and narrative comments. *Academic Medicine, 88*(10), 1539–1544.

Ginsburg, S., van der Vleuten, C., & Eva, K. (2017). The hidden value of narrative comments for assessment: A quantitative reliability analysis of qualitative data. *Academic Medicine, 92*(11), 1617–1621.

Govaerts, M., & van der Vleuten, C.P.M. (2013). Validity in work-based assessment: Expanding our horizons. *Medical Education, 47*, 1164–1174.

Guerrasio, J., Cumbler, E., Trosterman, A., Wald, H., Brandenburg, S., & Aagaard, E. (2012). Determining need for remediation through postrotation evaluations. *Journal of Graduate Medical Education, 4*(1), 47–51.

Hanson, J.L., Rosenberg, A.A., & Lane, J.L. (2013). Narrative descriptions should replace grades and numerical ratings for clinical performance in medical education in the United States. *Frontiers in Psychology, 4*, 1–10.

Hodges, B. (2013). Assessment in the post-psychometric era: Learning to love the subjective and collective. *Medical Teacher, 35*, 564–568.

Holmboe, E.S., Sherbino, J., Long, D.M., Swing, W.R., & Frank, J.R. (2010). The role of assessment in competency-based medical education. *Medical Teacher, 32*, 676–682.

Kane, M.T. (2013). Validating the interpretations and uses of test scores. *Journal of Educational Measurement, 50*(1), 1–73.

Kogan, J.R., Hatala, R., Hauer, K.E., & Holmboe, E. (2017). Guidelines: The do's, don'ts and don't knows of direct observation of clinical skills in medical education. *Perspectives on Medical Education, 6*, 286–305.

Littlefield, J.H., DaRosa, D.A., Paukert, J., Williams, R.G., Klamen, D.L., & Schoolfield, J.D. (2005). Improving resident performance assessment data: Numeric precision and narrative specificity. *Academic Medicine, 80*(5), 489–495.

McConnell, M.M., Harms, S., & Saperson, K. (2016). Meaningful feedback in medical education: Challenging the "failure to fail" using narrative methodology. *Academic Psychiatry, 40*, 377–379.

Messick, S. (1989). Validity. In R.L. Linn (Ed.), *Educational measurement* (3rd ed., pp. 13–103). New York: American Council on Education and Macmillan.

12

ASSESSMENT PORTFOLIOS

Daniel J. Schumacher, Ara Tekian, and Rachel Yudkowsky

When implemented appropriately, portfolios can improve students' ability to integrate theory with practice, can encourage their self-awareness and reflection, and can offer support for students facing difficult emotional situations. Portfolios can also enhance student-tutor relationships and prepare students for the rigours of . . . training.

(Buckley, Coleman, & Khan, 2010)

The word *portfolio* comes from the Latin word *portare* (to carry) and *folium* (leaf, sheet). In health professions education, an assessment portfolio is a collection of evidence documenting progress, accomplishments, and reflective thoughts over time. Portfolios comprise a vehicle for the longitudinal, multi-method, multi-source assessment of learner development. Portfolios can be used for both formative and summative purposes, and we will focus on both. We will also explore some challenges of portfolio use.

PORTFOLIO DESIGN

Portfolios in fact differ so much in their form and use that it is almost impossible to make general statements about them.

(Driessen, 2017)

As portfolios have matured, this quote from Erik Driessen has become increasingly true. Depending on the purposes of an individual portfolio effort, a portfolio may contain any artifact (written, audio, or video) that provides evidence of learning and development over time (Friedman Ben David et al., 2001). Table 12.1 provides two frameworks for thinking about portfolio content and structure: (1) McEwen, Griffiths, and Schultz (2015) describe content elements included in a portfolio for family medicine residents and (2) Webb et al. (2002) provide analogies for different structural models for nursing portfolios.

While models can inform possibilities, at its foundation the contents of a portfolio depend on its purpose. Roberts, Shadbolt, Clark, and Simpson (2014) and Driessen (2017) observe that

Table 12.1 Two Models of Portfolio Content and Structure

Portfolio Assessment Support System (McEwen et al., 2015)	Webb and Colleagues' Nursing Program Models (Webb et al., 2002)
• Reflection elements (e.g., individualized learning plans, reflections on care, significant incidents) • Learning module elements (e.g., self-paced, web-based learning activities) • Assessment elements (e.g., multi-source feedback, objective structured clinical exam results, work-based assessments, in-training exam reports, chart audits and care quality metrics) • Document elements (e.g., conference attendance, continuing medical education activities, procedure logs, curriculum vitae, published papers)	• "Shopping trolley": the student collects anything deemed relevant to demonstrate their learning and development process • "Toast rack": the portfolio is comprised of a number of "slots" that must be filled to consider a portfolio complete for a specified period of time (such as a semester in school or year of training); each "slot" is a type of data (e.g., critical incident reflection, performance assessments in various areas) • "Spinal column": the portfolio contains a list of competencies (vertebrae in the spinal column analogy) that must be assessed, and students gather data to address each of these elements • "Cake mix": students blend individual elements of the portfolio to form the whole of the portfolio with the resultant portfolio being more than the sum of the parts; an example is written reflection on performance assessments

portfolios are either *reflective*, comprising a distinct, formative component of the curriculum, or *comprehensive*, comprising a vehicle for assessment across curricular components and over time. As a vehicle to promote reflection, a formative or learning portfolio may include private, reflective responses to learning experiences, including reflection on errors and mistakes. These reflections may be reviewed and discussed with a mentor, tutor, or peers for the purpose of formative assessment and feedback. Summative, assessment, or comprehensive portfolios, on the other hand, consist of a public compilation of evidence of learning and/or work samples, sometimes reflecting a learner's best work, most typical work, or work on a theme (Paulson, Paulson, & Meyer, 1991; Davis et al., 2001; Rees, 2005; O'Sullivan, Reckase, McClain, Savidge, & Clardy, 2004). While an assessment portfolio may include reflections on its contents and selected entries from the reflective portfolio, the different purposes should be explicit, and the selection of reflective entries to be made public should be left to the learner (Pinsky & Fryer-Edwards, 2004; Pitts, 2007).

A portfolio can serve to document the accomplishment of a single curricular objective or competency, such as self-directed learning. Portfolios are especially suited to providing evidence for the achievement of competencies that are difficult to observe directly in controlled circumstances at a single point in time. By providing an annotated, reflective record of activities over time, portfolios can afford indirect observation of complex competencies such as practice-based learning and improvement or system-based practice. In addition, the process of selecting and justifying "best work" for an assessment portfolio allows the learner to demonstrate aspects of professionalism, such as the ability to reflect on and self-assess one's own work, and implies a deep understanding of the characteristics and criteria that determine the quality of the work (Pinsky & Fryer-Edwards, 2004).

Portfolios can also complement single-source, single-competency assessment by providing a rich multidimensional description of the learner's accomplishments over time and verifying the achievement of multiple and complex learning objectives. An "omnibus" or comprehensive assessment portfolio is a compilation of evidence from a variety of methods and sources. The omnibus portfolio can include entries across the spectrum of Miller's pyramid from "knows" to "does" (Chapter 1 and Figure 12.1). Entries can continue to accumulate in the portfolio until the

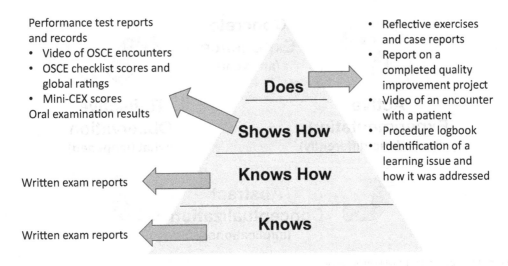

Performance test reports
and records
- Video of OSCE encounters
- OSCE checklist scores and
  global ratings
- Mini-CEX scores
Oral examination results

Does

Shows How

Knows How

Written exam reports

Knows

Written exam reports

- Reflective exercises
  and case reports
- Report on a
  completed quality
  improvement project
- Video of an encounter
  with a patient
- Procedure logbook
- Identification of a
  learning issue and
  how it was addressed

Figure 12.1 Portfolio elements from across Miller's pyramid

evidence is sufficient for the decision required. As faculty gain experience with assessment portfolios, patterns of precocious or delayed learning and performance, like "growth charts," can provide an opportunity for early intervention and remediation. Comprehensive assessment portfolios can be critical components of programmatic assessment systems (see Chapter 16).

FORMATIVE PURPOSES OF PORTFOLIOS: LEARNER DRIVEN, MENTOR SUPPORTED

Competency-based health professions education, the prevailing contemporary approach in health professions education, argues that learners should be the driving force for their learning, supported by mentors who share in the responsibility for ensuring learning goals are met (Carraccio, Wolfsthal, Englander, Ferentz, & Martin, 2002). This focus on the learner having the locus of control is foundational to the formative purposes of portfolios. To facilitate this, portfolios need to be designed in a learner-centered fashion, ensuring design and functionality that not only achieves the stated goals of the portfolio but also fosters the development of lifelong learning skills (Gordon & Campbell, 2013; Tochel et al., 2009). For example, electronic portfolios (compared to non-electronic) may be better at promoting reflection (Tochel et al., 2009). Furthermore, too much or too little structure in portfolio design can disengage learners (Van Tartwijk & Driessen, 2009). Ideally, a portfolio provides a framework to focus a learner's goals and reflections in areas that are important to their development but offers flexibility in how they are able to document their learning and development in those areas (Driessen, van der Vleuten, Schuwirth, Van Tartwijk, & Vermont, 2005; Moores & Parks, 2010). For example, professionalism could be a required focus in a portfolio, but development in this area could be documented through a variety of methods, such as a multi-source feedback assessment from a patient or an interprofessional colleague, a written reflection about an encounter with an abusive patient or co-worker, or the results of completing a conflict mode inventory to gain insight into striving for effective and professional communication during difficult conversations.

Consistent with a learner-centered approach that fosters the development of lifelong learning skills, a distinctive aspect of a portfolio is the reflective component, an opportunity for the learner to provide a commentary on the included items and explicate their meaning to the reader. As

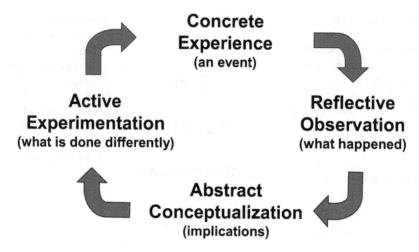

Figure 12.2 Kolb's experiential learning cycle

such, it is a unique and individual creation and a dynamic record of personal and professional growth. A portfolio can serve as both a *vehicle* to promote reflective learning and as *evidence* of that reflection and of other learning. The use of portfolios to facilitate learning is based on the experiential/reflective learning models of Kolb (1984) and Schön (1987) (Figure 12.2). These models emphasize the need to reflect on an experience, often together with a coach or mentor, in order for the experience to be incorporated effectively as new learning. The process of portfolio development promotes this reflection: writing about experiences is itself a tool that forces thinking, structuring thoughts and reflection, thus supporting professional development (Pitkala & Mantyranta, 2004).

THE IMPORTANCE OF MENTORS IN PORTFOLIO-FACILITATED LIFELONG LEARNING

> Self-directed learning usually takes place in association with various kinds of helpers, such as teachers, tutors, mentors, resource people and peers.
>
> (Knowles, 1975)

Humans possess limited ability to identify and address gaps in knowledge and performance (Eva & Regehr, 2008; Regehr, 2006). Therefore, external assessments from mentors, peers, and other sources can, and should, inform self-assessment and defining learning goals. With the learner in the driver's seat to seek and gather this information, Eva and Regehr (2008) have aptly named this activity *self-directed assessment seeking*. When considering portfolios, mentors or coaches become a central source of external calibration of learners' self-assessment of performance, definition of learning goals, and reflections. As they work with learners, mentors should be sure they attend to learners' senses of competence, relatedness, and autonomy (i.e., ability to act of one's own volition), because these factors play a role in learners' desire to learn (Ryan, 2000). Attending to learners' sense of relatedness with their mentors promotes their remaining open and in "learning mode" as a colleague rather than in "defensive mode" as an outsider (Ryan, 2000). Learners have a tendency to fear external information that does not match their self-assessments and even discount feedback from supervisors (Epstein, Siegel, & Silberman, 2008; Mann et al., 2011; Sargeant et al., 2010; Watling, van der Vleuten, & Lingard, 2012). With this in mind, a supportive, collegial relationship that places learners and mentors at the same level cannot be emphasized enough. The required balance can be likened to a dance between points of vulnerability, which threaten the learner-mentor relationship, and points of adaptability, which enhance learner-mentor engagement (Arntfield, Parlett, Meston, Apramian, & Lingard, 2016).

SUMMATIVE PURPOSES OF PORTFOLIOS: LEARNER DRIVEN, SUPERVISOR EVALUATED

The primary challenge of assessment portfolios is how to move from a collection of evidence to a single summative decision. As an example, imagine an omnibus portfolio consisting of four components: annual written exam scores, annual performance test (OSCE) scores, monthly end-of-rotation clinical evaluations with quantitative (e.g., ratings) and qualitative (e.g., written comments) assessment data, and semi-annual reflections by the learner. Some possibilities for scoring the portfolio are:

- Assess each component separately, assign a rating for each, and average the scores across components for the final portfolio score (*compensatory scoring*). In such situations, good performance on one or more components will compensate for the poor performance on other components. For example, if a student performs poorly on the monthly end-of-rotation clinical evaluation, the good performance of the other three components will compensate for the poor performance on this component. In a compensatory system, it is difficult to give feedback about each component, because the score is an aggregate of several components.
- Assess each component separately and assign a rating for each; the learner must reach a minimum standard in each component in order to pass (*conjunctive scoring*). For example, if a student performs poorly on the monthly end-of-rotation clinical evaluation, irrespective of the good performance on the other three components, he/she still will not get a passing rating because the ratings for each component do not compensate for each other.
- Rate the portfolio as a whole using an analytic or primary trait-rating rubric (see Chapter 9). For example, the portfolio as a whole could be rated on characteristics such as organization, completeness, or quality of reflection. Alternatively, the portfolio as a whole could be rated on the quality of evidence provided for each of the individual competencies such as communication, knowledge, or professionalism.
- Rate the portfolio as a whole using a single global rating rubric; for example, a five-point scale ranging from definite pass to definite fail.

One of the challenges inherent to evaluating the portfolio is how to integrate quantitative and qualitative assessment data. Historically, qualitative assessment data has been undervalued because psychometric data cannot support its validity and reliability. However, recent efforts have shown the value of applying qualitative research approaches to this data to ensure its credibility and dependability (Driessen et al., 2005). Work by Ginsburg and colleagues has demonstrated the inter-rater reliability of written comments on assessment forms (Ginsburg, van der Vleuten, & Eva, 2017). As the evidence base for qualitative assessment data has grown, so too has the description of value that those rendering summative assessment decisions ascribe to such data (Govaerts, van der Vleuten, Schuwirth, & Muijtjens, 2007; Oudkerk Pool, Govaerts, Jaarsma, & Driessen, 2017; Schumacher, Michelson et al., 2018). At their core, the value of both quantitative and qualitative assessment data underscores the value of expert human judgment in making summative assessment decisions that incorporate "numbers" and "words" to provide a holistic picture of performance and development.

ADDRESSING THREATS TO VALIDITY

Portfolios face the same threats to validity as other assessment methods (Chapter 2 and Table 12.2). Because of these challenges, portfolios are best used as part of a comprehensive assessment system that can triangulate on learner competence (Chapter 16) (Melville, Rees, Brookfield, & Anderson, 2004; Webb et al., 2002; Tochel et al., 2009).

The contents of the portfolio should systematically sample the learning objectives to be assessed. A portfolio intended to assess the self-directed learning of nurse practitioners, whose entries include only a log of textbook reading, is an example of a *construct underrepresentation* (CU) or undersampling validity challenge (see Chapter 2). CU can be avoided by providing learners with a portfolio structure and guidelines that specify the learning objectives to be documented, the types of desirable evidence, and the amount of evidence required, sampling work *over time* and *over tasks*. For example, guidelines for a portfolio intended for the assessment of self-directed learning might specify:

Table 12.2 Threats to Validity: Portfolios

	Problem	Remedy
Construct Underrepresentation (CU)	Not enough evidence of learning is presented	Provide learners with guidelines for type and quantity of evidence needed Formative review with preceptor
	Evidence is not presented for all learning objectives	Specify portfolio structure based on blueprint of learning objectives Formative review with preceptor
Construct-Irrelevant Variance (CIV)	Examiner bias	Provide scoring rubric Train examiners to use rubric Rater consensus discussion
	Systematic rater error: halo, severity, leniency, central tendency	Benchmarks, frame of reference training for examiners Rater consensus discussion
	Ability to reflect may be confounded with writing ability	Oral discussion/defense of portfolio Formative review of portfolio for correct writing and presentation before official submission
	Insincere reflective entries because of confidentiality and privacy concerns	Separate formative and summative functions of portfolio Give learners control over which reflective entries to include
Reliability Indicators	Generalizability Inter-rater reliability or agreement Reproducibility of pass/fail decisions Credibility Dependability	

- an explanation of two new learning objectives initiated by critical incidents;
- learning plans to achieve these objectives;
- a description of the educational activities undertaken; or
- a reflective self-appraisal of learning showing that growth and professional development is taking place.

Construct-irrelevant variance (CIV) can be due to either learner or rater factors. Learners may be reluctant to reflect honestly on errors or to expose their weaknesses in the context of an assessment. Separating the formative and summative functions of the portfolio and allowing learners to select the "best work" or "best evidence" entries to make public in the assessment portfolio can help minimize this problem (Pinsky & Fryer-Edwards, 2004).

Portfolio raters are subject to the same biases and errors as raters for oral exams and performance exams (see Table 12.2 and Chapters 8 and 9) (Ward, Gruppen, & Regehr, 2002; Roberts, Newble, & O'Rourke, 2002). One approach to the rater (dis)agreement challenge is to standardize the contents of the portfolio and to use multiple raters whenever possible—parallel to the approach for standardizing oral and performance exams. An example would be to have various portfolio entries scored by different raters, resulting in multiple "observations" by multiple raters. As with other subjective judgments, benchmarks for acceptable entries, frame-of-reference rater training, and rater consensus through discussion can improve rater agreement (Chapter 9; O'Sullivan, Cogbill, McClain, Reckase, & Clardy, 2002; O'Sullivan et al., 2004; Rees & Sheard, 2004; Pitts, Coles, Thomas, & Smith, 2002). Roberts et al. (2014) provides a good example of a study of the reliability and validity of a programmatic assessment portfolio in a clinical placement.

When addressing threats to validity raised by the inclusion of qualitative assessment data, the concept of applying qualitative research methods seems to be a good fit for purpose (Driessen et al., 2005). The *credibility* of an assessment can be improved by employing triangulation (combining different information sources—analogous to multiple raters), prolonged engagement (e.g., multiple formative reviews of the portfolio over time—analogous to multiple observations), and member checking (reviewing and discussing the assessment with the learner). *Dependability* is enhanced by audit (quality assurance procedures with external auditors) and audit trail (documentation of the assessment process to enable external checks). These qualitative approaches to the summative assessment and quality assurance of portfolios can help avoid reductionism and preserve an integrated, holistic view of the learner as a unique individual developing over time.

Beyond decisions focused on how to make valid and reliable summative assessment decisions using portfolios is the question of who should be making these decisions. Clearly, these decisions should ultimately reside in assessors who are not the learner of interest. However, given the significant formative purpose of portfolios and their ability to foster and develop lifelong learning skills, we believe even the summative purposes of portfolios should be learner-driven (O'Brien, Sanguino, Thomas, & Green, 2016; Schmitz, Whitson, Van Heest, & Maddaus, 2010; Sklansky, Frohna, & Schumacher, 2017). Case Example 12.1 provides an example of a learner-driven portfolio.

Figure 12.3 shows how an oral "defense" of the portfolio may allow learners to compile and present the contents of the portfolio to allow examiners to probe for additional information and understanding, promote discussions between examiners to reach a consensus grade, and facilitate requesting additional information and/or rating by additional examiners for marginal or borderline students. The middle of Figure 12.3 focuses on what and how evaluators review. Clinical competency committees are groups that review assessment data and make summative decisions (see, for example, Accreditation Council for Graduate Medical Education, 2017). Recent work suggests variability in both the review processes and the content of what CCC members prioritize in their reviews. Individual members' review processes and their roles in the assessment system may influence the summative decisions that are made (Friedman, Raimo, Spielmann, & Chaudhry, 2016; Nabors et al., 2017; Schumacher, King et al., 2018). Reviewing more residents, being involved

---

Case Example 12.1 Learner-Driven Synthesis of Assessment Data (Sklansky et al., 2017)

In this example from post-graduate training in the United States, the primary responsibility for synthesizing the information in the portfolio and recommending summative decisions resides with the learner. The role of the learner as primary driver of assessment is emphasized. The need for self-assessments to be calibrated by external assessments is met through presentation and discussion at the clinical competency committee (CCC), where final decisions are made regarding any areas of concern.

"Milestones" refers to a developmental, behaviorally anchored approach to assessment promoted by the US Accreditation Council for Graduate Medical Education (ACGME); see Chapter 1 and Holmboe, Edgar, & Hamstra (2016).

Steps in the resident-driven assessment program:

1. Resident completes a self-assessment based on milestones.
2. Resident reviews his/her portfolio of external assessment data (e.g., milestones-based ratings from rotations, multi-source feedback from nurses and families, written comments) from program.
3. Resident assembles assessment data into a synthesized (organized, summarized) format to support milestone level assignments for himself/herself.
4. Resident reflects on missing data that is needed to assign milestone levels for all competencies and determines if he/she possesses data/information that can inform those milestone assignments, adding this data to the portfolio as needed.
5. Resident documents progress in completing program requirements that fall outside traditional rotations (e.g., scholarly projects, quality improvement projects, advocacy work).
6. Resident reviews self-assessment (step 1) and adjusts based on external assessment data and then constructs a statement summarizing progress from the last review cycle, accomplishments, areas of notable development, areas for future development, and specific plans for improvement.
7. Resident presents his/her synthesis to the clinical competency committee and makes additional modifications as needed.
8. With CCC, resident determines overall classification of current developmental progress and goals for the future.

---

in more review cycles, and providing feedback to residents after the review have all been shown to lead to more stringent summative assessments (Schumacher, King et al., 2018). CCC members may have personally-preferred data they use as anchors for their reviews; for example, qualitative assessment data seems to be highly valued by many reviewers (Oudkerk Pool et al., 2017; Schumacher, Michelson et al., 2018). With this in mind, it is important to encourage CCC members to consider data that goes beyond their preferred data type, to ensure that data used to inform summative decisions comes from a variety of sources (Kinnear, Warm, & Hauer, 2018).

POTENTIAL CHALLENGES OF PORTFOLIO USE

While portfolios offer several benefits for formative and summative assessment, they can also present challenges. First, their use for summative purposes may hamper their use for formative

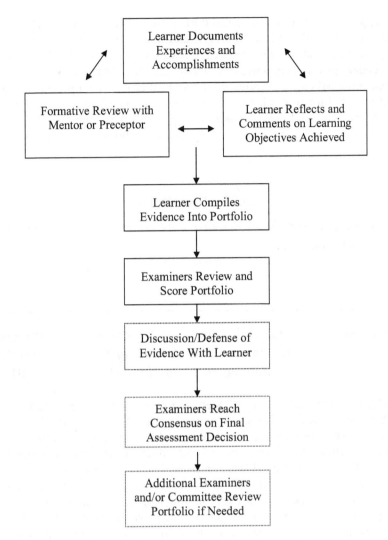

Figure 12.3 Assessment portfolio

purposes (Nagler, Andolsek, & Padmore, 2009). Mentors must attend to the manner in which they provide feedback in order to strike the best possible balance between helping learners improve and ensuring that their sense of competence is not overly threatened. This underscores the importance of faculty development in building a portfolio system (Chertoff et al., 2016). Another potential challenge is that portfolios can be time consuming for both learners and mentors (Gadbury-Amyot, Bray, & Austin, 2014; Van Tartwijk & Driessen, 2009). Taking adequate time to reflect simply cannot be reduced beyond a certain point without losing value in the activity. Thus, it is important to take measures to maximize utility, including optimizing feasibility, so that the portfolio does not become just another bureaucratic hurdle for learners to overcome (Driessen, Van Tartwijk, van der Vleuten, & Wass, 2007; van der Vleuten, 1996; Driessen, 2017). Beyond tending to the time constraints of learners and mentors with portfolios, it is important to remain sensitive to the time and resources of administrative leaders employing a portfolio in their schools and programs as well. Ensuring adequate information technology support is fundamental in these efforts (Chertoff et al., 2016). Finally, medico-legal concerns can present a challenge. Portfolios can, and should, include reflection on experiences with actual patients, including when these experiences do not go as intended or even involve errors. Thus, patient privacy is important (Nagler et al., 2009). Individuals should be sure they understand institutional and legal privacy policies as they develop a portfolio. Legal discoverability and potential for professional liability exposure should also be understood (Nagler et al., 2009). By intent, portfolios are focused on improvement and should not be discoverable, and measures (e.g., hospital policies) preventing discoverability should be taken to ensure this intention is preserved.

CASE EXAMPLES

The following case studies illustrate three creative adaptations of portfolios for the assessment of learners in the health professions.

Case Example 12.2: Vanderbilt University Competency Milestones for Medical Students: A Learner-Centered, Developmentally Focused Portfolio (Lomis et al., 2017)

The Vanderbilt University School of Medicine developed a milestones-based portfolio system for medical students, beginning in 2012. Milestones are developmental steps that a student is expected to progress through in a range of competency areas. At Vanderbilt, milestones-based assessment is introduced in the first, non-clinical, year of medical school and continued into the clinical years. Milestones are rated by designated faculty with responsibility for direct observation of the students. Milestones serve as one source of assessment data for students, to be used alongside other evidence of performance, such as course grades. The power of the milestones-based program of assessment is that all competency domains, with the same metrics, are assessed across the entire curriculum. The portfolio system that houses this data can clearly display development in specific areas as well as overall, over time, in a visual fashion. Rather than calculating scores at a single point in time, the portfolio focuses on developmental trends.

Student reflection on their milestones-based performance data is a hallmark of the Vanderbilt system. At defined points, students review their portfolio with a coach to identify areas of relative strength, areas of focus for future development, and individualized learning plans focused on taking the next steps in their development. Students and coaches evaluate the relative value and importance of each data point to determine which points offer signal and which are adding noise. For areas of concern, promotion actions are only taken after this review.

Several characteristics of the Vanderbilt system make it noteworthy. First, it places a focus on development rather than judgment. Second, it is highly learner-centered, but includes a portfolio coach or mentor. Students are in the driver's seat of reviewing their data, and concerning performance is only called out once students have identified it with their portfolio coach.

Case Example 12.3 Psychiatry Residents: A Showcase or "Best Work" Portfolio (O'Sullivan et al., 2002, 2004)

Psychiatry residents were asked to exhibit their "best work" in five of 13 essential topic areas each year, including topics such as initial evaluation and diagnosis, treatment course, self-directed learning, working with teams, crisis management, legal issues, and presentation/teaching skills. Residents could choose four of the topics to present; an entry in the area of bio/psycho/social formulation was mandatory. Resident guidelines specified the meaning of each topic, what to include in the entry, and the rubric showing how the entry would be evaluated. For each entry, residents selected a case or experience to showcase their "best work" in that topic. Entries were not developed specifically for the portfolio. Residents submitted copies of (de-identified) patient documentation that they had produced, and wrote a brief reflective self-assessment explaining how this case and the supporting documentation demonstrated their competency.

Rating the Portfolio

Two external examiners who were unfamiliar with the residents and their patients rated each of the portfolio entries. Program faculty developed topic-specific, six-point scoring rubrics in which the low end indicated a lack of knowledge or skill that could place patients at risk, and the high end indicated an ability to deal with complex problems effectively and creatively. Raters were trained by scoring benchmark entries. Portfolio entries were sorted by topic, and raters scored all entries within a given topic (across residents) before moving to the next topic

Sample Scoring Rubric for "Legal Issues" Topic

1. Important legal knowledge missing to adequately deal with the case.
2. Appropriate approach to legal issues, but weaknesses that could lead to potential problems.
3. Competent to successfully deal with legal issues following standard approach with little collateral information necessary.
4. Able to apply standard approach with fairly complex legal issues.
5. Well-integrated knowledge of legal issues that shows ability to integrate information. Aware of legal documentation needed.
6. Wide breadth of knowledge of legal issues and well integrated from numerous and varied sources to resolve very complex cases. Thorough presentation; acknowledges short-term outcomes.

Overall portfolio scores tended to increase with year of training. Scores were moderately correlated with a national, in-training written exam, but not with clinical rotation ratings. A generalizability analysis and D study showed that five entries scored by two raters provided sufficient reliability for norm-referenced (relative) decisions with G = .81, and that five entries scored by three raters or six entries scored by two raters would provide sufficient reliability for criterion-referenced (absolute) decisions. As an unintended consequence, the portfolios identified poor performance across residents in certain topic areas, resulting in an almost immediate change in the curriculum.

Case Example 12.4 Nursing Professional Portfolio for Practicing Nurses: A Portfolio to Support the Ongoing Development of Health Professionals in Practice After Training (Williams & Jordan, 2007)

Portfolios are not just for trainees. Continuing professional development is essential in the fast-evolving domain of health care. To promote the ongoing development of their nurses, Texas Children's Hospital developed a nursing professional portfolio with the following purposes:

1. Establish career goals.
2. Showcase professional accomplishments.
3. Illustrate specific areas of expertise.
4. Enhance knowledge and skills.
5. Plan for additional career opportunities.
6. Help gain admission to school in order to advance academic preparation.
7. Apply to participate in the hospital's clinical ladder program.

The portfolio provides a structure to organize and track formal and informal activities and accomplishments including certifications, continuing education activities, precepting/ mentoring, committee participation, notes of appreciation from patients and family, and exemplary innovations or practice improvements.

The authors believe that attention to informal activities and accomplishments in particular helps drive exploration of new directions for growth. Capturing these often-overlooked successes and the value that nurses brings to their professional role can help nurses realize their creative potential and define career paths. Each nurse's portfolio is submitted prior to their annual performance evaluation. Portfolio review with the supervisor facilitates a more comprehensive picture of the nurse that aids in the selection of candidates for future growth opportunities, including committee appointments and leadership positions.

On the whole, the Texas Children's Hospital Nursing Professional Portfolio is an excellent example of using portfolios to support and enhance ongoing professional development after training.

SUMMARY

Portfolios provide a useful structure for gathering multi-method, multi-source, reflection-annotated evidence about the achievements of learners over time, beneficial for both formative and summative assessment purposes. Portfolios are subject to the same validity threats as other types of qualitative or holistic assessments. Mentoring, scoring, feedback, and feasibility issues must be addressed; learner-centered approaches, learner input, and appropriate coaching are crucial to prevent portfolios from becoming bureaucratic hurdles. Comprehensive portfolios are a key component of programmatic assessments (Chapter 16) and can assist in moving from single point-assessments to a developmentally oriented, holistic approach.

Table 12.3 provides a summary of guidelines for the successful implementation of assessment portfolios in the health professions.

Note: Additional material and resources may be available at the UIC AHPE website: https://go.uic.edu/AHPE

Table 12.3 Practical Guidelines for Assessment Portfolios

Introducing the portfolio
- Introduce portfolios slowly with input and feedback from learners and faculty
- Clarify goals
- Separate formative and summative performance portfolio functions
- Provide support and training in the use of portfolios for both learners and mentors

Implementing the portfolio
- Provide learners with a standard structure and guideline for the type and quantity of material to be included the portfolio—provide structure but do not be overly prescriptive
- Sample learners' work over tasks and over time
- Provide frequent formative feedback and mentoring in a supportive educational climate
- Provide time for creating portfolio entries within the structure of existing activities

Assessing the portfolio
- Provide benchmarks and frame-of-reference training to raters
- Allow raters to discuss scores and reach a consensus
- Use both qualitative and quantitative approaches to assessment and quality assurance
- Triangulate the results of the portfolio assessment with other assessment methods

---

REFERENCES

Accreditation Council for Graduate Medical Education: Clinical Competency Committees: A Guidebook for Programs. (2017). Accreditation council for graduate medical education (2nd ed.), www.acgme.org/What-We-Do/Accreditation/Milestones/Resources accessed 21 Feb 2019.

Arntfield, S., Parlett, B., Meston, C.N., Apramian, T., & Lingard, L. (2016). A model of engagement in reflective writing-based portfolios: Interactions between points of vulnerability and acts of adaptability. *Medical Teacher*, *38*(2), 196–205.

Buckley, S., Coleman, J., & Khan, K. (2010). Best evidence on the educational effects of undergraduate portfolios. *Clinical Teacher*, *7*(3), 187–191.

Carraccio, C., Wolfsthal, S.D., Englander, R., Ferentz, K., & Martin, C. (2002). Shifting paradigms: From Flexner to competencies. *Academic Medicine*, *77*(5), 361–367.

Chertoff, J., Wright, A., Novak, M., Fantone, J., Fleming, A., Ahmed, T., . . . Zaidi, Z. (2016). Status of portfolios in undergraduate medical education in the LCME accredited US medical school. *Medical Teacher*, *38*(9), 886–896.

Davis, M.H., Friedman Ben-David, M., Harden, R.M., Howe, P., Ker, J., McGhee, C., Pippard, M.J., & Snadden, D. (2001). AMEE medical education guide # 24: Portfolios as a method of student assessment. *Medical Teacher*, *23*, 535–551.

Driessen, E. (2017). Do portfolios have a future? *Advances in Health Sciences Education Theory and Practice*, *22*(1), 221–228.

Driessen, E., van der Vleuten, C., Schuwirth, L., Van Tartwijk, J., & Vermont, J. (2005). The use of qualitative research criteria for portfolio assessment as an alternative to reliability evaluation: A case study. *Medical Education*, *39*, 214–220.

Driessen, E., van Tartwijk, J., van der Vleuten, C., & Wass, V. (2007). Portfolios in medical education: Why do they meet with mixed success? A systematic review. *Medical Education*, *41*(12), 1224–1233.

Epstein, R.M., Siegel, D.J., & Silberman, J. (2008). Self-monitoring in clinical practice: A challenge for medical educators. *The Journal of Continuing Education in the Health Professions*, *28*(1), 5–13.

Eva, K.W., & Regehr, G. (2008). "I'll never play professional football" and other fallacies of self-assessment. *The Journal of Continuing Education in the Health Professions*, *28*(1), 14–19.

Friedman Ben-David, M., Davis, M.H., Harden, R.M., Howie, P.W., Ker, J., & Pippard, M.J. (2001). AMEE medical education guide no. 24: Portfolios as a method of student assessment. *Medical Teacher*, *23*(6), 535–551.

Friedman, K.A., Raimo, J., Spielmann, K., & Chaudhry, S. (2016). Resident dashboards: Helping your clinical competency committee visualize trainees' key performance indicators. *Medical Education Online*, *21*, 29838.

Gadbury-Amyot, C.C., Bray, K.K., & Austin, K.J. (2014). Fifteen years of portfolio assessment of dental hygiene student competency: Lessons learned. *Journal of Dental Hygiene*, *88*(5), 267–274.

Ginsburg, S., van der Vleuten, C.P., & Eva, K.W. (2017). The hidden value of narrative Comments for assessment: A quantitative reliability analysis of qualitative data. *Academic Medicine*, *92*(11), 1617–1621.

Gordon, J.A., & Campbell, C.M. (2013). The role of ePortfolios in supporting continuing professional development in practice. *Medical Teacher*, *35*(4), 287–294.

Govaerts, M.J., van der Vleuten, C.P., Schuwirth, L.W., & Muijtjens, A.M. (2007). Broadening perspectives on clinical performance assessment: Rethinking the nature of in-training assessment. *Advances in Health Sciences Education Theory and Practice*, *12*(2), 239–260.

Holmboe, E.S., Edgar, L., & Hamstra, S. (2016). *The milestones guidebook*. Chicago, IL: Accreditation Council for Graduate Medical Education. Retrieved from www.acgme.org/What-We-Do/Accreditation/Milestones/Resources. Accessed July 2, 2019.

Kinnear, B., Warm, E.J., & Hauer, K.E. (2018). Twelve tips to maximize the value of a clinical competency committee in postgraduate medical education. *Medical Teacher*, *40*(11), 1110–1115.

Knowles, M. (1975). *Self-directed learning: A guide for learners and teachers*. New York: Associated Press.

Kolb, D. (1984). *Experiential learning: Experience as a source of learning and development*. Englewood Cliffs, NJ: Prentice Hall.

Lomis, K.D, Russell, R.G., Davidson, M.A., Fleming, A.E., Pettepher, C.C., Cutrer, W.B., Fleming, G.M., & Miller, B.M. (2017). Competency milestones for medical students: Design, implementation, and analysis at one medical school. *Medical Teacher*, *39*(5), 494–504.

Mann, K., van der Vleuten, C., Eva, K., Armson, H., Chesluk, B., Dornan, T., . . . Sargeant, J. (2011). Tensions in informed self-assessment: How the desire for feedback and reticence to collect and use it can conflict. *Academic Medicine*, *86*(9), 1120–1127.

McEwen, L.A., Griffiths, J., & Schultz, K. (2015). Developing and successfully implementing a competency-based portfolio assessment system in a postgraduate family medicine residency program. *Academic Medicine*, *90*(11), 1515–1526.

Melville, C., Rees, M., Brookfield, D., & Anderson, J. (2004). Portfolios for assessment of pediatric specialist registrars. *Medical Education*, *38*, 1117–1125.

Moores, A., & Parks, M. (2010). Twelve tips for introducing e-Portfolios with undergraduate students. *Medical Teacher*, *32*(1), 46–49.

Nabors, C., Forman, L., Peterson, S.J., Gennarelli, M., Aronow, W.S., DeLorenzo, L., . . . Frishman, W.H. (2017). Milestones: A rapid assessment method for the clinical competency committee. *Archives of Medical Science*, *13*(1), 201–209.

Nagler, A., Andolsek, K., & Padmore, J.S. (2009). The unintended consequences of portfolios in graduate medical education. *Academic Medicine*, *84*(11), 1522–1526.

O'Brien, C.L., Sanguino, S.M., Thomas, J.X., & Green, M.M. (2016). Feasibility and outcomes of implementing a portfolio assessment system alongside a traditional grading system. *Academic Medicine*, *91*(11), 1554–1560.

O'Sullivan, P.S., Cogbill, K.K., McClain, T., Reckase, M.D., & Clardy, J.A. (2002). Portfolios as a novel approach for residency evaluation. *Academic Psychiatry*, *26*, 173–179.

O'Sullivan, P.S., Reckase, M.D., McClain, T., Savidge, M.A., & Clardy, J.A. (2004). Demonstration of portfolios to assess competency of residents. *Advances in Health Sciences Education*, *9*, 309–323.

Oudkerk Pool, A., Govaerts, M.J.B., Jaarsma, D.A.D.C., & Driessen, E.W. (2017). From aggregation to interpretation: How assessors judge complex data in a competency-based portfolio. *Advanves in Health Sciences Education: Theory and Practice*, *23*(2), 275–287.

Paulson, F.L., Paulson, P.P., & Meyer, C.A. (1991). What makes a portfolio a portfolio? *Educational Leadership*, *48*, 60–63.

Pinsky, L.E., & Fryer-Edwards, K. (2004). Diving for PERLS: Working and performance portfolios for evaluation and reflection on learning. *Journal of General Internal Medicine*, *19*, 582–587.

Pitkala, K., & Mantyranta, T. (2004). Feelings related to first patient experiences in medical school: A qualitative study on students' personal portfolios. *Patient Education and Counseling*, *54*, 71–177.

Pitts, J. (2007). Portfolios, personal development and reflective practice. Pages 1–24. Association for the Study of Medical Education (ASME) Edinburgh.

Pitts, J., Coles, C., Thomas, P., & Smith, F. (2002). Enhancing reliability in portfolio assessment: Discussions between assessors. *Medical Teacher*, *24*(2), 197–201.

Rees, C. (2005). The use (and abuse) of the term "portfolio". *Medical Education*, *39*, 436–437.

Rees, C., & Sheard, C. (2004). The reliability of assessment criteria for undergraduate medical students' communication skills portfolios: The Nottingham experience. *Medical Education*, *38*, 138–144.

Regehr, G.E.K. (2006). Self-assessment, self-direction, and the self-regulating professional. *Clinical Orthopedics and Related Research*, *449*, 34–38.

Roberts, C., Newble, D., & O'Rourke, A. (2002). Portfolio-based assessments in medical education: Are they valid and reliable for summative purposes? *Medical Education*, *36*, 899–900.

Roberts, C., Shadbolt, N., Clark, T., & Simpson, P. (2014). The reliability and validity of a portfolio designed as a programmatic assessment of performance in an integrated clinical placement. *BMC Medical Education, 14*, 197.

Ryan, R.D.E. (2000). Self-Determination Theory and the Facilitation of Intrinsic Motivation, Social Development, and Well-Being. *American Psychologist, 55*(1), 68–78.

Sargeant, J.A.H., Chesluk, B., Dornan, T., Eva, K., Holmboe, E., Lockyer, J., Loney, E., Mann, K., & van der Vleuten, C. (2010). The processes and dimensions of informed self-assessment: A conceptual model. *Academic Medicine, 85*, 1212–1220.

Schmitz, C.C., Whitson, B.A., Van Heest, A., & Maddaus, M.A. (2010). Establishing a usable electronic portfolio for surgical residents: Trying to keep it simple. *Journal of Surgical Education, 67*(1), 14–18.

Schön, D.A. (1987). *Educating the reflective practitioner.* San Francisco: Jossey-Bass Publishers.

Schumacher, D.J., King, B., Barnes, M.M., Elliott, S.P., Gibbs, K., McGreevy, J.F., de Rey, J.G., Michelson, C., Schwartz, A., and Members of the APPD LEARN CCC Study Group. (2018). Influence of clinical competency committee review process on summative resident assessment decisions. *The Journal of Graduate Medical Education, 10*(4), 429–437.

Schumacher, D.J., Michelson, C., Poynter, S., Barnes, M.M., Li, S.T., Burman, N., . . . the APPD LEARN CCC Study Group. (2018). Thresholds and interpretations: How clinical competency committees identify pediatric residents with performance concerns. *Medical Teacher, 40*(1), 70–79.

Sklansky, D.J., Frohna, J.G., & Schumacher, D.J. (2017). Learner-driven synthesis of assessment data: Engaging and motivating residents in their milestone-based assessments. *Medical Science Educator, 27*(2), 417–421.

Tochel, C., Haig, A., Hesketh, A., Cadzow, A., Beggs, K., Colthart, I., & Peacock, H. (2009). The effectiveness of portfolios for post-graduate assessment and education: BEME guide no 12. *Medical Teacher, 31*(4), 299–318.

van der Vleuten, C. (1996). The assessment of professional competence: Developments, research and practical implications. *Advances in Health Sciences Education, 1*, 41–67.

Van Tartwijk, J., & Driessen, E.W. (2009). Portfolios for assessment and learning: AMEE guide no. 45. *Medical Teacher, 31*(9), 790–801.

Watling, C.D.E., van der Vleuten, C.P.M., & Lingard, L. (2012). Learning from clinical work: The roles of learning cues and credibility judgements. *Medical Education, 46*, 192–200.

Ward, M., Gruppen, L., & Regehr, G. (2002). Measuring self-assessment: Current state of the art. *Advances in Health Sciences Education: Theory and Practice, 7*, 63–80.

Webb, C., Endacott, R., Gray, M., Jasper, M., Miller, C., McMullan, M., & Scholes, J. (2002). Models of portfolios. *Medical Education, 36*(10), 897–898.

Williams, M., & Jordan, K. (2007). The nursing professional portfolio. *Journal for Nurses in Staff Development, 23*(3), 125–131.

PART III

SPECIAL TOPICS

PART III

SPECIAL TOPICS

13

KEY FEATURES APPROACH

Georges Bordage and Gordon Page

Based on research from Elstein and Shulman (1978) that showed that medical problem solving is case specific, the key features (KFs) approach was introduced as a means of "focusing assessment on the unique and challenging decisions in each clinical situation" (Norman et al., 1985). The KFs approach is not meant to assess the underlying knowledge or reasoning processes of the candidates, but rather to focus solely on the critical, case-specific decisions or actions. Advantages of KF-based questions include the fact that they can be formulated using different types of question formats to best fit the nature of the clinical task assessed and can allow for multiple correct answers depending on the complexity of the task being assessed. We begin by describing the process of developing and scoring KF cases and end by discussing how the KFs approach can address two major threats to validity, namely construct underrepresentation and construct-irrelevant variance.

A KF case generally begins with a scenario that includes the patient's age and gender and the clinical situation, for example, "An unknown man in his thirties is brought to the emergency room by ambulance because he collapsed on to the sidewalk while waiting for the bus. After falling, he began to twitch for a short while . . . etc." The scenario is followed by two or three questions to specifically assess the unique challenging decisions and actions in the resolution of the problem at hand, the problem's KFs. Typically, one question is used to test one KF; occasionally, one question may test two KFs, for example, asking, "What will you do next?" can test simultaneously an investigation KF and a treatment KF. The development of KF cases and questions goes through three separate and sequential steps, that is, selecting clinical problems, defining KFs, and preparing test material (i.e., clinical scenarios, test questions, and scoring keys).

SELECTING KF PROBLEMS

The goal of selecting clinical problems for an exam is to have a representative and adequate number of problems from the domain for which the candidates are held accountable (Bordage, 1987; Page & Bordage, 1995). For example, the domain for graduating medical students seeking qualification to practice in Canada is defined in a set of objectives listed as clinical presentations (e.g., chest pain, abdominal-pelvic mass, falls, seizures, family violence, etc.) (Medical Council of

Canada, 2018a). The selection of problems is guided by a test blueprint, either by selecting problems randomly from the domain or according to one or a number of organizing dimensions such as medical disciplines or organ systems, focus of care (Touchie & Streefkerk, 2018), or patient age groups (Bordage, 1987). The number of problems to be included on the exam can be estimated using the Spearman-Brown prophecy formula that would best yield a specified level of reliability (internal consistency), for example 0.70 for a locally developed test or 0.80 or 0.90 for a high-stakes, certification, or licensing exam (see Chapter 3); in the latter case, that would mean about 35 to 40 cases (Bordage & Page, 2018).

DEFINING KFS

Developing a KF-based examination typically entails working with a committee of clinician item writers. Once the clinical problems have been selected based on the test blueprint, one or two committee members are asked to define the KFs for a set of problems as a homework assignment, using the literature and their own experience and that of colleagues. Note that given the same problem, the KFs can be different depending on the level of knowledge and experience of the candidates being tested, for example medical students compared to residents or specialists. The unique KFs for a given problem also depend on the clinical situation in which the problem occurs (Bordage, 1987). For example, different KFs will be generated depending on whether one is assessing the management of congestive heart failure as an undifferentiated complaint compared to a multisystem event or preventive care.

KFs can be viewed as the difficult aspects of a case in practice or the actions most likely to cause errors (Page, Bordage, & Allen, 1995); for example, where do interns go wrong in this situation? These are the unique critical decisions that will best discriminate among varying levels of ability from stronger to weaker examinees (Bordage & Page, 2018). Box 13.1 contains an example of the KFs defined for a problem of seizures, cast as a life-threatening situation in an adult, and intended for assessing graduating medical students.

Research indicates that two to three KFs per case maximizes test score reliability (Norman, Bordage, Page, & Keane, 2006); fewer KFs per case reduces testing information and lowers test score reliability, whereas using more than three KFs provides only redundant measurement information, resulting in a waste of testing time.

Box 13.1 Example of the KFs for a Problem of Seizures

Given an adult brought to the emergency room with multiple seizures and without having regained full consciousness, the graduating medical student (new intern) will:

1. Generate a provisional diagnosis of status epilepticus;
2. Begin immediate initial management: secure airways, vitamin complex, bolus of hypertonic glucose, and anti-epileptic medication; and
3. Order immediate investigation to identify potentially treatable causes of the seizures: alcohol level, arterial blood gases, brain CT or MRI, serum calcium, serum, and drug screening. Note: Although appropriate, electrolytes and serum glucose were not included in the KF because they are part of routine orders in this situation and not likely to discriminate among interns.

Source: Adapted, with permission, from an example from the Medical Council of Canada's *Guidelines for the Development of Key Feature Problems and Test Cases, 2012*

The initial, draft KFs are then presented to the test committee as a whole, or to colleagues, for possible refinement and approval. KFs are defined in relation to the range of cases related to the clinical problem selected and not solely based on one particular case that an item writer might have seen recently. Writing a test case and questions are done as a separate and subsequent step, taking into consideration the problem and KFs selected for assessment.

PREPARING KF TEST MATERIAL

With KFs in hand, the item writer is then asked to prepare the test material, that is: (i) an opening clinical scenario, as dictated by the KFs to be tested, (ii) test questions to assess only the KFs, (iii) a scoring key for each KF, and (iv) one or two references from the literature to support the KFs tested. The selection and training of item writers is a key contributor to the quality of the test material. Selection criteria include the established clinical expertise of the item writers and their ongoing experience with the specific type of candidates being assessed (e.g., medical students, residents, fellows, family physicians, or specialists).

The initial scenario must contain the kind of information, and in sufficient amount, that prompts the candidates to interpret the information in order to make decisions. Eva, Wood, Riddle, Touchie, and Bordage (2010), in their study of the effect of lay versus medical terms in the scenario, also recommend the use of lay terms to maximize test score reliability and testing time.

RESPONSE FORMATS

Answers to test questions can be obtained using a variety of constructed- or selected-response formats, for example, short-answer, written, or oral responses (e.g., *What is your leading working diagnosis(es) at this point in time? You may not list more than two.*), multiple-choice short menus with as few as three or four options or as many as 25–30 options depending on the task (e.g., *What lab test(s), if any, will you order at this time? You may not select more than six.*), or computerized, dialogue-box long menus (Rotthoff et al., 2006). The selection of a particular response format depends on the nature of the assessment task; for example, using a short menu or actual order forms when requesting laboratory tests or imaging, as would occur normally in practice, or using a write-in format when eliciting a working diagnosis. Write-in responses are especially useful for diagnosis and management questions that require short answers (e.g., two–three words) and are more discriminating, especially around the pass-fail cut score (Page, Boulais, Blackmore, & Dauphinee, 2000; Bordage & Page, 2018).

Although the KFs approach was developed initially for paper-and-pencil exams, the approach can be used just as well for other test formats, such as multiple-choice questions, OSCEs, or structured oral exams (Jacques, Sindon, Bourque, Bordage, & Ferland, 1995). In the case of OSCEs and when selecting checklist items for a clinical task, the item writer, instead of seeking thoroughness, can focus exclusively on items that would best discriminate among the performance levels of the candidates sitting the OSCE. Hence, this type of focused, discriminating checklist "improve[s] the reliability of checklist scores and reduce[s] the number of stations needed for acceptable reliability" (Daniels, Bordage, Gierl, & Yudkowsky, 2014).

SCORING

A KF may have a single or multiple correct answers "depending on the complexity of the challenge involved" (Bordage & Page, 2018); for example, an initial management may include intubation and the administration of hypertonic glucose, vitamin B, and anti-epileptic medication. Each KF can be scored using dichotomous (0/1) scoring (i.e., having all the correct answers) or a partial-credit (fraction) scoring (e.g., getting 0.75 when giving three out of four correct answers). The use of partial credit will maximize test score reliability because it contains more assessment information than a dichotomous score (Page & Bordage, 1995; Hrynchak, Glover Takahashi, & Nayer, 2014).

Write-in responses can be scored by human raters or by automated systems. Studies have shown that these automated systems produce results as good as, if not better than, human raters (Gierl, Latifi, Lai, Boulais, & de Champlain, 2014; Latifi, Gierl, Boulais, & de Champlain, 2016).

KF TEST SCORES

The unit of measurement for a KF exam is the case, not the questions or KFs, because from a psychometric perspective, items on an exam must be independent of one another (Bordage & Page, 2018). Hence, the response to any given question, in a KF case with multiple questions, may influence the response to other questions in the case, thus violating the principle of item independence.

The scores for the KFs within each case are averaged and given equal weight to produce a case score (e.g., for a case containing three KFs: (1 + .75 + .60) / 3 = 0.78). Equal weights are used since "[d]ifferential weighting does not improve test score reliability" (Norcini & Guille, 2002; Bordage & Page, 2018) and takes up a lot of unproductive test committee time. Schuwirth (1998) also found no empirical objection to "simply adding the scores of all the items without adjustment or weighting for the different number of alternatives in a question" (Bordage & Page, 2018).

For a KF-based exam as a whole, the case scores are also averaged, giving equal weight to each case (e.g., for a test containing 36 cases: (.67 + .75 ...) / 36 = .78, that is, this candidate mastered on average 78% of the KFs for each of the 36 cases on the test). The pass/fail cut score for a KF test can be set using a criterion, item-centered method, such as a straight or modified Angoff procedure (Chapter 6; Page & Bordage, 1995) or a bookmark method (Medical Council of Canada, 2018b).

The last step in preparing each KF case is to include one or two references from the literature to provide evidence for the appropriateness of the KFs. This is illustrated in Box 13.2 that contains an example of a multi-part KF case for graduating medical students, along with the scoring key and a reference. The questions presented in this case assess the three KFs presented as examples earlier in this chapter.

Box 13.2 Example of a Multi-Part Key Feature Case (Three Sections, Three Questions) and Its Scoring Key

Clinical Scenario

An unknown man in his thirties is brought to the emergency room by ambulance because he collapsed on to the sidewalk while waiting for the bus. A witness immediately called an ambulance and reported that before falling to the ground, the man seemed confused, agitated, and arguing with himself. After falling, he began to twitch for a short while, his face became blue, and then he began to have jerky movements all over his body for about a minute. He then partly recovered consciousness but remained confused. During the 12-minute ambulance ride, he presented a similar incident, without recovering full consciousness, and was given lorazepam 2 mg IV by the ambulance personnel who also installed a normal saline IV line.

On arrival in the emergency room, he had a third incident that you witnessed. His vital signs are: Pulse is 74/minute, regular; respiration rate is 16/minute, non-labored; blood pressure is 122/74 mmHg; temperature is 37.8 °C; and an oxygen saturation of 89% on room air. He looks neglected and is unconscious. No relatives or friends accompanied him. His capillary glucose level is 4.6 mmol/l.

Part 1

Question 1: What is (are) your leading working diagnosis(es) at this point in time? You may not list more than two.

1. _____
2. _____

STOP: Once you advance to the next section, you cannot come back and change your answers in the current section.

Part 2

Question 2: What is your immediate management (excluding investigation) at this point in time? Be specific; you may not list more than six.

1. _____
2. _____
3. _____
4. _____
5. _____
6. _____

STOP: Once you advance to the next section, you cannot come back and change your answers in the current section.

Part 3

Question 3: You have not been able to contact anyone who might know him. What investigation will you order at this point? You may select as many as you feel appropriate. Select option 35 if you do not wish to order any investigation at this time.

1. Alanine aminotransferase (ALT)
2. Alcohol level
3. Aldolase, serum
4. Alkaline phosphatase, serum
5. Amylase, serum
6. Arterial blood gases (ABG)
7. Aspartate aminotransferase (AST)
8. Brain CT-scan
9. Brain MRI
10. Brain PET-scan
11. Calcium, serum
12. Carotid US-doppler
13. Cerebral angiography
14. Cerebro-spinal fluid examination
15. Complete blood count (CBC)

16. C-Reactive protein
17. Creatine phosphokinase, serum
18. Creatinine, serum
19. Drug screening, serum
20. Drug screening, urine
21. Echovirus, serology
22. EEG recording
23. Electrolytes (Na, K, Cl)
24. g-Glutamyl transferase
25. Glucose, serum
26. Lactate dehydrogenase, serum
27. Lyme disease, serology
28. Protein electrophoresis, plasma
29. T4, Free
30. Temporal artery biopsy
31. Thyroid-stimulating hormone
32. Total protein, plasma
33. Urea, serum
34. VDRL (Venereal Disease Research Laboratory), serum
35. No investigation needed at this point in time

End of the case.

Scoring Key

Note: Correct answers to each element of a key feature receive partial credit. Over-treatment, over-investigation, harmful decisions, or going over the stated response limit results in 0 points for the entire key feature.

Question 1: KF-1: *Given an adult brought to the emergency room with multiple seizures and without having regained full consciousness, the graduating medical student (new intern) will generate a provisional diagnosis of status epilepticus.*

Points	Keyed responses
1	Status epilepticus. Note: Both elements are required; epilepsy alone is not acceptable.
0	Wrote more than two diagnoses.

Note: If the KF case is presented via computer or by an examiner in an oral examination situation, either the computer or the examiner may or may not allow a candidate to list more than the permitted number of responses.

Question 2: KF-2: *Begin immediate initial management: secure airways, vitamin B complex, bolus hypertonic glucose, and anti-epileptic medication.*

Points	Keyed responses
0.25	Intubation, mechanical ventilation, or secure airways. Note: Oxygen alone is *not* acceptable.

0.25	Vitamin B, B1, or thiamine.
0.25	Glucose, hypertonic, bolus. Note: All three elements are required.
0.25	[lorazepam or diazepam or clonazepam] AND [phenytoin *or valproate sodium or levetiracetam*]
0	Listed more than five responses or wrote "none."

Question 3: KF-3: *Order immediate investigation to identify potentially treatable causes of the seizures: Alcohol level, ABG, brain CT or MRI, drug-screening test, and serum calcium.*

Points	Keyed responses
0.20	2. Alcohol level
0.20	6. Arterial blood gases (ABG)
0.20	8. Brain CT or 9. Brain MRI
0.20	11. Calcium, serum
0.20	19. Drug screening, serum or 20. Drug screening, urine
0	Selected more than eight options (i.e., over-investigation) or selected option 35.

Reference

Brophy, G.M., Bell, R., Claassen, J., Alldredge, B., Bleck, T.P., Glauser, T., Laroche, S.M., Riviello, J.J., Jr., Shutter, L., Sperling, M.R., Treiman, D.M., Vespa, P.M. (2012). Neurocritical Care Society Status Epilepticus Guideline Writing Committee. Guidelines for the Evaluation and Management of Status Epilepticus. *Neurocritical Care, 17,* 3–23.

Source: Adapted, with permission, from an example from the Medical Council of Canada's *Guidelines for the Development of Key Feature Problems and Test Cases, 2012*

Once the test material is ready, it is presented to the committee as a whole or a group of colleagues for discussion and approval. These peer-reviewed verifications of the KFs and test material and corresponding revisions will contribute greatly to ensuring the high quality of the exam. It is also highly recommended to pilot test the cases before actually using them. The item analysis data and reliability estimates and the candidates' comments from the pilot test or information from prior administrations can be used to revise ambiguous or non-discriminating items.

KF-based tests have been used for assessment purposes at various levels of training, including medical students (e.g., Hatala & Norman, 2002), residents (e.g., Hinchy & Farmer, 2005), and practicing health professionals (e.g., Trudel, Bordage, & Downing, 2008), either to make pass/fail decisions about candidates, to provide formative feedback, or to rank candidates for selection purposes. KF cases have also been used for research and instructional purposes. Guidelines for the development of KF cases and exams have also been published (e.g., Farmer & Page, 2005; Kopp, Möltner, & Fischer, 2006 [in German]; MCC Guidelines, 2012 [in French and English]). See Bordage and Page (2018) for detailed listings of uses and guidelines.

If the test results are used for formative purposes, then more detailed post-test information can be provided to the examinees and their supervisors to help prepare a learning plan. Information may contain the candidate's performance regarding each case as captured in the information-rich scoring keys, including the number of potentially harmful actions taken for the set of cases on the test.

The KFs approach was developed to address major threats to validity, namely construct underrepresentation and construct-irrelevant variance.

CONSTRUCT UNDERREPRESENTATION

Three measures can be taken to address construct underrepresentation when preparing KF cases and exams. First, KF cases shift the object of assessment from clinical reasoning and problem-solving skills in general to "focusing only on the most challenging clinical decisions and actions in each case, resulting in tests with many short, focused cases" (Bordage & Page, 2018). Second, KF exams can be built to contain the required number of cases to obtain reliability coefficients in the 0.7 to 0.9 range, depending on the stakes of the exam. Accordingly, KF exams contain a broad range and variety of cases to yield a more representative sample of cases from the domain to be assessed, compared to oral exams for example.

CONSTRUCT-IRRELEVANT VARIANCE

Two measures can be taken specifically to address construct-irrelevant variance. First, item writers can use a variety of response formats to better fit the nature of the clinical task assessed. Furthermore, cueing can be minimized by using written response questions or short menus that resemble order forms in practice. Second, each decision or action is scored only in relation to the case's KFs, whereas in the past, scoring overly rewarded thoroughness, despite the fact that thoroughness is a poor predictor of performance (Elstein & Shulman, 1978; Bordage & Page, 2018).

More generally speaking and using the unitary framework of construct validity as presented in the *Standards for Educational and Psychological Testing* (AERA, APA, & NCME, 2014), Bordage and Page (2018) provide a detailed analysis of the validity evidence gathered to date regarding the KFs approach. The validity evidence gathered strongly supports the KFs approach.

In summary, the KFs approach is aimed at assessing applied knowledge, "knows how" in Miller's pyramid, for case-specific decisions and actions. It is not an item or test format as such or an assessment of clinical reasoning. A KF test contains an adequate and representative sample of clinical problems and a scoring procedure that only rewards mastery of critical, challenging decisions or actions for the candidates taking the test. The varied response formats of a KF question or examination are selected to best fit the nature of the clinical task being assessed. Finally, a criterion, item-centered approach to setting cut scores results in defensible pass/fail decisions.

ACKNOWLEDGEMENTS

We are grateful to the Medical Council of Canada for their permission to adapt one of their examples of a KF case and to Drs. M.R. Nendaz, M.D., MHPE (Geneva, Switzerland) and G. Bandiera, M.D., MEd (Toronto, Canada) for their contribution to the example of a KF case.

Note: Additional material and resources may be available at the UIC AHPE website: https://go.uic.edu/AHPE

REFERENCES

American Educational Research Association AERA, American Psychological Association APA, Joint Committee on Standards for Educational, Psychological Testing (US), & National Council on Measurement in Education NCME. (2014). *Standards for educational and psychological testing*. Washington, DC: American Educational Research Association.

Bordage, G. (1987). An alternative approach to PMPs. The "key features" concept. In I.R. Hart & R.M. Harden (Eds.), *Further developments in assessing clinical competence* (pp. 59–75). Montreal: Can-Heal Publications.

Bordage, G., & Page, G. (2018). The key-features approach to assess clinical decisions: Validity evidence to date. *Advances in Health Sciences Education*, 1–32.

Daniels, V.J., Bordage, G., Gierl, M.J., & Yudkowsky, R. (2014). Effect of clinically discriminating, evidence-based checklist items on the reliability of scores from an Internal Medicine residency OSCE. *Advances in Health Sciences Education*, 19(4), 497–506.

Elstein, A., Shulman, L., & Sprafka, S.A. (1978). *Medical problem solving.* Cambridge, MA: Harvard University Press.

Eva, K.W., Wood, T.J., Riddle, J., Touchie, C., & Bordage, G. (2010). How clinical features are presented matters to weaker diagnosticians. *Medical Education, 44*(8), 775–785.

Farmer, E.A., & Page, G. (2005). A practical guide to assessing clinical decision-making skills using the key features approach. *Medical Education, 39*(12), 1188–1194.

Gierl, M.J., Latifi, S., Lai, H., Boulais, A.P., & de Champlain, A. (2014). Automated essay scoring and the future of educational assessment in medical education. *Medical Education, 48*(10), 950–962.

Hatala, R., & Norman, G.R. (2002). Adapting the key features examination for a clinical clerkship. *Medical Education, 36*(2), 160–165.

Hinchy, J., & Farmer, E. (2005). Assessing general practice clinical decision making skills: The key features approach. *Australian Family Physician, 34*(12), 1059.

Hrynchak, P., Glover Takahashi, S., & Nayer, M. (2014). Key-feature questions for assessment of clinical reasoning: A literature review. *Medical Education, 48*(9), 870–883.

Jacques, A., Sindon, A., Bourque, A., Bordage, G., & Ferland, J.J. (1995). Structured oral interview. One way to identify family physicians' educational needs. *Canadian Family Physician, 41*, 1346.

Kopp, V., Möltner, A., & Fischer, M.R. (2006). Key-Feature-Probleme zum Prüfen von prozeduralem Wissen: Ein Praxisleitfaden. *GMS Zeitschrift Für Medizinische Ausbildung, 23*(3), 2006–2023.

Latifi, S., Gierl, M.J., Boulais, A.P., & de Champlain, A.F. (2016). Using automated scoring to evaluate written responses in English and French on a high-stakes clinical competency examination. *Evaluation & the Health Professions, 39*(1), 100–113.

Medical Council of Canada. (2012). *Guidelines for the development of key feature problems and test cases.* Ottawa, ON: Medical Council of Canada. Retrieved from http://mcc.ca/wp-content/uploads/CDM-Guidelines.pdf.

Medical Council of Canada. (2018a). *Exam objectives overview.* Retrieved from http://mcc.ca/objectives/.

Medical Council of Canada. (2018b). *MCCQE part I annual technical report.* Canada, 2016. Retrieved from http://mcc.ca/wp-content/uploads/MCCQE-Part-I-Annual-Technical-Report-2016-EN.pdf.

Norcini, J.J., & Guille, R. (2002). Chapter 25: Combining tests and setting standards. In: G.R. Norman, C.P.M. van der Vleuten, & D.I. Newble (Eds.), *International handbook of research in medical education.* Springer International Handbooks of Education. New York: Springer-Verlag.

Norman, G., Bordage, G., Curry, L., et al. (1985). Review of recent innovations in assessment. In R. Wakeford (Ed.), *Directions in clinical assessment.* Report of the Cambridge Conference on the Assessment of Clinical Competence. Cambridge: Office of the Regius Professor of Physic.

Norman, G., Bordage, G., Page, G., & Keane, D. (2006). How specific is case specificity? *Medical Education, 40*(7), 618–623.

Page, G., & Bordage, G. (1995). The Medical Council of Canada's key features project: A more valid written examination of clinical decision-making skills. *Academic Medicine: Journal of the Association of American Medical Colleges, 70*(2), 104–110.

Page, G., Bordage, G., & Allen, T. (1995). Developing key-feature problems and examinations to assess clinical decision-making skills. *Academic Medicine, 70*(3), 194–201.

Page, G., Boulais, A.P., Blackmore, D., & Dauphinee, D. (2000). *Justifying the use of short answer questions in the KF problems of the MCCC's qualifying exam.* Proceedings of the 9th Ottawa Conference on Medical Education, Cape Town.

Rotthoff, T., Baehring, T., Dicken, H.D., Fahron, U., Richter, B., Fischer, M.R., & Scherbaum, W.A. (2006). Comparison between long-menu and open-ended questions in computerized medical assessments. A randomized controlled trial. *BMC Medical Education, 6*(1), 50.

Schuwirth, L.W.T. (1998). *An approach to the assessment of medical problem solving: Computerised Case-based Testing.* Doctoral dissertation. Maastricht, The Netherlands: Maastricht University.

Touchie, C., & Streefkerk, C. (2018). *Blueprint project—qualifying examinations blueprint and content specifications.* Ottawa, ON. Retrieved from http://mcc.ca/wp-content/uploads/Blueprint-Report.pdf.

Trudel, J.L., Bordage, G., & Downing, S.M. (2008). Reliability and validity of key feature cases for the self-assessment of colon and rectal surgeons. *Annals of Surgery, 248*(2), 252–258.

14

SIMULATIONS IN ASSESSMENT

Luke A. Devine, William C. McGaghie, and Barry Issenberg

INTRODUCTION

This chapter addresses the role of simulation in the assessment of training and practicing health professionals. It amplifies, but does not duplicate, the lessons of Chapter 9, which discusses performance tests, and Chapter 10 on workplace-based assessment methods. This chapter is about how to design and implement simulation-based assessments (SBAs) to assess learners. In many institutions and programs, simulations have become an essential component of health professions education. Simulations give context to assessments by engaging learners in professional situations that resemble "in vivo" conditions.

This chapter focuses on the use of simulation in summative assessment. It should be noted, however, that simulation is a powerful teaching tool that is also commonly used in formative assessment. When used for formative assessment, feedback and debriefing are essential components of simulation (Issenberg, McGaghie, Petrusa, Gordon, & Scalese, 2005). Feedback is specific information that is provided to a learner about gaps between desired and observed performance, with the goal of improving future performance (van de Ridder, McGaghie, Stokking, & ten Cate, 2015). Feedback derives from various sources, including a simulator, a standardized patient (SP), peers and instructors, and can occur during or after a simulation activity (Motola, Devine, Chung, Sullivan, & Issenberg, 2013). Debriefing involves an interaction that prompts learner reflection to improve future learning and performance (Cheng et al., 2014).

This chapter has six sections. The first two sections discuss key background matters: (1) what is simulation and why use it? and (2) when to use simulation for assessment. The next section provides educators practical advice on (3) how to use simulation in assessment to achieve their assessment goals. This is followed by a discussion of (4) threats to the validity of SBAs, (5) faculty development needed to implement SBAs and (6) the consequences and educational impact of SBAs. We assume that readers have covered the introductory chapter to this book and have a basic understanding of the concepts of validity (Chapter 2), reliability (Chapter 3) and standard setting (Chapter 6). Familiarity with assessment principles discussed in these and other chapters will make it easier for educators to determine how to use simulation in their assessment plans.

WHAT IS SIMULATION AND WHY USE IT?

A common definition of simulation comes from Gaba (2007, p. 126): "Simulation is a technique—not a technology—to replace or amplify real experiences with guided experiences that evoke or replicate substantial aspects of the real world in a fully interactive manner." It is important to note that *simulation* is a technique to represent real-word conditions in an authentic manner, while a *simulator* is a device used in simulation. The examples used in this chapter will focus primarily on technology-based simulation modalities such as part-task trainers, responsive mannequins and virtual reality devices. Simulations can also be as simple as paper or computer-based patient problems or can involve the use of SPs. When simulation is discussed in broad terms throughout this chapter, the principles described also apply to the use of SPs and other forms of simulation. SPs also are discussed in detail in Chapter 9.

The use of simulation has become widespread for many reasons. Simulation allows for learners to train, receive feedback and be assessed without putting patients at risk of harm (Ziv, Wolpe, Small, & Glick, 2006). Simulators can be used at any time, including after hours, for self-directed learning (Brydges, Nair, Ma, Shanks, & Hatala, 2012) and can represent a range of clinical conditions, including rare and life-threatening conditions. A large study conducted by the US National Council of State Boards of Nursing demonstrated that up to 50% of traditional clinical hours could be replaced by simulation-based training (Hayden, Smiley, Alexander, Kardong-Edgren, & Jeffries, 2014). The use of simulation has also expanded, because improving technology has allowed for an increasing number of clinical contexts to be mimicked. Most importantly, simulation-based healthcare education (SBHE) is an impactful educational tool that research has shown to be effective (Cook, Brydges, Zendejas, Hamstra, & Hatala, 2013; McGaghie, Issenberg, Cohen, Barsuk, & Wayne, 2011).

WHEN TO USE SIMULATION IN ASSESSMENT

There are many benefits to simulation in the assessment of healthcare professionals. SBA is an excellent way to assess (a) procedural skills, (b) critical thinking and responses to changing circumstances, (c) behavior under stress, (d) communication skills and (e) teamwork. Although SBA can be used to assess at the "knows" and "knows how" levels of Miller's pyramid, it is best suited to assess performance at the "shows how" level. Similar to performance assessments using SPs, SBAs can consistently and repeatedly present clinical situations to learners in a standardized way. Standardization is important because to improve reliability, we must minimize variation or error related to factors (e.g., the patient, simulator or the examiner) other than the performance of the candidate being assessed. Simulators can often collect performance data that can be used alone or in combination with examiner observations to score an assessment. Simulations can now imitate countless clinical situations, allowing a broad range of content to be sampled within an SBA program.

SBAs are increasingly being incorporated into "high-stakes" assessments in certification and licensing examinations, including in internal medicine in Canada (Hatala, Kassen, Nishikawa, Cole, & Issenberg, 2005), in anesthesiology in Israel (Berkenstadt, Ziv, Gafni, & Sidi, 2006) and for nurses in many jurisdictions (Ziv, Berkenstadt, & Eisenberg, 2013). SBAs are also used for candidate selection into health professions education programs (Eva et al., 2012), for promotion to subsequent levels of training (Papadakis, 2004), in maintenance of certification programs (Holmboe, Rizzolo et al., 2011) and in retraining and remediation activities (Levine, Schwartz, Bryson, & DeMaria Jr, 2012).

HOW TO USE SIMULATION IN ASSESSMENT

Groups developing SBAs must have relevant expertise and work together to design appropriate and effective assessments. Education experts and psychometricians must collaborate with content experts and simulation experts to ensure that solid measures of performance are created. We endorse a seven-step plan for assessment design drawn from several sources to create an assessment program's architecture (Downing, 2006; Nehring & Lashley, 2010; Scalese & Issenberg, 2008). The steps in this plan are not always sequential and are often iterative. The plan is a practical guide for faculty and program directors who aim to match educational assessment goals with suitable SBAs. Table 14.1 lists the seven assessment planning steps. The discussion following amplifies each step.

Determine Learning Outcome(s)

The most important step in designing an assessment is determining and defining what learning outcomes are to be assessed. These outcomes are statements that describe what the successful learner can demonstrate at the end of or at a predefined point in training, and they must align with the overall goals and objectives of the curriculum (Dent, Harden, & Hunt, 2017). Health professions educators need to have one or more learning outcomes clearly articulated before selecting and using SBA methods. *The outcomes-methods match is the most important message of this chapter.* Educators should not use simulation modalities for learner assessment without understanding the assessment goals and outcomes, context, and consequences.

Like other assessments, the content of an SBA is best captured by a blueprint (Chapter 2) that identifies the cases, tasks or other content to be included (and, by inference, excluded) in an assessment and how they will elicit the response to be evaluated. Responses might include making a diagnosis, performing a procedure, formulating a management plan or knowing when to get help.

Table 14.1 Seven Steps for Planning a Simulation-Based Assessment

Step	Features
Determine Learning Outcome(s)	• Determine what is to be assessed • Align with curriculum • Blueprint appropriately
Choose an Assessment Method	• Determine if simulation is most appropriate method for a given outcome • Consider validity, reliability, educational impact, cost, acceptability (van Der Vleuten, 1996)
Choose a Simulation Modality	• Part-task trainer with normal and/or abnormal findings • Responsive mannequins • Virtual or augmented reality • Standardized patients • Multi-modal
Develop Assessment Scenario	• Outline necessary equipment, environment, simulator • Create prompts, scripts, scenario flow diagrams • Pilot test
Score the Assessment	• Determine how data will be obtained from the simulation activity and develop data collection method • Can be checklist or global rating data, automatically recorded process data or data from assessment of the "product" of an activity
Set Standards for the Assessment	• Apply standard-setting procedures appropriate for the stakes of the assessment (Chapter 6) • Consider examinee-based standards where appropriate
Standardize Test Conditions	• Standardize components of the simulation/scenario and examiner rating • Pilot test to determine likely range of examinee behavior to plan appropriate simulator and SP responses within the SBA

An example of a blueprint for an SBA for an end-of-year objective structured clinical examination (OSCE, see Chapter 9) for post-graduate year 3 internal medicine residents is shown in Tables 14.2 and 14.3. For illustrative purposes, we have included only four stations on this OSCE; however, depending upon the purpose and stakes of the assessment, additional stations and content would need be included to improve reliability and ensure adequate sampling of content. Table 14.2 outlines the core competencies expected of the resident, based upon the CanMEDS Framework (Frank, Snell, & Sherbino, 2015) and details that are assessed in a given station. SBA content may also be blueprinted based upon other criteria, including certain tasks (history taking, physical examination, performing a procedure, etc.), and specific content areas. The blueprint will depend upon desired outcomes and the existing curriculum. Table 14.3 outlines the SBA stations that were designed, using the seven-step approach, to assess the desired outcomes.

Table 14.2 Simulation-Based Assessment Blueprint Mapping the Four Stations of an OSCE Onto CanMEDS Competencies

Station	Medical Expert	Communicator	Collaborator	Leader	Health Advocate	Scholar	Professional
1	X	X			X		X
2	X	X					X
3	X	X	X				
4		X	X	X	X	X	

Table 14.3 Outcomes to Be Assessed and Description of the Four Stations of a Simulation-Based OSCE

Station	Outcome	Description	Type of Simulation/ Simulator
1	Lead a discussion with an acutely ill patient's substitute decision maker regarding advanced directives and goals of care. Demonstrate an understanding of principles substitute decision makers must use when making a decision on a patient's behalf.	Learner is provided patient's background information: it is an elderly patient with advanced dementia and multiple medical comorbidities and has been admitted with severe sepsis. His preexisting quality of life would be considered low and he has a < 5% chance of surviving this admission and returning to his recent quality of life. The learner meets with the patient's spouse (who is the substitute decision maker for health decisions) to discuss prognosis and determine his goals of care and advanced directives for this admission.	Standardized patient (SP) (in this case, a standardized caregiver or decision maker—the patient's partner)
2	Demonstrate effective performance of knee arthrocentesis. Demonstrate ability to obtain informed consent for a procedure. Maintain awareness of, and attend to, patient comfort.	Part-task trainer is an ultrasound compatible knee for arthrocentesis. Simulator is positioned next to the SP on a bed, and the SP is draped so the simulated knee appears to be his (Stroud & Cavalcanti, 2013). The SP portrays the role of a 42-year-old male with an acute monoarthritis of the right knee; a diagnosis of septic arthritis is suspected. The learner must obtain informed consent for the procedure, and then conduct the entire procedure while interacting with the SP. The SP has anxiety about the procedure.	Multi-modal simulation involving an SP and part-task trainer

(Continued)

Table 14.3 (continued)

Station	Outcome	Description	Type of Simulation/ Simulator
3	Perform an integrated cardiac physical examination. Identify abnormal cardiac findings. Communicate clinical information and recommend management plan to surgical colleagues.	Learner is provided background information regarding a patient presenting for pre-operative assessment before elective knee replacement surgery. The learner must integrate information from the stem and from physical examination of a cardiopulmonary simulator in order to make recommendations to the surgeon and anesthetist involved in the patient's care. After examining the simulator, the learner will dictate a brief note.	Part-task trainer—cardiopulmonary simulator capable of displaying the components of an integrated precordial examination
4	Supervise a junior trainee and provide feedback regarding her use of a structured handover tool when providing handover to an on-call resident.	The learner is provided background material outlining clinical information on three patients admitted to the gastroenterology service. She is asked to supervise a final year medical student providing handover about these patients to the resident on call. She is asked to provide feedback and teaching to this student about handover skills using the framework used in their local training context.	SP-based with the scripted roles of a medical student providing handover and resident receiving handover played by SPs

SBA also permits training and assessment of teamwork skills, key competencies in the modern healthcare setting (Capella et al., 2010). A team composed of competent individuals does not automatically function as a competent team (Lingard, 2012). Specific leadership and teamwork must be taught and assessed (Salas, Rosen, & King, 2007). Simulation-based team training and assessment allow for these complex skills to be measured and observed in a more controlled manner than would be possible in a real-world situation. When designing scenarios involving teams, it is important to determine the outcomes of interest and ensure the scenario is designed to elicit the behavior to be assessed. The goal is not to assess individual competencies that can be evaluated outside of a complex team interaction. Instead, the assessment focus is teamwork skills such as communication, situational awareness, leadership and others (Gaba, Howard, Fish, Smith, & Sowb, 2001). If assessing the teamwork skills of an individual, the other team members in a simulation may be confederates (embedded participants in the simulation) aware of its outcomes and scripted to help guide the scenario and add realism to ensure a standardized experience for the individual being assessed (Nestel, Mobley, Hunt, & Eppich, 2014). SBA also allows the more complex assessment of entire teams to determine potential teamwork deficiencies and facilitating training and education targeted to improved team function (Box 14.1).

Choose an Assessment Method

The reliability, validity, acceptability, educational impact and cost of an assessment method must be considered when judging the utility of that method for assessing a given outcome (van der Vleuten, 1996). Educators must ensure that SBAs are used when they will have the most impact and be cost effective. SBAs are well suited to assess events that may be difficult to assess with workplace-based assessments (WBAs), such as rare and life-threatening situations, difficult communication or teamwork situations and procedural skills.

Box 14.1 Example of Teamwork-Focused Scenarios Using a Responsive Mannequin Simulator

Outcome (team)—demonstrate the ability for the team to efficiently assemble, establish leadership, demonstrate effective communication and provide mutual support.

Outcome (individual/team leader)—ensure a shared mental model of the patient's issues and care plan exist and maintain appropriate situational awareness.

Description—a multidisciplinary trauma team composed of the same team members that typically respond to the trauma are called to the trauma-bay to assess a 24-year-old female who presents with a gunshot wound to the right upper quadrant of the abdomen. Her vital signs upon transfer from the ambulance service are heart rate = 140/min., blood pressure = 84/62 mm Hg, respiratory rate = 16/min and O_2 saturation = 91% on 30% FiO_2.

The team members arrive to find the responsive mannequin in the trauma bay with the vital signs programmed as above and moulage (applying mock injuries using makeup or other means) demonstrating the gunshot wound entry site. The scenario is planned to have the patient respond realistically to provided medical interventions. Three minutes into the scenario, a deterioration in the patient condition is scripted to provide an additional challenge for the team to demonstrate appropriate teamwork skills.

The scenario can be conducted in the simulation laboratory or in the actual clinical environment in a scheduled or unannounced manner. Additional or alternative challenges can be planned to trigger situations in which desired behaviors can be assessed. For example, one of the team members can be a confederate who is scripted to distract the leader to impair their ability to maintain situational awareness or who creates communication challenges by not interacting in a collaborative manner with the team leader.

The international movement toward competency-based medical education (CBME) in health professions education has produced an increased focus on mechanisms for competence assessment. CBME is a mastery learning approach (see Chapter 18) that focuses on desired outcomes and recognizes that learners may require varying amounts of time to achieve these outcomes and develop competence (Frank et al., 2010). Although frequent formative WBAs are a cornerstone of assessment programs in CBME (see Chapter 10), other assessment methods, including simulation, continue to be important components in providing additional information about competency in various domains. SBAs are ideally suited to serve as part of the practice phase in a mastery learning model (Chapter 18).

As health professions education regulatory bodies and training programs implement competency-based training programs, they are defining competency domains and the outcomes within these domains that are expected of learners and professionals at various stages of training, such as the CanMEDS framework (Frank et al., 2015), ACGME milestones (Nasca, Philibert, Brigham, & Flynn, 2012) or the VetPro framework (Bok, 2015). In turn, educators within the various professions are working to determine which assessment methods (including simulation) are best suited to assess the required outcomes. One early example of the successful implementation of a competency-based curriculum was in an orthopedic surgery post-graduate education (residency) training program that used simulation as a key component in teaching and assessment (Ferguson et al., 2013). In this program, simulation is used in a "boot camp" to ensure all trainees can demonstrate basic technical skills before they complete other modules, which also regularly use simulation in formative and summative assessment of specific competencies (Nousiainen

---

Box 14.2 Toronto Orthopedic Boot Camp—An Example of Competency-Based Curriculum That Incorporates a Significant Simulation Component

The Division of Orthopedic surgery at the University of Toronto created a novel, comprehensive competency-based curriculum in 2010 for postgraduate trainees. All trainees complete a "boot camp" where basic surgical skills are learned. The boot camp incorporates five key principles (Mironova, Girardi, Burns, & Safir, 2018).

1. Flipped classroom
   - Increase engagement and maximize "hands-on" simulation time

2. Near-peer facilitators
   - More senior trainees provide guidance and feedback
   - This improves trainee-to-instructor ratios, improves socialization and reduces anxiety for the more junior trainees; staff physicians are also available to provide additional input and assistance

3. Graduated complexity
   - Start basic and build complexity to avoid cognitive overload

4. Case-based learning
   - Provide context for all simulations
   - Structured similar to oral certification exam cases

5. Formative feedback
   - Faculty development for instructors on how to provide feedback

In addition to frequent formative feedback, trainees complete a baseline objective structured assessment of technical skills (OSATS) and a comprehensive exit examination. Residents who do not meet the minimum passing standard undergo non-punitive remediation and retake the examination until the standard is met.

---

et al., 2016) (Box 14.2). The boot camp has been shown to greatly enhance knowledge and skills that are retained throughout training (Nousiainen et al., 2016).

Choose a Simulation Modality

Once it has been determined that an SBA is the best method to assess a learning outcome, educators must choose the type of simulation modality to be used. Simulation modalities include SPs, paper cases and other modalities that do not use specialized technology. One classification scheme for technology-enhanced simulation divides simulation modalities into part-task trainers, responsive mannequins and virtual and augmented reality devices. The distinction between these modalities is diminishing as many new simulators combine elements from more than one category.

Part-task trainers are anatomic models and single-task trainers (e.g., venipuncture arms and intubation mannequin heads) (Figure 14.1). These models generally provide limited performance

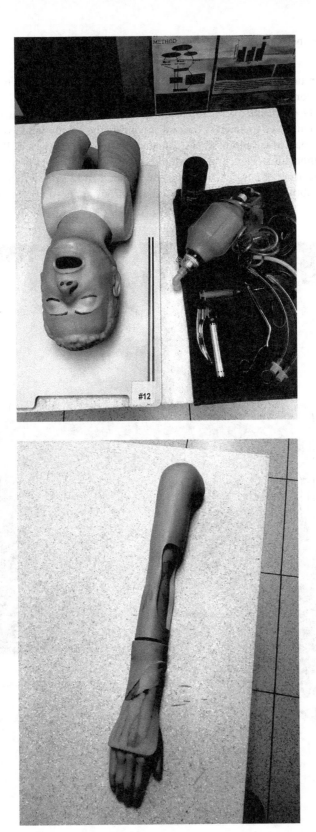

Figure 14.1 Part-task trainers for airway management and phlebotomy and intravenous catheter insertion simulation

Source: Photos courtesy of Surgical Skills Centre, University of Toronto

feedback, e.g., the return of blood after a vein has been successfully cannulated. Part-task trainers generally do not incorporate technologic components. Increasingly, certain features, such as ultrasound compatibility, or means to provide feedback on task performance, such as hand motion analysis, are being employed to increase the realism during the practice and assessment of certain tasks (Matsumoto, Hamstra, Radomski, & Cusimano, 2002; Perry, Bridges, & Burrow, 2015).

Responsive mannequins (Figure 14.2) are often life-sized and programmable to allow them to represent a wide array of clinical conditions on demand and respond dynamically to learner actions, such as defibrillation, administration of medications or anesthetic gases, or management

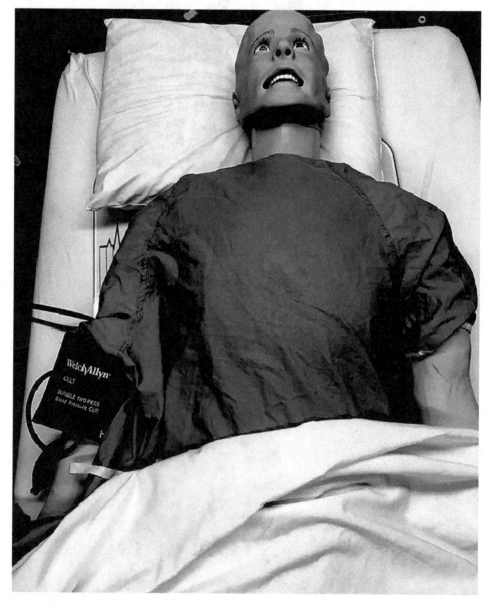

Figure 14.2 Responsive mannequin used for simulation-based education and assessment

Source: Photo courtesy of SimSinai, Mount Sinai Hospital, Toronto

of obstetrical emergencies (Scalese, 2018). They can be powerful tools to assess complex skills of individuals and teams, such as leadership, communication and critical thinking.

Virtual and augmented reality simulators involve digitally generated displays that simulate portions of the real world (Figure 14.3). Learners interact with them through various interfaces, such as more basic controllers similar to those used in video games to instruments used in actual clinical procedures. These simulators can provide audiovisual feedback as well as haptic feedback (e.g., touch, vibration, pressure, etc.) in response to learner actions. There are many examples of these simulators in medical training, including those used to train physicians to perform breast examination (Laufer et al., 2015) and surgeons to perform laparoscopic surgery (Grantcharov et al., 2004) and neurosurgical procedures (Yudkowsky et al., 2013). These simulators are used for teaching and assessment in many other fields, including the treatment of periodontal disease in dentistry (Steinberg, Bashook, Drummond, Ashrafi, & Zefran, 2007) and intravenous injection in veterinary medicine (Lee et al., 2013). Although often used to teach and assess procedural skills, these simulators can also be used to assess teamwork and other skills using entire virtual wards, operating rooms or emergency departments, with avatars controlled by one or more learners (Halvorsrud, Hagen, Fagernes, Mjelstad, & Romundstad, 2003).

In choosing a simulation modality, the bottom line is simple. The outcomes to be assessed govern decisions about the choice of assessment modality. A modality should be selected that is appropriate for learner level, is feasible and creates the desired context for the assessment to be conducted.

Increasingly, multiple simulators from different categories of modalities are being used together within a single simulation, in what is often termed hybrid or multi-modal simulation (Kneebone et al., 2005). Multi-modal simulation can draw on the strengths of various modalities and allow outcomes to be assessed in novel ways. For example, a part-task trainer that allows for ultrasound-guided insertion of a central venous catheter can be placed next to an SP who is located under a drape and is protected from accidental needle-stick by a Kevlar guard. The resident can be asked to perform an ultrasound-guided central venous catheter insertion while interacting with the SP prior to and during the procedure and with a nurse (Figure 14.4).

Develop Assessment Scenario

The next step in planning SBAs is development of a specific scenario that will elicit the assessment target behavior. A scenario is the clinical activity that the simulation replicates and includes consideration of the equipment (not only the simulator) to be included in the scenario, the personnel (including SPs, confederates or raters), the environment in which the simulation will be conducted and the expected way that the simulation will unfold over time. When developing a scenario, it is essential to start with well-defined outcomes appropriate for the level of the learner (see Box 14.3). Many templates for scenario creation exist in the literature (Benishek et al., 2015; Childs, Sepples, & Chambers, 2007) and are based upon established methodologies. One "best-practice" approach is event-based approach to training (EBAT), a means to introduce critical events into simulated activities to trigger behaviors that educators can observe and assess (Fowlkes, Dwyer, Oser, & Salas, 1998).

To assess certain outcomes, it may be desirable to use simulation in a context as similar to the real clinical setting as possible. This may be the only practical way to assess certain objectives when WBA cannot be conducted because of the infrequency of an event or because of potential risk of harm to patients. In these cases, the simulation setting can be designed to closely mimic the clinical setting. Alternatively, by bringing the necessary simulation devices into the actual clinical setting, the SBA can be conducted in situ—for example, conducting mock resuscitation events in a real hospital ward room. The in situ approach is a powerful way to assess how individuals and teams operate in their actual environments, which can uncover areas of strength or system and performance gaps that may not be uncovered in the simulation lab.

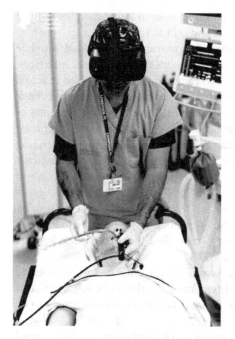

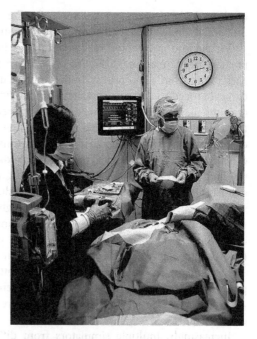

Figure 14.3 Trainee wearing a virtual reality (VR) headset and participating in a VR intubation exercise

Source: Photo courtesy of Collaborative Human Immersive Interaction Laboratory (CHISIL), Toronto

Figure 14.4 Multi-modal simulation of central venous catheter insertion. A part-task trainer is placed next to a standardized patient (SP), who is protected from accidental needle-stick by Kevlar. The learner must carry out the procedure while communicating with the SP and a nurse (a confederate embedded in the simulation) who is assisting with the procedure

Source: Photo courtesy of the HoPingKong Centre for Excellence in Education and Practice (CEEP), University Health Network, Toronto

---

Box 14.3 Scenario Development Steps

- Determine learning outcomes to be assessed
- Develop scenario overview
- Select environment where scenario will occur and equipment to be included
- Determine required additional personnel (confederates) and provide scripts
- Develop examinee prompts/instructions
- Plan progression/flow of scenario with identification of planned events/actions/triggers that will prompt specific actions and determine responses to possible trainee actions
- Outline instructions/notes for technician and instructor/assessor
- Program simulator (if necessary)
- Develop assessment instruments and debriefing questions (if applicable)

There are a number of practical considerations when implementing SBAs. Technical devices are not always reliable, and it is important to have a backup simulator or other plan in place should a simulator malfunction. Assessors should test all equipment in advance and on the day of an assessment. It is also necessary to determine if a given scenario requires a simulation technician to operate certain components or if these will be automated or controlled by the assessor. It is vital to pilot test a new SBA to ensure it elicits the behavior to be assessed. Unexpected events can happen in simulations where learners are free to make multiple decisions based upon their interpretation of the clinical scenario. An EBAT approach where specific events are embedded in the scenario can be employed to ensure that the desired outcomes of the scenario can be assessed. For example, if the objectives of an SBA are for a learner to recognize that a patient is experiencing an anaphylactic reaction and then to manage that reaction, a plan must be in place to ensure the learner is prompted about the presence of anaphylaxis if they do not identify it on their own. Absent the prompt, her ability to manage the reaction cannot be assessed. This can be done in several ways, such as having a confederate point out the presence of urticaria and remind the learner that the patient just received an antibiotic to which they had a known allergy (Dieckmann, Lippert, Glavin, & Rall, 2010). Obviously, although the learner may not score as well on her ability to recognize anaphylaxis as a learner who did not require prompts, this intervention will allow her to demonstrate ability to manage the condition. Finally, at the end of the assessment, it is important to make notes about any facets of the SBA that require modification before future use.

Score the Assessment

Data from an SBA can be numerical, categorical (e.g., meets expectations) or qualitative. In most evaluation settings, simulations rely on trained assessors to observe learners, record data and judge their performance. The data from these assessments are transformed into numerical scores or interpreted by appropriate experts in order to make assessment decisions based upon predetermined standards.

Some simulators automate data collection, recording and scoring, which makes the process faster and less prone to observer error. Automated data can provide highly accurate information about many things, including time to complete a procedure, efficiency of hand motion, damage to surrounding anatomic structures during a procedure, or strength and depth of motion (such as chest compressions). Depending upon the outcome being assessed, assessors are used in addition to, or in place of, simulator-based data to make overall judgements about learner performance and to assess skills that are not easily quantified or measured, such as leadership, communication and teamwork skills.

To obtain high-quality data, purpose-built assessment instruments such as checklists and global rating scales must often be created for a specific clinical scenario (Chapter 9). This can be done by bringing clinical and assessment experts together. For checklists, the relative importance (weighting) of items must be determined as well as whether any items are of such critical importance that missing them or completing them incorrectly could lead to automatic failure. The assessment instruments must also consider the specific attributes of the simulation and can be refined during pilot testing. It must then be determined if and how additional data from the simulator or products of the simulation will be combined with checklist and rating scale performance. For example, in an assessment of ability to follow an advanced cardiac life support (ACLS) protocol, a checklist with steps including called for help, started adequate CPR and attached defibrillator may be combined with information about adequacy (e.g., rate, depth, etc.) of chest compressions and time to defibrillation, which are obtained from the responsive mannequin simulator. Additional information about overall performance in the scenario, including assessment of overall approach, organization and problem solving, can also be collected via a global rating scale used by an expert assessor (Box 14.4).

The use of SBAs to assess teamwork creates additional challenges. The outcomes assessed must be clear and attention must be paid to distinguishing individual-level performance and team-level performance. Skills that are difficult to measure directly such as leadership, communication, situation awareness and mutual support are often the outcomes of interest. This requires use of multiple measures including expert judgments of performance using rating scales (for overall performance for each component of teamwork) with appropriate behavioral anchors. Several

Box 14.4 Example of Assessment Instrument That Integrates Data From the Simulator With Checklist and Global Rating Scale Measures

This instrument is used during a scenario that focuses on a trainee's ability to carry out the medical management of a patient in cardiac arrest secondary to ventricular fibrillation. The other members of the resuscitation team in the simulation are confederates that follow a script to ensure the teamwork skills of the trainees can be assessed in a standardized manner. The relative weighting of items, minimum passing score and manner in which data from this instrument is integrated as part of a broader assessment or assessment program would be determined based upon the specified outcomes.

Checklist	Correct	Not Correct
Check responsiveness	1	0
Get help	1	0
Call for AED/defibrillator	1	0
Check for a pulse	1	0
Initiate CPR	1	0
Ensure CPR quality	1	0
Open airway	1	0
Apply oxygen	1	0
Attach defibrillator	1	0
Check rhythm/identify Vfib	1	0
Charge to appropriate energy	1	0
Clear	1	0
Defibrillate	1	0
Immediately resume CPR	1	0
Ensure CPR quality	1	0
Establish IV access	1	0
Epinephrine 1 mg IV/IO push	1	0
Checklist Total		

Simulator-Based Data	Percentage of Time Target Achieved			
Rate of compressions (100–120/min)	<70%	70–80%	80–90%	>90%
Depth of compressions (2–2.4 inches)	<70%	70–80%	80–90%	>90%
Allows full chest recoil	<70%	70–80%	80–90%	>90%

Global Rating Scale	1	2	3	4	5
Leadership	Frequent loss of control, unable to make decisions.		Infrequent/brief loss of control of situation. Makes most decisions confidently and with minimal delay.		Remains in control throughout, efficiently and confidently makes decisions.

Global Rating Scale	1	2	3	4	5
Communication	Does not communicate with other team members or transmits information in a vague or unclear manner.		Generally provides specific, clear and concise information to team members. Occasionally uses SBAR and closed-loop communication.		Reliably provides specific, clear and concise information to team members. Consistently uses SBAR and closed-loop communication.
Situational Awareness	Fails to monitor the patient, team or environment or frequent failure to anticipate changes in the situation. Frequent fixation errors.		Infrequent loss of awareness of patient, team or environment changes. Infrequent fixation errors.		Maintains awareness of, and anticipates changes to, the patient, team or environment without cues. Avoids fixation errors.
Mutual Support	Fails to provide support and feedback directed at optimizing team function.		Provides intermittent support, feedback and directed assistance to the team.		Provides optimal supports to the team through provision of feedback and directed assistance.

Note: SBAR = situation, background, assessment, recommendation

scales such as the Trauma NOTECHS (Steinemann et al., 2012) and the Communication and Teamwork Skills Assessment (Frankel, Gardner, Maynard, & Kelly, 2007) have been created for this purpose. The EBAT approach to scenario design can be particularly valuable in teamwork SBAs, because critical events that require a team-based response can be introduced at a predetermined time in a simulation, allowing raters to focus their attention to determine if the team demonstrates the expected behaviors (Rosen et al., 2008). The TeamSTEPPS Team Performance Observation Tool is shown in Box 14.5.

Set Standards for the Assessment

Thoughtful standard setting is essential in making credible decisions. Standard setting is important because it specifies the minimum passing score (MPS) or standard for each assessment or program of assessment and sets expectations for students. Standard setting for SBAs requires similar considerations to those needed in general and for other performance-based tests (Chapters 6 and 9); however, SBAs have some specific standard-setting considerations. For example, a patient safety approach that identifies essential items that must be correctly completed in order for a trainee to receive a passing score should be considered when setting standards for procedural skills (Yudkowsky, Tumuluru, Casey, Herlich, & Ledonne, 2014). When using SBAs in a mastery learning model, rigorous standard-setting procedures are necessary to determine appropriate minimum passing standards (Chapter 18) (Barsuk, Cohen, Wayne, McGaghie, & Yudkowsky, 2018; Yudkowsky, Park, Lineberry, Knox, & Ritter, 2015).

Standard setting relies on systematic collection of expert judgments about expected learner performance (Downing, Tekian, & Yudkowsky, 2006; Norcini & Guille 2002). SBAs often involve experts skilled in the delivery of the SBA as assessors. Experts are also often experienced health professionals—frequently teaching faculty. This makes examinee-based standard-setting approaches, such as the contrasting groups and borderline group, particularly feasible for many

---

Box 14.5 Team Performance Observation Tool

Rating Scale (please comment if 1 or 2)

1= Very Poor, 2= Poor, 3= Acceptable, 4= Good, 5= Excellent

1. Team Structure	Rating
a. Assembles a team	
b. Assigns or identifies team members' roles and responsibilities	
c. Holds team members accountable	
d. Includes patients and families as part of the team	
Comments:	
Overall Rating—Team Structure	
2. Communication	
a. Provides brief, clear, specific and timely information to team members	
b. Seeks information from all available sources	
c. Uses check-backs to verify information that is communicated	
d. Uses SBAR, call-outs, and handoff techniques to communicate effectively with team members	
Comments:	
Overall Rating—Communication	
3. Leadership	
a. Identifies team goals and vision	
b. Utilizes resources efficiently to maximize team performance	
c. Balances workload within the team	
d. Delegates tasks or assignments, as appropriate	
e. Conducts briefs, huddles and debriefs	
f. Role models teamwork behaviors	
Comments:	
Overall Rating—Leadership	
4. Situation Monitoring	
a. Monitors the status of the patient	
b. Monitors fellow team members to ensure safety and prevent errors	
c. Monitors the environment for safety and availability of resources (e.g., equipment)	
d. Monitors progress toward the goal and identifies changes that could alter the plan of care	
e. Fosters communication to ensure team members have a shared mental model	
Comments:	
Overall Rating—Situation Monitoring	

5. Mutual Support	
a. Provides task-related support and assistance	
b. Provides timely and constructive feedback to team members	
c. Effectively advocates for patient safety using the Assertive Statement, Two-Challenge Rule or CUS (Concern, Uncomfortable, Safety)	
d. Uses the Two-Challenge Rule or DESC Script (Describe, Express, Suggest, Consequences) to resolve conflict	
Comments:	
Overall Rating—Mutual Support	
Team Performance Rating	

Source: Reproduced with permission from TeamSTEPPS® Instructor Manual (Agency for Healthcare Research and Quality, 2014)

SBAs. Determining how assessment data from SBAs is incorporated into a broader program of assessment must also be considered (Chapter 16).

There is no single best approach to standard setting for SBAs. Standard setting must be appropriate for the stakes of assessment and must be feasible given practical constraints such as required amount of faculty time. As for any assessment, the degree of rigor used to set standards should be commensurate with the stakes of the examination.

Standardize Assessment Conditions

The conditions for SBA, like other approaches to learner assessment, need to be standardized to yield best results. In an SBA, "fixed" conditions can include (a) patient (mannequin, SP), (b) trained examiner, (c) assessment instruments (checklist, rating scale), (d) room or laboratory space and (e) time allocation. In dynamic simulations with SPs, virtual reality and responsive mannequins, the simulator or SP needs to respond flexibly and realistically in response to examinee behaviors but should do so within set parameters. When implementing an SBA, it is also important to ensure the simulation is administered in a standardized way. This includes ensuring that the simulation begins in the same manner for each learner by ensuring all equipment is packaged and placed identically for each learner and that the simulator and confederates respond to learner actions uniformly. The elements that must be standardized become apparent by following the seven-step plan.

The reliability of assessment data depends on ruling out extraneous error (noise) by standardizing test conditions. There are two distinct types of assessment noise: random error or unreliability and systematic error or construct-irrelevant variance (Chapters 2 and 3). The goal, of course, is to reduce both types of noise (error) to improve the strength of inferences drawn from the assessment data.

THREATS TO VALIDITY OF SIMULATION-BASED ASSESSMENTS

Threats to the validity of SBAs are summarized in Table 14.4. Our discussion will focus on the main threats discussed in earlier chapters: construct underrepresentation (CU) and construct-irrelevant variance (CIV) (Chapter 2). CU and CIV issues related to performance tests (Chapter 9) are true in SBAs as well. We will also describe some additional considerations.

Construct underrepresentation can threaten SBAs if sufficient content is not sampled or if the selected samples do not systematically represent the domain being assessed. For example, if a lumbar puncture part-task trainer only represents one anatomic variation, the trainee's ability

Table 14.4 Threats to Validity of Simulation-Based Assessments (SBAs)

	Problem	Remedy
Construct Underrepresentation (CU) "Undersampling"	Simulator does not exist that is capable of simulating desired task or salient variations of the task	Reexamine the outcomes to determine if they can be adequately assessed using other assessment methods. Work with simulation experts to modify existing equipment or create new equipment suitable to meet needs.
	Standardized patients (SP) or simulators unable to portray certain abnormal clinical findings	Use multimodal simulation (e.g., SP combined with a simulator demonstrating an abnormal finding).
	Simulation does not recreate the challenges of performing a task in complex clinical environment	SBA can be carefully designed to create the appropriate realism and challenges for a given learner level or can be conducted in situ.
	Cost may limit ability to incorporate SBAs or limit the ability to include a sufficient number of SBAs for a reliable assessment	Simulation experts or technicians may be able to find creative ways to save money (e.g., reusing certain disposable equipment or creating lower cost simulators). Engage leadership by building a sound argument that SBAs are the best method for assessing certain outcomes.
Construct-Irrelevant Variance (CIV) "Systematic error"	Scenario difficulty not appropriate for level of learner	Pilot testing.
	Prior experience in simulation/ with a specific simulator/with similar technology	Embed simulation in the curriculum and ensure all learners are familiar with the simulation environment, simulators and simulation in general prior to assessment.
	"Performance anxiety" in simulation context	Ensure trainees have sufficient exposure to non-threatening simulation experiences regularly to make them comfortable being assessed with simulation.
	Rater errors	Adequate rater training including familiarization with simulation.

to perform a lumbar puncture on a patient with anatomic variation (e.g., a child, obese or elderly patient) cannot be inferred. This can compromise assessment validity if anatomic or other important aspects of the task are not adequately represented and the assessment of desired outcomes is limited.

As technology continues to evolve, simulators that can address such concerns and represent a broad range of clinical situations will be developed. In the interim, simulation educators should re-examine the seven-step plan to determine if there are other means to assess the outcome. An existing simulator or other equipment may be modified to allow it to serve the required need. Most simulation labs have skilled technicians and simulation experts who can devise ways to create simulators and scenarios that can elicit needed outcomes and create desired variation.

Another limitation to the inferences that we can draw from performance on an SBA is that SBAs are often conducted in settings that do not present all of the contextual performance challenges found in a real clinical environment, such as a busy emergency department or operating room. Real patients may not stay as still as a task trainer or be as easy to communicate with as an SP. These concerns can often be address by carefully developed simulations that employ strategies such as multi-modal and in situ simulation.

The cost of simulators and the time and effort required to conduct high-quality SBAs can be barriers to ensuring an adequate array of content for making valid decisions is sampled. The various elements (validity, reliability, educational impact, acceptability and cost) that determine an assessment's utility (van Der Vleuten, 1996) should be revisited to determine if the benefits of an SBA justify its potentially higher cost relative to other assessment methods. If an SBA is judged the best method based upon utility considerations, simulation educators and technicians may develop lower cost alternatives that serve the intended purpose. Otherwise, working with educational leadership to ensure the necessary resources are allocated is vital.

CIV too can occur in SBAs. Poorly designed scenarios that are not pilot tested may be too easy or difficult for the target group of learners. Scenarios may contain distractors that increase extraneous cognitive load, which diverts the focus of the learner other than by design and does not allow the construct of interest to be properly assessed (Fraser et al., 2012). Evaluation apprehension or anxiety about "performing" in the simulation environment may also impact assessments of performance (McGaghie, 2018). CIV can occur if some learners have extensive prior experience with a certain simulator or similar simulators and related equipment and others have not had any such exposure. In this case, the assessment may simply be measuring familiarity rather than the actual construct of interest. This impact can be mitigated by integrating the simulators that will be used in SBAs into the existing curriculum, or at minimum by providing sufficient orientation to the function of the simulator, the simulation environment and expected behavior within the simulation (pre-briefing) (Rudolph, Raemer, & Simon, 2014). Finally, SBAs may be prone to systematic or inconsistency rating errors. This may occur with raters who are experts in a specific content area but have not had sufficient preparation and orientation about the considerations specifically relevant to a given SBA, such as which behaviors should be conducted as they would in "real life" and which can be simulated and the limitations of simulator responses within an SBA. As discussed in Chapter 9, rater training is essential for SBA.

FACULTY DEVELOPMENT NEEDS

Despite the increasing use of simulation in health professions education, faculty training and development about effective use of simulation technology to promote learner achievement and to assess learning outcomes needs to be strengthened (Holmboe, Ward et al., 2011). Simple or sophisticated simulation technology will be ineffective or misused unless health professions faculty are prepared as simulation educators.

CONSEQUENCES AND EDUCATIONAL IMPACT

Implementation of low-stakes SBAs as part of educational programs can have substantial impact on learning. The development of simulation-based training and assessment programs based upon the principles of mastery learning (see Chapter 18) have demonstrated that performance can be improved, costs reduced and patient outcomes improved (Barsuk, Cohen, Feinglass, McGaghie, & Wayne, 2009; Barsuk, McGaghie, Cohen, O'Leary, & Wayne, 2009; McGaghie et al., 2011; Zendejas et al., 2011). The use of SBAs may also catalyze a more widespread adoption of SBHE and impact the overall educational and organizational culture regarding safety and quality (Siassakos, Crofts, Winter, Weiner, & Draycott, 2009).

When SBAs are used for summative assessments, even as a small part of a larger program of high-stakes assessment, the potential impact of simulation as a learning tool must be considered. Many educators who use simulation strive to ensure that SBHE occurs in a non-threatening but challenging climate where learners feel comfortable enough to suspend disbelief and engage fully in the simulation. They must feel safe enough to know they can make mistakes and that they will be supported in learning and not embarrassed or ridiculed by teachers (Rudolph et al., 2014). Maintaining this safe environment for learning can become more difficult when it is no longer true that "things that happen in the simulation stay in the simulation." It is imperative that educators find an optimal balance of simulation as a learning tool and as an assessment tool.

CONCLUSION

This chapter has covered the use of a variety of simulation technologies for learner assessment in the health professions. The emphasis has been on assessment planning and achieving a match between outcomes to be assessed and the method chosen to assess them, with the intent of rational integration of simulation technology into health science curricula. We argue that simulation is not a panacea for assessment or instruction. Instead, simulation is one of many tools available to health professions educators. Thoughtful use of these tools will increase the odds that educators and learners will reach their assessment goals.

Note: Additional material and resources may be available at the UIC AHPE website: https://go.uic.edu/AHPE

REFERENCES

Agency for Healthcare Research and Quality. (2014). *Team performance observation tool.* Retrieved from www.ahrq.gov/teamstepps/instructor/reference/tmpot.html.

Barsuk, J.H., Cohen, E.R., Feinglass, J., McGaghie, W.C., & Wayne, D.B. (2009). Use of simulation-based education to reduce catheter-related bloodstream infections. *Archives of Internal Medicine, 169*(15), 1420–1423.

Barsuk, J.H., Cohen, E.R., Wayne, D.B., McGaghie, W.C., & Yudkowsky, R. (2018). A comparison of approaches for mastery learning standard setting. *Academic Medicine, 93*(7), 1079–1084.

Barsuk, J.H., McGaghie, W.C., Cohen, E.R., O'Leary, K.J., & Wayne, D.B. (2009). Simulation-based mastery learning reduces complications during central venous catheter insertion in a medical intensive care unit. *Critical Care Medicine, 37*(10), 2697–2701.

Benishek, L.E., Lazzara, E.H., Gaught, W.L., Arcaro, L.L., Okuda, Y., & Salas, E. (2015). The template of events for applied and critical healthcare simulation (TEACH Sim): A tool for systematic simulation scenario design. *Simulation in Healthcare, 10*(1), 21–30.

Berkenstadt, H., Ziv, A., Gafni, N., & Sidi, A. (2006). Incorporating simulation-based objective structured clinical examination into the Israeli National Board Examination in Anesthesiology. *Anesthesia & Analgesia, 102*(3), 853–858.

Bok, H.G. (2015). Competency-based veterinary education: An integrative approach to learning and assessment in the clinical workplace. *Perspectives on Medical Education, 4*(2), 86–89.

Brydges, R., Nair, P., Ma, I., Shanks, D., & Hatala, R. (2012). Directed self-regulated learning versus instructor-regulated learning in simulation training. *Medical Education, 46*(7), 648–656.

Capella, J., Smith, S., Philp, A., Putnam, T., Gilbert, C., Fry, W., . . . Baker, D. (2010). Teamwork training improves the clinical care of trauma patients. *Journal of Surgical Education, 67*(6), 439–443.

Cheng, A., Eppich, W., Grant, V., Sherbino, J., Zendejas, B., & Cook, D.A. (2014). Debriefing for technology-enhanced simulation: a systematic review and meta-analysis. *Medical Education, 48*(7), 657–666.

Childs, J., Sepples, S., & Chambers, K. (2007). Designing simulations for nursing education. In N.L.F. Nursing (Ed.), *Simulation in nursing education.* New York: National League for Nursing.

Cook, D.A., Brydges, R., Zendejas, B., Hamstra, S.J., & Hatala, R. (2013). Mastery learning for health professionals using technology-enhanced simulation: A systematic review and meta-analysis. *Academic Medicine, 88*(8), 1178–1186.

Dent, J., Harden, R.M., & Hunt, D. (2017). *A practical guide for medical teachers.* Edinburgh: Elsevier Health Sciences.

Dieckmann, P., Lippert, A., Glavin, R., & Rall, M. (2010). When things do not go as expected: scenario life savers. *Simulation in Healthcare, 5*(4), 219–225.

Downing, S.M. (2006). Twelve steps for effective test development. In S.M. Downing & T.M. Haladyna (Eds.), *Handbook of test development* (pp. 3–25). Mahwah, NJ: Lawrence Erlbaum Associates.

Downing, S.M., Tekian, A., & Yudkowsky, R. (2006). Procedures for establishing defensible absolute passing scores on performance examinations in health professions education. *Teaching and Learning in Medicine, 18*(1), 50–57.

Eva, K.W., Reiter, H.I., Rosenfeld, J., Trinh, K., Wood, T.J., & Norman, G.R. (2012). Association between a medical school admission process using the multiple mini-interview and national licensing examination scores. *JAMA, 308*(21), 2233–2240.

Ferguson, P.C., Kraemer, W., Nousiainen, M., Safir, O., Sonnadara, R., Alman, B., & Reznick, R. (2013). Three-year experience with an innovative, modular competency-based curriculum for orthopaedic training. *The Journal of Bone and Joint Surgery. American Volume, 95*(21), e166(1)–e166(6).

Fowlkes, J., Dwyer, D.J., Oser, R.L., & Salas, E. (1998). Event-based approach to training (EBAT). *The International Journal of Aviation Psychology, P*(3), 209–221.

Frank, J.R., Snell, L., Sherbino, J. (2015). *CanMEDS 2015 physician competency framework.* Ottawa, ON: Royal College of Physicians and Surgeons of Canada.

Frank, J.R., Snell, L.S., ten Cate, O., Holmboe, E.S., Carraccio, C., Swing, S.R., … Harris, K.A. (2010). Competency-based medical education: theory to practice. *Medical Teacher, 32*(8), 638–645.

Frankel, A., Gardner, R., Maynard, L., & Kelly, A. (2007). Using the communication and teamwork skills (CATS) assessment to measure health care team performance. *Joint Commission Journal on Quality and Patient Safety, 33*(9), 549–558.

Fraser, K., Ma, I., Teteris, E., Baxter, H., Wright, B., & McLaughlin, K. (2012). Emotion, cognitive load and learning outcomes during simulation training. *Medical Education, 46*(11), 1055–1062.

Gaba, D., Howard, S., Fish, K., Smith, B., & Sowb, Y. (2001). Simulation-based training in Anaesthesia Crisis Resource Management (ACRM): A decade of experience. *Simulation 7 Gaming, 32*(2), 175–193.

Gaba, D.M. (2007). The future vision of simulation in healthcare. *Simulation in Healthcare, 2*(2), 126–135.

Grantcharov, T.P., Kristiansen, V.B., Bendix, J., Bardram, L., Rosenberg, J., & Funch-Jensen, P. (2004). Randomized clinical trial of virtual reality simulation for laparoscopic skills training. *The British Journal of Surgery, 91*(2), 146–150.

Halvorsrud, R., Hagen, S., Fagernes, S., Mjelstad, S., & Romundstad, L. (2003). Trauma team training in a distributed virtual emergency room. *Studies in Health Technology and Informatics, 94*, 100–102.

Hatala, R., Kassen, B.O., Nishikawa, J., Cole, G., & Issenberg, S.B. (2005). Incorporating simulation technology in a Canadian internal medicine specialty examination: A descriptive report. *Academic Medicine, 80*(6), 554–556.

Hayden, J.K., Smiley, R.A., Alexander, M., Kardong-Edgren, S., & Jeffries, P.R. (2014). The NCSBN national simulation study: A longitudinal, randomized, controlled study replacing clinical hours with simulation in prelicensure nursing education. *Journal of Nursing Regulation, 5*(2), C1–S64.

Holmboe, E., Rizzolo, M.A., Sachdeva, A.K., Rosenberg, M., & Ziv, A. (2011). Simulation-based assessment and the regulation of healthcare professionals. *Simulation in Healthcare, 6*(7), S58–S62.

Holmboe, E.S., Ward, D.S., Reznick, R.K., Katsufrakis, P.J., Leslie, K.M., Patel, V.L., … Nelson, E.A. (2011). Faculty development in assessment: The missing link in competency-based medical education. *Academic Medicine, 86*(4), 460–467.

Issenberg, S.B., McGaghie, W.C., Petrusa, E.R., Lee Gordon, D., & Scalese, R.J. (2005). Features and uses of high-fidelity medical simulations that lead to effective learning: A BEME systematic review. *Medical Teacher, 27*(1), 10–28.

Kneebone, R., Kidd, J., Nestel, D., Barnet, A., Lo, B., King, R., … Brown, R. (2005). Blurring the boundaries: Scenario-based simulation in a clinical setting. *Medical Education, 39*(6), 580–587.

Laufer, S., Cohen, E.R., D'Angelo, A.L., Yudkowsky, R., Boulet, J.R., McGaghie, W.C., & Pugh, C.M. (2015). Sensor technology in assessments of clinical skill. *The New England Journal of Medicine, 372*(8), 784–786.

Lee, S., Lee, J., Lee, A., Park, N., Song, S., Seo, A., … Eom, K. (2013). Augmented reality intravenous injection simulator based 3D medical imaging for veterinary medicine. *The Veterinary Journal, 196*(2), 197–202.

Levine, A.I., Schwartz, A.D., Bryson, E.O., & DeMaria Jr., S. (2012). Role of simulation in US physician licensure and certification. *Mount Sinai Journal of Medicine: A Journal of Translational and Personalized Medicine, 79*(1), 140–153.

Lingard, L. (2012). Rethinking competence in the context of teamwork. In B.D. Hodges & L. Lingard (Eds.), *The question of competence: Reconsidering medical education in the twenty-first century* (pp. 42–69). Ithaca: Cornell University Press.

Matsumoto, E.D., Hamstra, S.J., Radomski, S.B., & Cusimano, M.D. (2002). The effect of bench model fidelity on endourological skills: A randomized controlled study. *The Journal of Urology, 167*(3), 1243–1247.

McGaghie, W.C. (2018). Evaluation apprehension and impression management in clinical medical education. *Academic Medicine, 93*(5), 685–686.

McGaghie, W.C., Issenberg, S.B., Cohen, E.R., Barsuk, J.H., & Wayne, D.B. (2011). Does simulation-based medical education with deliberate practice yield better results than traditional clinical education? A meta-analytic comparative review of the evidence. *Academic Medicine, 86*(6), 706–711.

Mironova, P., Girardi, B., Burns, D., & Safir, O. (2018). Toronto Orthopaedic Boot Camp (TOBC). In O. Safir, R. Sonnadara, P. Mironova, & R. Rambani (Eds.), *Boot camp approach to surgical training* (pp. 19–29). Cham, Switzerland: Springer International Publishing.

Motola, I., Devine, L.A., Chung, H.S., Sullivan, J.E., & Issenberg, S.B. (2013). Simulation in healthcare education: A best evidence practical guide. AMEE Guide No. 82. *Medical Teacher*, *35*(10), e1511–e1530.

Nasca, T.J., Philibert, I., Brigham, T., & Flynn, T.C. (2012). The next GME accreditation system—Rationale and benefits. *New England Journal of Medicine*, *366*(11), 1051–1056.

Nehring, W.M., & Lashley, F.R. (2010). *High-fidelity patient simulation in nursing education*. Sudbury, MS: Jones & Bartlett Publishers.

Nestel, D., Mobley, B.L., Hunt, E.A., & Eppich, W.J. (2014). Confederates in health care simulations: Not as simple as it seems. *Clinical Simulation in Nursing*, *10*(12), 611–616.

Norcini, J., & Guille, R. (2002). Combining tests and setting standards. In G.R. Norman, C.P.M. van der Vleuten, & D.I. Newble (Eds.), *International handbook of research in medical education* (pp. 811–834). Dordrecht, The Netherlands: Kluwer Academic Publishers.

Nousiainen, M.T., McQueen, S.A., Ferguson, P., Alman, B., Kraemer, W., Safir, O., . . . Sonnadara, R. (2016). Simulation for teaching orthopaedic residents in a competency-based curriculum: Do the benefits justify the increased costs? *Clinical Orthopaedics and Related Research*, *474*(4), 935–944.

Papadakis, M.A. (2004). The step 2 clinical-skills examination. *New England Journal of Medicine*, *350*(17), 1703–1705.

Perry, S., Bridges, S.M., & Burrow, M.F. (2015). A review of the use of simulation in dental education. *Simulation in Healthcare*, *10*(1), 31–37.

Rosen, M.A., Salas, E., Wilson, K.A., King, H.B., Salisbury, M., Augenstein, J.S., . . . Birnbach, D.J. (2008). Measuring team performance in simulation-based training: Adopting best practices for healthcare. *Simulation in Healthcare*, *3*(1), 33–41.

Rudolph, J.W., Raemer, D.B., & Simon, R. (2014). Establishing a safe container for learning in simulation: The role of the presimulation briefing. *Simulation in Healthcare*, *9*(6), 339–349.

Salas, E., Rosen, M., & King, H. (2007). Managing teams managing crises: Principles of teamwork to improve patient safety in the emergency room and beyond. *Theoretical Issues in Ergonomics Science*, *8*(5), 381–394.

Scalese, R.J. (2018). Simulation-based assessment. In E.S. Holmboe, S.J. Durning, & R.E. Hawkins (Eds.), *Evaluation of clinical competence* (pp. 215–255). Philadelphia: Elsevier.

Scalese, R.J., and Issenberg, S.B. (2008). Simulation-based assessment. In E.S. Holmboe & R.E. Hawkins (Eds.), *Practical guide to the evaluation of clinical competence* (pp. 179–200). Philadelphia: Elsevier.

Siassakos, D., Crofts, J., Winter, C., Weiner, C., & Draycott, T. (2009). The active components of effective training in obstetric emergencies. *BJOG: An International Journal of Obstetrics & Gynaecology*, *116*(8), 1028–1032.

Steinberg, A.D., Bashook, P.G., Drummond, J., Ashrafi, S., & Zefran, M. (2007). Assessment of faculty perception of content validity of Periosim©, a haptic-3D virtual reality dental training simulator. *Journal of Dental Education*, *71*(12), 1574–1582.

Steinemann, S., Berg, B., DiTullio, A., Skinner, A., Terada, K., Anzelon, K., & Ho, H.C. (2012). Assessing teamwork in the trauma bay: Introduction of a modified "NOTECHS" scale for trauma. *The American Journal of Surgery*, *203*(1), 69–75.

Stroud, L., & Cavalcanti, R.B. (2013). Hybrid simulation for knee arthrocentesis: Improving fidelity in procedures training. *Journal of General Internal Medicine*, *28*(5), 723–727.

van de Ridder, J.M., McGaghie, W.C., Stokking, K.M., & ten Cate, O.T. (2015). Variables that affect the process and outcome of feedback, relevant for medical training: A meta-review. *Medical Education*, *49*(7), 658–673.

van der Vleuten, C.P. (1996). The assessment of professional competence: Developments, research and practical implications. *Advances in Health Sciences Education*, *1*(1), 41–67.

Yudkowsky, R., Luciano, C., Banerjee, P., Schwartz, A., Alaraj, A., Lemole Jr., G.M., . . . Byrne, R. (2013). Practice on an augmented reality/haptic simulator and library of virtual brains improves residents' ability to perform a ventriculostomy. *Simulation in Healthcare*, *8*(1), 25–31.

Yudkowsky, R., Park, Y.S., Lineberry, M., Knox, A., & Ritter, E.M. (2015). Setting mastery learning standards. *Academic Medicine*, *90*(11), 1495–1500.

Yudkowsky, R., Tumuluru, S., Casey, P., Herlich, N., & Ledonne, C. (2014). A patient safety approach to setting pass/fail standards for basic procedural skills checklists. *Simulation in Healthcare*, *9*(5), 277–282.

Zendejas, B., Cook, D.A., Bingener, J., Huebner, M., Dunn, W.F., Sarr, M.G., & Farley, D.R. (2011). Simulation-based mastery learning improves patient outcomes in laparoscopic inguinal hernia repair: A randomized controlled trial. *Annals of Surgery*, *254*(3), 502–511.

Ziv, A., Berkenstadt, H., & Eisenberg, O. (2013). Simulation for licensure and certification. In A.I. Levine, S. DeMaria Jr., A.D. Schwartz, & A.J. Sim (Eds.), *The comprehensive textbook of healthcare simulation* (pp. 161–170). New York: Springer.

Ziv, A., Wolpe, P.R., Small, S.D., & Glick, S. (2006). Simulation-based medical education: An ethical imperative. *Simulation in Healthcare*, *1*(4), 252–256.

15

SITUATIONAL JUDGMENT TESTS

Harold I. Reiter and Christopher Roberts

PROLOGUE

Many have believed, and some continue to believe, that personal competencies can be measured accurately using personal statements, reference letters, file review, and traditional one-on-one or panel interviews. The truth lies elsewhere. Personal statements, reference letters, and traditional interviews show no predictive validity in literature reviews of selection to medicine (Albanese, Snow, Skochelak, Huggett, & Farrell, 2003) and allied healthcare (Salvatori, 2001), while file review worsens predictive validity when added to simple formulaic approaches (Burgess, 1928; Sarbin, 1943; Grove & Meehl, 1996). Yet many schools continued to hope, using debunked selection methods (Edwards, Johnson, & Molidor, 1990), while others embraced despair with implementation of a grade-weighted lottery (Netherlands medical schools). With the advent of the multiple mini-interview (MMI) (Eva, Rosenfeld, Reiter, & Norman, 2004) (see Chapter 8), a third option presented itself. Newer methods like the MMI, more in line with accepted psychometric principles, might have the capacity to provide a valid measure of personal competencies without demanding the resources of the MMI. Over the last 15 years, the focus of many groups around the world has centered on situational judgment test (SJT) development. This chapter is written for those who hope—hope to implement, modify, or interpret SJTs.

EXERCISE 15.1

Situational judgment test items have three parts—a situation presentation, question(s) asked, and response required. There is great variety in each of these three parts. Two examples of SJT items are provided. Consider how the key components differ between the two examples.

SJT Example 1

You are a physician's assistant covering inpatient care at a surgical ward on the first day of a three-day weekend. A patient asks you for the results of a lung biopsy, which might be benign or cancer. She tells you that she must make plans for her business, as soon as possible, contingent upon her availability in the coming months. You are aware that her physician, who would be expected to provide the biopsy results, returns in three days' time. You are also aware that the results unfortunately do show cancer. The patient is becoming increasingly strident in requesting the results. What should be done? Rank the following options, in order of most preferred action to least preferred action.

a. Inform the patient that the biopsy reveals cancer.
b. Tell the patient that the results are expected in three days' time.
c. Contact the patient's physician at home and request that s/he reveal the results to the patient that day.
d. Explain to the patient that the results did arrive, but that according to protocol, only the physician can share that information with the patient.
e. "Accidentally" leave a paper copy of the biopsy report by the patient's bedside.
f. Without specifically stating the result, describe in great detail the process of further investigation and therapy that typically follow a biopsy report positive for lung cancer.

SJT Example 2

Boilerplate statement displayed for ten seconds prior to commencement of video, stating, "You are an employee of NewWorld Inc., sitting in a coffee shop with two close friends."

> [Fade in. Interior shot, coffee shop. Camera shot from the angle of someone seated at a small round table for three. Two others seated at the table. Both in their mid-twenties, casual dress, sipping coffee. Female "Georgina" is on the left, male "Marcus" is on the right. Marcus and Georgina are turned to face each other.]

Marcus: How is the job hunt going?

Georgina: I got an offer last week from Puppies are Forever, but it's not exactly the kind of job I'm looking for. I'm a lot more excited about the interview I had last week at New-World. It would be a perfect fit for what I want. I think the interview went really well, and they're supposed to get back to me in a few days. [Georgina turns to face the camera.] Thank you so much for suggesting my name to your company. Your boss is so cool, and it would be so great to work together.

Marcus: When do you have to respond to Puppies are Forever?

Georgina: [Turns to Marcus.] That's my problem. They want to know by the end of today, and if I don't accept their offer, they're going to move on to their next preferred candidate. [Georgina turns to the camera.] Do you know whether your boss is likely to offer me the position?
[Fade out]

You have a total of five minutes to type responses to all three questions:

Question 1. You are aware that your boss is strongly leaning towards offering the NewWorld position to a different candidate. Company policy is that you may not communicate anything regarding internal discussions about hiring. What do you tell your friend Georgina, and what are the factors that most influence you to do so?

Question 2. You are aware that your boss *is* planning to offer the position to your friend Georgina. However, the management team has confidentially informed company employees that there is likely to be a corporate change soon that may well cause the offered position to cease to exist within months. None of this information is to be shared outside of the company. What do you tell Georgina, and what are the factors that most influence you to do so?

Question 3. Does the presence of your other close friend Marcus at the same table change any of your responses to the previous two questions? Why or why not?

EXERCISE 15.2

Review the three case studies, and consider the issues involved. How would you address each challenge? Keep these case studies in mind as you read through the chapter.

Case Study 1

You are the admissions dean for an undergraduate medical school receiving over 10,000 applications annually for 200 available seats. Over the last five years, the school's position in media rankings of medical schools nationally has dropped 15 spots, and the deanery has expressed deep concern that this change has driven a severe drop in funding from alumni, placing several core school activities at risk. At the same time, the student affairs office has noted a slow but steady increase in reports of student lapses in professionalism over the last ten years and is advocating for changes in student selection. Separate from all that, pipeline program integration just two years earlier has already begun to bear fruit, with a modest increase in class diversity, a gain that community stakeholders adamantly wish to safeguard. Grades, standardized tests of cognition, personal statements, reference letters, and file review have been used to generate 800 invitations to interview annually. Recent consideration has been given to switch from traditional interview to MMI, but this would require additional resources at a time that the school's discretionary funds are dropping. Some have suggested an SJT, but what would that ideally look like, and would it address the rising concerns?

Case Study 2

You are the dean of an undergraduate nursing program financially dependent upon recruitment of foreign, as well as domestic, students. Partly due to cultural differences, a small number of episodes of inappropriate conduct have been reported that, fairly or unfairly, have brought your school into disrepute and negatively impacted upon the employability of your graduates. You are asked whether an SJT taken by your admitted students early during their first year might help identify the handful of students most likely to benefit from additional training and support, to better hasten their acculturation.

Case Study 3

You are the program director for an inner-city hospital's family medicine residency program. Your program receives 100 applications annually for 20 positions. Regional counties have long experienced a shortage of family medicine graduates willing to make service of the underserved their career focus. You have identified some demographic characteristics that correlate with that endpoint, but you are also aware that your publicly broadcast mission statement to serve the underserved has inclined many applicants to falsely distort their application responses in line with that message, in personal statements and in interviews. You are wondering whether an SJT might be more reflective of applicants' true intent.

RECENT HISTORY OF SJT DEVELOPMENT FOR ASSESSMENT IN HEALTH PROFESSIONS EDUCATION

A Need Is Recognized

The breadcrumb trail of complaints against physicians, predominantly due to lapses of professionalism, had been available since the 1950s (Stokes, 1952) but remained peripheral to the tasks of selection and training, simply because of a lack of hard data to demand our attention. If patients were to be better protected, and learners were to be funneled to careers most compatible with their individual set of personal strengths (or lack thereof), the literature on lapses in professionalism would need to be objectified. With Medical Board of California quarterly reports of disciplinary actions against graduates of medical schools as both the impetus and the starting point, a research agenda led by Maxine Papadakis turned those isolated data points into a larger narrative—bad behavior in medical school portends for bad behavior in practice (Papadakis, Hodgson, Teherani, & Kohatsu, 2004); further, greater attention on personal competencies is deserved, with close to 95% of identifiable disciplinary actions against physicians found to be due to lapses in professionalism (Papadakis et al., 2005), with the financial toll of those actions exceeding $50 billion annually in the United States alone (Mello, Chandra, Gawande, & Studdert, 2010).

These findings prompted larger movement towards greater accountability, accelerated by healthcare regulators, using competency-based models: Medical Council of Canada (MCC)—roles of the physician (Physicians & Canada, 2000), Accreditation Council for Graduate Medical Education (ACGME) in the United States—core competencies (Reisdorff, Hayes, Carlson, & Walker, 2001), General Medical Council in the United Kingdom—Good Medical Practice (General Medical Council, 2017), and Global Minimum Essential Requirements from the Institute for International Medical Education (Schwarz & Roy, 2000). In a changing world, there arose a desire for "fundamental changes in order to select physicians with both the academic and interpersonal and intrapersonal competencies necessary to operate in the health care system of the future" (Mahon, Henderson, & Kirch, 2013).

Two Worlds Collide

The generation of SJTs in assessment for healthcare professional education has arisen independently from two separate sets of literature—personnel psychology and medical education. With the passage of time and increased dissemination of research results, SJTs arising from these two origins have gradually shifted closer to one another, sharing more middle ground.

From the personnel psychology literature, SJTs were seen, in contrast to more resource-intensive assessment centers, as a series of lower fidelity simulations of the workplace. Used historically for selection into civil service and the military (Lievens, Peeters, & Schollaert, 2008) and more recently for human resources, this type of SJT aligned with the theory of implicit behavior (Motowidlo, Hooper, & Jackson, 2006; Koczwara et al., 2012), in which prosocial elements of behavior are driven by beliefs of those behaviors' importance to work effectiveness and for which job analysis is critical. The hallmarks of SJTs emerging from this approach include (1) a focus on behavior and on procedural knowledge (Motowidlo & Beier, 2010), (2) selected responses (e.g., multiple choice, rank order, or rate individual merit of each proffered option), (3) response options assigned degree of correctness scores prior to test administration, (4) as judged by subject matter experts (SMEs), and (5) situations that tend to be task-specific (work-specific) rather than skill-specific (Krumm et al., 2015). More recently, the SJTs for healthcare professions assessment emerging from this literature have shifted more toward the skill-specific, lining up more closely with the competency-based models espoused by the regulators (Patterson et al., 2017; Roberts et al., 2018).

From the medical education literature, the creation of the objective structured clinical examination (OSCE) (Harden & Gleeson, 1979) and the MMI (Eva et al., 2004) demonstrated that historical failure to accurately measure clinical and personal competencies was due not to subjectivity but to lack of adequate sampling. Subjectivity alone neither precludes nor guarantees test validity. Further, based on a literature review of medical resident ethical decision-making (Ginsburg et al., 2000), it was concluded that trainees' behavioral choices were less important than the reasons expressed for making those choices. This would align with the integrated model of the theory of planned behavior (Fishbein, Hennessy, Yzer, & Douglas, 2003)—each individual exercises self-control over his/her behavior in potentially predictable ways, but not necessarily in

Table 15.1 Two Approaches to Situational Judgment Tests

Personnel Psychology Approach to SJTs	Medical Education Approach to SJTs
Focus on behavior and on procedural knowledge	Focus on the combination of behavior, personal attitude, and social context
Selected responses (e.g., multiple choice, rank order, or rate individual merit of each proffered option)	Constructed responses (typed or audio or audiovisual recordings)
Response options assigned degree of correctness scores prior to test administration	Situational equipoise (no right or wrong answer but rather a balance of intrinsic values)
Judged by subject matter experts (SMEs)	Test scores generated by human raters provided with background insights into the intrinsic values encompassed within the situation
Situations that tend to be task-specific (work-specific) rather than skill-specific	Situations that tend to be skill-specific rather than task-specific

ways tied to the workplace. The hallmarks of SJTs emerging from this approach include (1) a focus on the combination of behavior, personal attitude, and social context (Jha, Brockbank, & Roberts, 2016; Rees & Knight, 2007), (2) constructed responses (typed or audio or audiovisual recordings), (3) situational equipoise (no right or wrong answer but rather a balance of intrinsic values), (4) post-test scores generated by human raters provided with background insights into the intrinsic values encompassed within the situation, and (5) situations that tend to be skill-specific rather than task-specific. See Table 15.1.

DEFINING KEY COMPONENTS OF SJTS AND DESIRED OUTCOMES

Converting Research Data Into Practice

As more groups develop and research SJTs for healthcare professional assessment, research findings drive proponents of both sets of literature towards more common ground. The emerging symbiotic literature can present a fairly demanding journey for the uninitiated and is further complicated by a fundamental dissonance between researcher and practitioner. A researcher may seek a better theoretical understanding by asking the question, "if I change certain aspects of an SJT, what will be the outcome?" whereas an end user of SJTs is more likely to ask, "if I want a specific outcome, what aspects of an SJT should I prefer?" The researcher's approach is beautifully captured in a review of the personnel selection literature (Lievens & Sackett, 2017), which argues that single changes in any of a test's key components may have a dramatic and independent or interdependent effect on outcomes. Based upon the modular approach described in that paper, this chapter will take the opposite approach. Given desired outcomes, what key components should you prefer in an SJT?

Key Components

Assessment tools fundamentally are composed of a series of stimuli, responses, and scores. The key components of stimuli in SJTs are related to the stem (situation presented) and to the question, and include stem format, context, degree of contextualization, and stimulus consistency. The key components of responses and scores in SJTs are related to response instructions, response format, and scoring consistency.

Stimulus (stem) format in SJTs are almost always either written or audiovisual (video clips).
Stem contexts in SJTs are typically either task-based (e.g., simulation of a critical incident arising in the workplace of interest) or skill-based (simulation challenging one or more regulator-defined competencies, typically in a non-workplace setting).

Degree of contextualization reflects the level of fidelity, or realism, of the situation presented. For instance, a video clip with a detailed and highly realistic setting would have greater degree of contextualization than a written stem.

Stimulus consistency is high when all test-takers are equivalently challenged. SJTs can be fixed, pseudo-branched, or branched. In a fixed SJT, each question is independent of each other, each generating independent scores, and this holds true whether there is only one or multiple questions arising from a stem. In a pseudo-branched SJT, multiple interdependent questions are used for each stem, with a single overall score generated from all responses within that single stem. In a branched SJT, multiple interdependent questions are used for each stem, with test-takers' different possible responses to the first question triggering different secondary questions. Stimulus consistency is high for fixed and pseudo-branched SJTs, low for branched SJTs. There is little research published on branched SJTs.

Response instructions in SJTs can be behavioral (e.g., "describe a situation when you were part of a group struggling to work together to achieve a common goal, and how you dealt with it") or situational and personalized (e.g., "given this specific situation, what would you do?") or situational and depersonalized (e.g., "given this specific situation, what should be done?").

Response format in SJTs utilize selected responses or constructed responses. Examples of selected responses are choosing the single best option from a list of options (multiple choice), rank ordering all listed options from most preferable to least preferable, or rating each option independently on a scale anchored from not at all preferable to highly preferable. Constructed responses may be written/typed, audio recorded, or audiovisually recorded.

Scoring consistency for selected response SJTs requires high concordance between SMEs judging degree of correctness of each possible response, after which post-test scoring is automated. The situation and question must be straightforward enough to get high SME concordance, but not so straightforward as to allow all test-takers to score highly. Scoring consistency for constructed-response SJTs requires high scorer agreement between post-test human ratings. This would require extensive attention to rater recruitment, training, accreditation, and provision of background and theory and ability to benchmark (compare different test-taker responses and adjust scores accordingly, on the fly) for each stem.

Refer to Table 15.2 to compare SJT Example 1 with SJT Example 2 in terms of the key components described. Both examples were designed as sample items assessing ethics, communication, and teamwork. While the first example is more reflective of an SJT item emerging from the Personnel Psychology literature, and the second example is more reflective of an SJT item emerging from the Medical Education literature, test designers from both schools of thought continue to adapt SJT key components as more research results become available, blurring the progenitor lines between the two.

Table 15.2 Answers to Exercise 15.1

	SJT Example 1	SJT Example 2
Stimulus Format	Written	Audiovisual
Stem Context	Task-based (clinical setting)	Skill-based (non-clinical setting)
Degree of Contextualization	Moderately high	Very high
Stimulus Consistency	Fixed	Pseudo-branched
Response Instructions	Situational—depersonalized	Situational—personalized
Response Format	Selected—rank order	Constructed—written
Scoring Consistency	Subject matter expert concordance	Scorer agreement

DESIGNING A SITUATIONAL JUDGMENT TEST

When designing an SJT, the first step is defining the constructs to be assessed. When creating content, test designers must ensure that the items are mapped to the desired constructs and that there are enough items to appropriately sample the constructs of interest. If parallel tests are being conducted at separate times, efforts should be made to make the delivery of the separate tests equitable.

Desirable Outcomes

As an end user, your desired outcomes are quite modest. Simply put, you want assessment tools that will (1) potentiate greater diversity and (2) identify better and worse trainees (3) in a manner that is affordable financially, politically, and legally. Analogically, you can think of these three as you would clinical trials. Phase I, how toxic is it? (i.e., is it going to impede diversity goals?) Phase II, does it work? (i.e., does it identify the trainees I want?) Phase III, should I use it? (i.e., can I afford to? can I afford not to?). Phase I and II trials ask biologic questions, questions that investigate the general principles of the science of assessment, and so from their theoretical groundings capture the greatest attention of researchers. Contrarily, Phase III trials ask pragmatic questions, questions relevant to individual schools "on the ground" and remain orphaned to a somewhat greater extent in the SJT literature.

Research reports on implications for diversity and for differentiating between better and worse trainees can be a tough row to hoe but can be simplified by thinking of them in terms of construct specificity and construct sensitivity, respectively, where "construct" is the thing you want to measure. In the case of SJTs, the construct of interest is typically personal competencies such as ethics, professionalism, teamwork, communication, and cultural competency.

Phase I—How Toxic Is It? Potentiating Diversity, aka Construct Specificity

Have you ever seen a test of cognitive skills show no significant subgroup differences? Even when bias is ruled out, subgroup differences persist (Young, 2001). The most commonly cited cause is variability in educational opportunity between those who have and those who have not. Due consideration to cognitive testing key components, like using constructed responses rather than selected responses (Arthur Jr, Edwards, & Barrett, 2002), can shrink but not eliminate those subgroup differences.

Have you ever seen a test of personal competencies show no significant subgroup differences? They do exist (Terregino, McConnell, & Reiter, 2015; Lievens, Sackett, Dahlke, Oostrom, & De Soete, 2018), albeit inconsistently for SJTs (McDaniel, Psotka, Legree, Yost, & Weekley, 2011; Juster et al., in press; Lievens, Patterson, Corstjens, Martin, & Nicholson, 2016; Work Psychology Group, 2017). It is therefore possible, unlike cognitive skills, that there might be no significant difference in average level of personal competencies between those who have and those who have not. If true, then any assessment tool that specifically tests only personal competencies and minimizes the influence of cognitive skills would ideally show no significant subgroup differences.

There are many ways in which tests intended to measure personal competencies face contamination from construct irrelevancies (see Table 15.3) because they simultaneously and unintentionally measure other constructs. To best avoid these intrusions, consider undue influence from different test key components.

Stimulus format—written stems measure reading skills that audiovisual stems do not (Weekley & Jones, 1997; Chan & Schmitt, 1997; Christian, Edwards, & Bradley, 2010). Audiovisual stems also prompt more positive applicant perceptions among members of underrepresented groups than do written stems (Chan & Schmitt, 1997; Richman-Hirsch, Olson-Buchanan, & Drasgow, 2000; Schmitt, Gilliland, Landis, & Devine, 1993; Kanning, Grewe, Hollenberg, & Hadouch,

Table 15.3 Threats to Validity: Situational Judgment Tests

	Problem	Remedy
Construct Underrepresentation (CU)	Too few questions to sample domain adequately	Increase number of situations
	Unrepresentative sampling of domain	Blueprint to be sure examinations systematically sample the domain
	Increase fidelity (make more realistic)	Audiovisual stems rather than written stems Audiovisual rather than written constructed responses
	Ensure adequate level of test difficulty	Selected response: increase question complexity to lowest acceptable limit of subject matter expert concordance Constructed response: provide background and theory to raters, let them benchmark against other applicants
Construct-Irrelevant Variance (CIV)	Coaching effect	Make situations complex, inhibit simple strategies for responses
	Flawed or inappropriate case scenarios or other prompts	Pilot test cases and prompts
	Measuring reading skills	Audiovisual stems rather than written stems
	Measuring procedural knowledge	Skill-based rather than task-based stems Ask personalized rather than depersonalized questions
	Measuring ability to distort responses (fake values)	Speeded testing
	Measuring according to overly narrow cultural values	Use item response theory (see Chapter 19)
	Measuring test-taking ability	Constructed response rather than selected response
	Measuring writing skills	For constructed response, use audiovisual rather than written responses

Note: For more about CU and CIV threats to validity, see Chapter 2.

2006). Positive correlations have been found between positive test perception and better test performance (Hausknecht, Day, & Thomas, 2004).

Stem context—task-based items measure familiarity with the job and its associated procedural knowledge that skill-based items do not (Lievens & Patterson, 2011; Stegers-Jager, 2018). Test results are tied to familiarity with the national culture, heightening the importance of depicting the situations in line with the national culture relevant to the schools using the SJT (Rockstuhl, Ang, Ng, Lievens, & Van Dyne, 2015; Stegers-Jager, 2018). For instance, SJT Example 1 would be culturally dissonant in a country which did not have physician assistants, or (gulp) did not allow females to run businesses.

Degree of contextualization—when cognitive-related task-based context is avoided, there is no compelling evidence to determine whether degree of realism of the situation impacts upon subgroup differences. There is one hypothetical consideration, however, that would favor a high degree of contextualization. Repeat test-taking often results in higher mean scores, a practice effect that is more beneficial for those who have (and can better afford retesting) than those who have not, for both cognitive tests (Koenig & Leger, 1997) and selected-response SJTs (Lievens, Buyse, & Sackett, 2005a), but which is not present in one study of an online video-stem constructed-response SJT (Dore, Reiter, Kreuger, & Norman, 2017). If practice effect is a function of test familiarity, then higher degree of variation in contextualization might lessen test familiarity acquisition, because of the general inability of individuals to transfer between one context and another (Salomon & Perkins, 1989), thus counteracting the contamination of personal competencies construct with test-taking skills.

Stimulus consistency—perhaps because stimulus consistency tends to be high in all common uses of SJTs (fixed or pseudo-branched), there is no clear evidence to indicate whether one has smaller subgroup differences than the other.

Response instructions—depersonalized situational questions—asking "what should be done" correlates more strongly with cognitive skills (McDaniel, Hartman, Whetzel, & Grubb III, 2007), presumably based on its coherence with procedural knowledge, compared to personalized situational questions—asking "what would you do?" Changing from personalized to depersonalized instructions can be associated with increases in subgroup differences (Work Psychology Group, 2014, 2017). Speeded testing has been found to decrease subgroup differences generally for cognitive tests (Arthur, Glaze, Villado, & Taylor, 2009), perhaps by adding cognitive load, constraining the time allowable for test-takers to use their cognitive skills to credibly distort their responses to personal competency questions.

Response format—due to higher associated cognitive load, selected-response tests tend to have significantly higher subgroup differences as compared to constructed-response tests (Arthur et al., 2002; Lievens et al., 2018). Additionally, any gainful coaching effect of test-prep courses more available to those who have than to those who have not, is countered when coaches cannot impart simple strategy and when the SJT response demands a complex approach (Cullen, Sackett, & Lievens, 2006), even to the point of completely reversing subgroup differences. Within constructed-response format options, written responses have larger subgroup differences than audiovisual responses (Lievens et al., 2018), perhaps due to the contamination of personal competencies construct with writing skills. At least one study randomizing between more interactive (branched) versus less interactive (fixed) response format concluded that more interactive was perceived more positively by members of underrepresented groups (Kanning et al., 2006). Positive correlations have been found between positive test perception and better test performance (Hausknecht et al., 2004).

Scoring consistency—sometimes initial scores may discriminate unintentionally against one particular group; scoring systems can be explored using item response theory (IRT) (Tiffin, Finn, & McLachlan, 2011) to help identify items to avoid (see Chapter 19). There is further indirect information supporting an association between greater scoring consistency and lowering subgroup differences. A meta-analysis in personnel psychology has demonstrated that perceptions of greater fairness and consistency have salutary effects on job interest levels of members of underrepresented groups (Hausknecht et al., 2004), with positive correlations found between test perception and test performance (Hausknecht et al., 2004).

Phase II—Does It Work? Identifying Better- and Lower-Performing Learners aka Construct Sensitivity

SJTs are not necessarily specific to the measurement of personal competencies. Rather, it is a test format that can be used to measure different constructs. Given the expertise and resources required to mount an SJT, it would make little sense to use it to measure constructs more easily measured using other means. Grade point average (GPA) and standardized tests like the Medical College Admissions Test (MCAT) are simpler options for assessing cognitive skills; OSCE is a simpler option for assessing clinical skills. SJTs are therefore typically reserved for assessment of the construct of personal competencies, as are traditional interviews and MMIs. The breadth of coverage of the personal competencies construct, the overarching construct sensitivity, should ideally translate into the ability to predict future personal competency performance—predictive validity. Any failure in breadth of coverage would be considered construct underrepresentation (see Table 15.3).

Predictive validity includes both convergent (positive) and discriminant (absent) correlations with future performance (Messick, 1995). If there are different assessment tool options for the same or overlapping construct, how can they be integrated to gain the greatest predictive advantage? It is insufficient to know just the degree of predictive validity provided. GPA and MCAT both predict for future cognitive assessment performance and correlate well with each other. Adding MCAT scores to GPA provides strong incremental predictive validity, whereas adding GPA to MCAT scores provides only a small amount of incremental predictive validity. This section describes how different key components of SJT influence predictive validity and incremental validity for the assessment of personal competencies. For correlations with cognitive assessment scores, some SJTs have demonstrated results that are strongly convergent, other SJTs strongly divergent; the same holds true for correlation with other assessment tools for personal competencies. Beyond that, what is its incremental value? For instance, if an SJT and an MMI correlate convergently, do both provide independent, incremental predictive validity to later performance outcomes, meriting use of both? To date, research results provide answers to all but that last question of score integration. Until research results of the relative contribution of SJT and MMI are known, a school deliberating use of both may well be driven more by Phase III, real-world considerations.

Stimulus format—audiovisual stems have demonstrated higher predictive validity than written stems on SJTs (Lievens & Sackett, 2006).

Stem context—both task-based and skill-based SJTs can provide small to moderate strength predictive validity (see "Response format" immediately below for full list of references).

Degree of contextualization—at least one study (Krumm et al., 2015) concluded that the degree of contextualization is not critical to achieve predictive validity.

Stimulus consistency—consistency in stimuli between test administrations—parallel test forms— is easier to achieve when that specific SJT has a long enough track record to allow use of item response theory (Tiffin et al., 2011) to ensure that parallel underlying constructs are being measured from one test to the next, an approach equally applicable to fixed or pseudo-branched format.

Response instructions—depersonalized situational questions—asking "what should be done?"— are less strongly associated with response distortion (ability to fake) than personalized situational questions—asking "what would you do?" (Whetzel & McDaniel, 2009). To maintain higher test reliability and so optimize potential predictive validity, opportunities for response distortion should ideally be eliminated. Using depersonalized situational questions is one way to do that but carries with it greater subgroup differences; if that is a concern, other means of combatting response distortion, like speeded testing, might be considered instead of using depersonalized questions.

Response format—both constructed-response SJTs and selected-response SJTs, when appropriately designed, have demonstrated predictive validity for future performance, with direct comparison showing better results with constructed response (Funke & Schuler, 1998). In the SJT literature specific to healthcare professions assessment, selected-response SJTs produce correlations with personal competency measures in the range $r = 0.09–0.57$ (Lievens, Buyse & Sackett, 2005b; Lievens & Sackett, 2012, 2006; Husbands, Rodgerson, Dowell, & Patterson 2015; Lievens & Patterson, 2011; Patterson, Baron, Carr, Plint, & Lane, 2009; Patterson, Knight, McKnight, & Booth, 2016; Patterson et al., 2009; Patterson et al., 2016; Cousans et al., 2017; Patterson, Roe, & Parsons, 2017; Patterson, Lievens, Kerrin, Munro, & Irish, 2013) and with cognitive competency measures in the range of $r = -0.11$–0.53 (Lievens et al., 2005b; Lievens & Sackett, 2012; Lievens & Coetsier, 2002; Lievens & Sackett, 2006; Husbands et al., 2015; Lievens & Patterson, 2011; Patterson et al., 2009, 2013, 2016; Koczwara et al., 2012; Work Psychology Group, 2013, 2014, 2015). In indirect comparison, constructed-response SJTs produce correlations with personal competency measures in the range of $r = 0.30$–0.51 (Dore et al., 2009, 2017), and with cognitive competency measures in the range of $r = -0.45$–0.17 (Dore et al., 2017). It is not at all clear, however, that selected-response and constructed-response SJTs are measuring the same thing. Rockstuhl et al. (2015) hypothesized that "adding an assessment of how people perceive and interpret situations (situational judgment) to SJTs will provide incremental information beyond the typical focus on choosing the best response (response judgment)." In a series of studies, they demonstrated the incremental and relatively equal value of each in predicting for future performance (with the exception of performance in organizational citizenship behavior, for which only constructed-response "situational judgment" proved predictive). Further, within constructed-response format options, audiovisual responses have generated higher predictive validity than written/typed responses (Lievens, De Corte, & Westerveld, 2015; Lievens et al., 2018).

Scoring consistency—SME concordance is difficult to achieve with situations that are not straightforward (Ginsburg, Regehr, & Lingard, 2004; Beesley et al., 2017). Because structured response SJTs depend upon SME concordance, it is challenging to construct items that are sufficiently straightforward to attain SME agreement but complex enough to separate between test-takers at the high end of the score distribution curve. Score distribution curves for selected-response SJTs therefore tend to be skewed to the right, with mean test scores in the 75%–86% range (Patterson et al., 2017; Patterson, Roe, & Parsons, 2017); items less able to discriminate between medium- to high-performing test-takers (Strahan, Fogarty, & Machin, 2005) result in that ceiling effect. In contrast, constructed-response SJT score distribution tends to approximate a bell-shaped curve with mean test scores of 50% (Dore et al., 2009).

Phase III—Should I Use It? Real-World Considerations

Because many of the real-world considerations lie outside theory and psychometric principles that drive research, and because these considerations tend to be driven more by locoregional than universal concerns, there is relatively less available in the literature to drive conclusions. Instead, this section presents far more in the way of questions than answers.

Resources—would SJT implementation require more, less, or the same resource requirements, relative to what you are presently using? If created locally, you will need psychometricians, test platform developers, test content developers, and scoring generated either from SMEs pre-test or human raters post-test. If a national or commercial SJT is available, who pays for students to take the test, does the construct of that test align with your program's mission statement, how are the resulted scores communicated? Does a national option correlate sufficiently well with an existing local assessment of personal competencies, like MMI (Dore et al., 2009), that SJT implementation would allow a decrease in a portion of existing admissions processes and save on local resources (Yingling, Park, Curry, Monson, & Girotti, 2018)?

Test and score integration—can you reasonably garner enough political buy-in from external stakeholders, faculty, and governance bodies to implement? Are there administrative or legal hurdles too high to clear? Is the applicant-to-seat ratio sufficiently high to commend an additional selection tool like an SJT? How might SJT scores be integrated to best match the local mission statement? One study modelled 12 different formulaic approaches to integrate SJT scores together with GPA and MCAT scores, comparing simulated results with historic benchmarks of diversity and resource usage, and identified those models most in alignment with the local mission statement (Juster, Baum, Ly, Risucci, & Dore, 2017; Juster et al., in press). Between local SJT development and national SJT usage, which would serve better? A national SJT might not reflect unique personal competencies most critical to individual schools. A locally developed SJT would not allow data comparisons across schools.

ANSWERS TO EXERCISE 15.2

Case Study 1

The demands in this case are from all sides. No recidivism on the gains made to diversity or on cognitive measures that drive school rankings would be considered acceptable, but there is a need to enhance personal competencies of selected students, with no change or decrease in resource utilization. To hold the line on diversity, as a minimum, consider SJT key components associated with high construct specificity—stems that are audiovisual, skill-based, high fidelity, and demanding personalized, constructed responses. Integrate SJT scores using a simulated model that will suggest solutions to at least maintain mean entering class GPA and MCAT scores. Consider an SJT with both audiovisual stems and responses, to get higher predictive validity. For both resource conservation and further enhancement of predictive validity for future professionalism, look for an SJT that correlates well with MMIs, allowing you to switch from traditional interview system with 800 interview slots to MMI format with far fewer interview slots. Using an SJT that correlates well with MMI scores, those less likely to do well enough on the MMI to commend their selection can be culled from the invitation list based upon their lower SJT scores—fewer interviewees, less cost. Alternatively, with SJT-induced range restriction of interviewee personal competencies at the high end, you could choose to keep the cost the same, but have fewer interviewees and increased MMI station number, driving up MMI test reliability and predictive validity for convergent correlation with future personal competency performance.

Case Study 2

You have one critical issue to address—the early identification of students most unused to your domestic culture. Any highly contextualized SJT, either locally or nationally created, should identify those with inherent challenges in acculturation. Outside of those key components, your decision should be driven by local considerations of resources and test integration. In contrast to the gateway to the profession in Case Study 1, the stakes here are moderate rather than high, and the willingness to expend resources should be judged accordingly.

Case Study 3

You have one critical issue to address—identify those applicants most likely to make service of the underserved the focal point of their career. If a review of the national SJT options does not support correlation with that construct, you may have to consider a locally created SJT. Applicants to the program know the kind of trainee values you are looking for, and many might try to convince you (and themselves) that they truly wish to serve the underserved, so you would have to minimize opportunities for response distortion—consider constructed-response, speeded testing, and highly contextualized test components, using situational contexts that allow you to disguise the skills you wish to assess (e.g., bury the value of serving the underserved in a question that involves other values and forces the applicant to demonstrate which value(s) they consider most quintessential). Because members of the underrepresented in medicine groups have a greater tendency to serve the underserved (Xierali & Nivet, 2018), you may wish to consider SJT key components associated with high construct specificity/stronger diversity—stems that are audiovisual, skill-based, high fidelity, and demanding personalized, constructed responses.

EPILOGUE

The story of situational judgment tests for assessment in healthcare professions education remains very much in flux. Much remains to be learned before the key components can be optimized for each of the different purposes (selection, advancement), program mission statements, and regional and national realities, for which SJTs can be implemented. Given preliminary successes achieved for better predictive validity and diversity, albeit with variable levels of consistency, it seems highly likely that they will be with us increasingly over the coming years.

Note: Additional material and resources may be available at the UIC AHPE website: https://go.uic.edu/AHPE

REFERENCES

Albanese, M.A., Snow, M.H., Skochelak, S.E., Huggett, K.N., & Farrell, P.M. (2003). Assessing personal qualities in medical school admissions. *Academic Medicine, 78*(3), 313–321.

Arthur Jr., W., Edwards, B.D., & Barrett, G.V. (2002). Multiple-choice and constructed response tests of ability: Race-based subgroup performance differences on alternative paper-and-pencil test formats. *Personnel Psychology, 55*(4), 985–1008.

Arthur, W., Glaze, R.M., Villado, A.J., & Taylor, J.E. (2009). Unproctored Internet-based tests of cognitive ability and personality: Magnitude of cheating and response distortion. *Industrial and Organizational Psychology, 2*(1), 39–45.

Beesley, R., Sharma, A., Walsh, J.L., Wilson, D.J. (2017). Situational judgment tests: Who knows the right answers? *Medical Teacher, 39*(12), 1293–1294.

Burgess, E.W. (1928). Factors determining success or failure on parole. *The Workings of the Indeterminate Sentence Law and the Parole System in Illinois,* 221–234.

Chan, D., & Schmitt, N. (1997). Video-based versus paper-and-pencil method of assessment in situational judgment tests: Subgroup differences in test performance and face validity perceptions. *Journal of Applied Psychology, 82*(1), 143.

Christian, M.S., Edwards, B.D., & Bradley, J.C. (2010). Situational judgment tests: Constructs assessed and a meta-analysis of their criterion-related validities. *Personnel Psychology, 63*(1), 83–117.

Cousans, F., Patterson, F., Edwards, H., Walker, K., McLachlan, J.C., & Good, D. (2017). Evaluating the complementary roles of an SJT and academic assessment for entry into clinical practice. *Advances in Health Sciences Education, 22*(2), 401–413.

Cullen, M.J., Sackett, P.R., & Lievens, F. (2006). Threats to the operational use of situational judgment tests in the college admission process. *International Journal of Selection and Assessment, 14*(2), 142–155.

Dore, K.L., Reiter, H.I., Eva, K.W., Krueger, S., Scriven, E., Siu, E., . . . Norman, G.R. (2009). Extending the interview to all medical school candidates—Computer-Based Multiple Sample Evaluation of Noncognitive Skills (CMS-ENS). *Academic Medicine, 84*(10), S9–S12.

Dore, K.L., Reiter, H.I., Kreuger, S., & Norman, G.R. (2017). CASPer, an online pre-interview screen for personal/professional characteristics: prediction of national licensure scores. *Advances in Health Sciences Education, 22*(2), 327–336.

Edwards, J.C., Johnson, E.K., & Molidor, J.B. (1990). The interview in the admission process. *Academic Medicine, 65*(3), 167–177.

Eva, K.W., Rosenfeld, J., Reiter, H.I., & Norman, G.R. (2004). An admissions OSCE: The multiple mini-interview. *Medical Education, 38*(3), 314–326.

Fishbein, M., Hennessy, M., Yzer, M., & Douglas, J. (2003). Can we explain why some people do and some people do not act on their intentions? *Psychology, Health & Medicine, 8*(1), 3–18.

Funke, U., & Schuler, H. (1998). Validity of stimulus and response components in a video test of social competence. *International Journal of Selection and Assessment, 6*(2), 115–123.

General Medical Council. (2017). Good medical practice. General Medical Council, UK. Retrieved from www.gmc-uk.org/-/media/documents/good-medical-practice—english-1215_pdf-51527435.pdf. Accessed March 15, 2019.

Ginsburg, S., Regehr, G., Hatala, R., McNaughton, N., Frohna, A., Hodges, B., . . . Stern, D. (2000). Context, conflict, and resolution: A new conceptual framework for evaluating professionalism. *Academic Medicine, 75*(10), S6–S11.

Ginsburg, S., Regehr, G., & Lingard, L. (2004). Basing the evaluation of professionalism on observable behaviors: A cautionary tale. *Academic Medicine, 79*(10), S1–S4.

Grove, W.M., & Meehl, P.E. (1996). Comparative efficiency of informal (subjective, impressionistic) and formal (mechanical, algorithmic) prediction procedures: The clinical—Statistical controversy. *Psychology, Public Policy, and Law, 2*(2), 293.

Harden, R.M., & Gleeson, F.A. (1979). Assessment of clinical competence using an objective structured clinical examination (OSCE). *Medical Education, 13*(1), 41–54.

Hausknecht, J.P., Day, D.V., & Thomas, S.C. (2004). Applicant reactions to selection procedures: An updated model and meta-analysis. *Personnel Psychology, 57*(3), 639–683.

Husbands, A., Rodgerson, M.J., Dowell, J., & Patterson, F. (2015). Evaluating the validity of an integrity-based situational judgement test for medical school admissions. *BMC Medical Education, 15*(1), 144.

Jha, V., Brockbank, S., & Roberts, T. (2016). A framework for understanding lapses in professionalism among medical students: Applying the theory of planned behavior to fitness to practice cases. *Academic Medicine, 91*(12), 1622–1627.

Juster, F., Baum, R., Ly, A., Risucci, D., & Dore, K.L. (2017). In H.I. Reiter (Ed.), *How a Hybrid holistic-formulaic approach using situational judgment tests may promote diversity and lessen resource expenditure*. Poster presented at the Association of American Medical Colleges (AAMC), Boston.

Juster, F., Baum, R.C., Reiter, H., Zou, C., Risucci, D., Anhphan, T., Miller, D.D., & Dore, K. Addressing the diversity-validity dilemma using situational judgment tests. *Academic Medicine*, in press.

Kanning, U.P., Grewe, K., Hollenberg, S., & Hadouch, M. (2006). From the Subjects' point of view. *European Journal of Psychological Assessment, 22*(3), 168–176.

Koczwara, A., Patterson, F., Zibarras, L., Kerrin, M., Irish, B., & Wilkinson, M. (2012). Evaluating cognitive ability, knowledge tests and situational judgement tests for postgraduate selection. *Medical Education, 46*(4), 399–408.

Koenig, J.A., & Leger, K.F. (1997). A comparison of retest performances and test-preparation methods for MCAT examinees grouped by gender and race-ethnicity. *Academic Medicine, 72*(10 Suppl 1), S100–S102

Krumm, S., Lievens, F., Hüffmeier, J., Lipnevich, A.A., Bendels, H., & Hertel, G. (2015). How "situational" is judgment in situational judgment tests? *Journal of Applied Psychology, 100*(2), 399.

Lievens, F., Buyse, T., & Sackett, P.R. (2005a). Retest effects in operational selection settings: Development and test of a framework. *Personnel Psychology, 58*(4), 981–1007.

Lievens, F., Buyse, T., & Sackett, P.R. (2005b). The operational validity of a video-based situational judgment test for medical college admissions: Illustrating the importance of matching predictor and criterion construct domains. *Journal of Applied Psychology, 90*(3), 442.

Lievens, F., & Coetsier, P. (2002). Situational tests in student selection: An examination of predictive validity, adverse impact, and construct validity. *International Journal of Selection and Assessment, 10*(4), 245–257.

Lievens, F., De Corte, W., & Westerveld, L. (2015). Understanding the building blocks of selection procedures: Effects of response fidelity on performance and validity. *Journal of Management, 41*(6), 1604–1627.

Lievens, F., & Patterson, F. (2011). The validity and incremental validity of knowledge tests, low-fidelity simulations, and high-fidelity simulations for predicting job performance in advanced-level high-stakes selection. *Journal of applied psychology, 96*(5), 927.

Lievens, F., Patterson, F., Corstjens, J., Martin, S., & Nicholson, S. (2016). Widening access in selection using situational judgement tests: Evidence from the UKCAT. *Medical Education, 50*(6), 624–636.

Lievens, F., Peeters, H., & Schollaert, E. (2008). Situational judgment tests: A review of recent research. *Personnel Review, 37*(4), 426–441.

Lievens, F., & Sackett, P.R. (2006). Video-based versus written situational judgment tests: A comparison in terms of predictive validity. *Journal of applied psychology, 91*(5), 1181.

Lievens, F., & Sackett, P.R. (2012). The validity of interpersonal skills assessment via situational judgment tests for predicting academic success and job performance. *Journal of Applied Psychology, 97*(2), 460.

Lievens, F., & Sackett, P.R. (2017). The effects of predictor method factors on selection outcomes: A modular approach to personnel selection procedures. *Journal of Applied Psychology, 102*(1), 43.

Lievens, F., Sackett, P.R., Dahlke, J., Oostrom, J., & De Soete, B. (2018). Constructed response formats and their effects on minority-majority differences and validity. *Journal of Applied Psychology, 104*(5), 715–726.

Mahon, K.E., Henderson, M.K., & Kirch, D.G. (2013). Selecting tomorrow's physicians: The key to the future health care workforce. *Academic Medicine, 88*(12), 1806–1811.

McDaniel, M.A., Hartman, N.S., Whetzel, D.L., & Grubb III, W.L. (2007). Situational judgment tests, response instructions, and validity: A meta--analysis. *Personnel Psychology, 60*(1), 63–91.

McDaniel, M.A., Psotka, J., Legree, P.J., Yost, A.P., & Weekley, J.A. (2011). Toward an understanding of situational judgment item validity and group differences. *Journal of Applied Psychology, 96*(2), 327.

Mello, M.M., Chandra, A., Gawande, A.A., & Studdert, D.M. (2010). National costs of the medical liability system. *Health Affairs, 29*(9), 1569–1577.

Messick, S. (1995). Validity of psychological assessment: Validation of inferences from persons' responses and performances as scientific inquiry into score meaning. *American Psychologist, 50*(9), 741.

Motowidlo, S.J., & Beier, M.E. (2010). Differentiating specific job knowledge from implicit trait policies in procedural knowledge measured by a situational judgment test. *Journal of Applied Psychology*, 95(2), 321.

Motowidlo, S.J., Hooper, A.C., & Jackson, H.L. (2006). A theoretical basis for situational judgment tests.

Papadakis, M.A., Hodgson, C.S., Teherani, A., & Kohatsu, N.D. (2004). Unprofessional behavior in medical school
is associated with subsequent disciplinary action by a state medical board. *Academic Medicine*, 79(3), 244–249.

Papadakis, M.A., Teherani, A., Banach, M.A., Knettler, T.R., Rattner, S.L., Stern, D.T., . . . Hodgson, C.S. (2005).
Disciplinary action by medical boards and prior behavior in medical school. *New England Journal of Medicine*,
353(25), 2673–2682.

Patterson, F., Baron, H., Carr, V., Plint, S., & Lane, P. (2009). Evaluation of three short-listing methodologies for
selection into postgraduate training in general practice. *Medical Education*, 43(1), 50–57.

Patterson, F., Carr, V., Zibarras, L., Burr, B., Berkin, L., Plint, S., . . . Gregory, S. (2009). New machine-marked tests
for selection into core medical training: Evidence from two validation studies. *Clinical Medicine*, 9(5), 417–420.

Patterson, F., Cousans, F., Edwards, H., Rosselli, A., Nicholson, S., & Wright, B. (2017). The predictive validity of a
text-based situational judgment test in undergraduate medical and dental school admissions. *Academic Medicine*, 92(9), 1250–1253.

Patterson, F., Knight, A., McKnight, L., & Booth, T.C. (2016). Evaluation of two selection tests for recruitment into
radiology specialty training. *BMC Medical Education*, 16(1), 170.

Patterson, F., Lievens, F., Kerrin, M., Munro, N., & Irish, B. (2013). The predictive validity of selection for entry into
postgraduate training in general practice: Evidence from three longitudinal studies. *British Journal of General
Practice*, 63(616), e734–e741.

Patterson, F., Roe, V., & Parsons, W. (2017). *A Situational Judgement Test for Admission to the Faculty of Medicine at
Memorial University of Newfoundland*. Oral Presentation, Canadian Conference on Medical Education, Win-
nipeg, Manitoba.

Patterson, F., Rowett, E., Hale, R., Grant, M., Roberts, C., Cousans, F., & Martin, S. (2016). The predictive validity of
a situational judgement test and multiple-mini interview for entry into postgraduate training in Australia. *BMC
Medical Education*, 16(1), 87.

Physicians, R.C.O., & Canada, S.o. (2000). CanMEDS 2000: Extract from the CanMEDS 2000 project societal needs
working group report. *Medical Teacher*, 22, 549–554.

Rees, C.E., & Knight, L.V. (2007). The trouble with assessing students' professionalism: Theoretical insights from
sociocognitive psychology. *Academic Medicine*, 82(1), 46–50.

Reisdorff, E.J., Hayes, O.W., Carlson, D.J., & Walker, G.L. (2001). Assessing the new general competencies for resident education: a model from an emergency medicine program. *Academic Medicine*, 76(7), 753–757.

Richman-Hirsch, W.L., Olson-Buchanan, J.B., & Drasgow, F. (2000). Examining the impact of administration
medium on examinee perceptions and attitudes. *Journal of Applied Psychology*, 85(6), 880.

Roberts, C., Khanna, P., Rigby, L., Bartle, E., Llewellyn, A., Gustavs, J., . . . Thistlethwaite, J. (2018). Utility of selection
methods for specialist medical training: A BEME (best evidence medical education) systematic review: BEME
guide no. 45. *Medical Teacher*, 40(1), 3–19.

Rockstuhl, T., Ang, S., Ng, K.Y., Lievens, F., & Van Dyne, L. (2015). Putting judging situations into situational judgment tests: Evidence from intercultural multimedia SJTs. *Journal of Applied Psychology*, 100(2), 464.

Salomon, G., & Perkins, D.N. (1989). Rocky roads to transfer: Rethinking mechanism of a neglected phenomenon.
Educational Psychologist, 24(2), 113–142.

Salvatori, P. (2001). Reliability and validity of admissions tools used to select students for the health professions.
Advances in Health Sciences Education, 6(2), 159–175.

Sarbin, T.R. (1943). A contribution to the study of actuarial and individual methods of prediction. *American Journal of Sociology*, 48(5), 593–602.

Schmitt, N., Gilliland, S.W., Landis, R.S., & Devine, D. (1993). Computer-based testing applied to selection of sec-
retarial applicants. *Personnel Psychology*, 46(1), 149–165.

Schwarz, A.W., Roy, M. (2000). Minimum essential requirements and standards in medical education. *Medical
Teacher*, 22(6), 555–559.

Stegers-Jager, K.M. (2018). Lessons learned from 15 years of non-grades-based selection for medical school. *Medical Education*, 52(1), 86–95.

Stokes, W. (1952). The complaints that reach our grievance committee. *The Medical Annals of the District of Columbia*, 21(3), 157.

Strahan, J., Fogarty, G.J., & Machin, M.A. (2005). *Predicting Performance on a Situational Judgement Test: The Role of
Communication Skills, Listening Skills, and Expertise*. Paper presented at the Proceedings of the 40th Australian
Psychological Society Annual Conference: Past Reflections, Future Directions.

Terregino, C.A., McConnell, M., & Reiter, H.I. (2015). The effect of differential weighting of academics, experiences,
and competencies measured by multiple mini interview (MMI) on race and ethnicity of cohorts accepted to
one medical school. *Academic Medicine*, 90(12), 1651–1657.

Tiffin, P.A., Finn, G.M., & McLachlan, J.C. (2011). Evaluating professionalism in medical undergraduates using selected response questions: Findings from an item response modelling study. *BMC Medical Education, 11*(1), 43.

Weekley, J.A., & Jones, C. (1997). Video-based situational testing. *Personnel Psychology, 50*(1), 25–49.

Whetzel, D.L., & McDaniel, M.A. (2009). Situational judgment tests: An overview of current research. *Human Resource Management Review, 19*(3), 188–202.

Work Psychology Group. (2013). Technical report—*Analysis of the situational judgement test for selection to the Foundation Programme*: 2013. Retrieve from https://isfporguk.files.wordpress.com/2017/04/fy1-sjt-2013-technical-report.pdf.

Work Psychology Group. (2014). Technical report—*Analysis of the situational judgement test for selection to the Foundation Programme*: 2014. Retrieve from https://isfporguk.files.wordpress.com/2017/04/fy1-sjt-2014-technical-report.pdf.

Work Psychology Group. (2015). Technical report—*Analysis of the situational judgement test for selection to the Foundation Programme*: 2015. Retrieve from https://isfporguk.files.wordpress.com/2017/04/fy1-sjt-2015-technical-report.pdf.

Work Psychology Group. (2017). Technical report—*Analysis of the situational judgement test for selection to the Foundation Programme*: 2017. Retrieve from file:///C:/Users/hreit/Downloads/FY1_SJT_Technical_Report_2016–17_FINAL.pdf.

Xierali, I.M., & Nivet, M.A. (2018). The racial and ethnic composition and distribution of primary care physicians. *Journal of Health Care for the Poor and Underserved, 29*(1), 556.

Yingling, S., Park, Y.S., Curry, R.H., Monson, V., & Girotti, J. (2018). Beyond cognitive measures: Empirical evidence supporting holistic medical school admissions practices and professional identity formation. *MedEdPublish, 7*.

Young, J.W. (2001). Differential validity, differential prediction, and college admission testing: A comprehensive review and analysis. Research report no. 2001–6. New York: College Entrance Examination Board.

16

PROGRAMMATIC ASSESSMENT: AN AVENUE TO A DIFFERENT ASSESSMENT CULTURE

Cees van der Vleuten, Sylvia Heeneman, and Suzanne Schut

In 1996, van der Vleuten published a paper in which the utility of any assessment was expressed as a compromise among the quality characteristics of reliability, validity, educational consequences and cost (van der Vleuten, 1996). This list of quality characteristics can be easily extended, as has been done in the literature (Baartman, Bastiaens, Kirschner, & van der Vleuten, 2006; Norcini et al., 2011); assessment is always a compromise between such criteria. Different compromises will need to be made depending on the context and the purpose of an assessment. For example, very different compromises will be made in the context of a licensing exam as compared to an in-training assessment. In a licensing exam, no compromises will be made on the reliability of the assessment, while in an in-training assessment, reliability is less critical and more attention might be given to the educational value of the assessment. Thus, assessment is also an optimization problem—and the question is when to optimize what? In van der Vleuten and Schuwirth (2005), quality characteristics may be improved by combining assessments into a program of assessment at the level of a whole curriculum. A framework was developed for addressing quality at the program level (Dijkstra, van der Vleuten, & Schuwirth, 2010), followed by a set of generic guidelines for setting up a program of assessment (Dijkstra et al., 2012). A model was proposed for what was termed programmatic assessment (van der Vleuten et al., 2012; Schuwirth & van der Vleuten, 2011) following best practices from assessment research (van der Vleuten, Schuwirth, Scheele, Driessen, & Hodges, 2010). This chapter will describe what programmatic assessment entails, present the experiences with programmatic assessment in practice and discuss the research within the literature on this topic so far.

THE TRADITIONAL APPROACH TO ASSESSMENT

Most assessment practices are characterized by their modular approach. An educational module (session, course, semester, clerkship) is closed with a final assessment; after passing the assessment, a learner moves on to the next educational module. When all modules are completed, the learner is finished and qualified as 'competent'. In some cases, additional end-of-year assessments or final assessments are also conducted. This is in line with a traditional view on learning: when mastery of the components is demonstrated, the learner is competent. Learners move from hurdle to hurdle and demonstrate short-term mastery of the specific area or topic that is being assessed at that moment. Contemporary education is moving away from this model of learning to a more constructivist approach, in which learners construct their knowledge and competence by working on challenging, authentic tasks or while learning in the workplace.

> Constructivist theories on learning suggest that learning is an interpretive, recursive, non-linear building process by active learners interacting with their surroundings, and the physical and social world. It describes how structures, language, activity and meaning-making come about, rather than simply characterising the structure and stages of thought, or isolating behaviours learned through reinforcement.
> (Berkhout, Helmich, Teunissen, van der Vleuten, & Jaarsma, 2018, p. 37)

Education programs are moving from a time-based model to an outcome-based model. Competency-based education is an answer to this paradigm shift; competency frameworks have been developed in many countries around the world. These competency frameworks focus on mastery of complex behavioural skills such as professionalism, collaboration and communication, in addition to the focus on medical knowledge and expertise. The desired outcomes are developed by giving them explicit attention in the curriculum, as longitudinal strands addressed over time, with appropriate feedback in safe learning environments (van den Eertwegh, van Dalen, van Dulmen, van der Vleuten, & Scherpbier, 2014). These complex skills are typically assessed through direct observation of the behaviour in context (Kogan, Hatala, Hauer, & Holmboe, 2017). For this purpose, non-standardized assessment technology is rapidly emerging for workplace-based assessments (Kogan, Holmboe, & Hauer, 2009) (see Chapter 10). Education is also moving from teacher-controlled education to learner-controlled education, in which the learner has an active self-directed role in learning and progressing. These trends in education are seen in undergraduate medical training as well as in postgraduate training. Programmatic assessment is targeted towards this type of competency-based education.

Traditional assessment programs often lead to poor learning strategies (Cilliers, Schuwirth, Adendorff, Herman, & van der Vleuten, 2010) and to reductionism (Harrison, Könings, Schuwirth, Wass, & van der Vleuten, 2017). In a traditional summative approach, little information is available for the learner. Information about the learner is primarily expressed in the form of grades; however, grades form a relatively poor source of feedback (Shute, 2008). Particularly when assessing complex skills, narrative information conveys much more meaning than do numeric scores (Govaerts & van der Vleuten, 2013; Ginsburg, Eva, & Regehr, 2013; Ginsburg, van der Vleuten, & Eva, 2017). When feedback is provided in traditional summative assessment systems, learners frequently do not engage with or utilize the feedback (Harrison, Könings, Schuwirth, Wass, & van der Vleuten, 2015)—passing the test lowers the motivation for feedback use. The summative focus hinders the formative function of assessment. Programmatic assessment attempts to address these problems and proposes a different perspective on assessment.

PROGRAMMATIC ASSESSMENT

In programmatic assessment, an overarching competency framework is chosen, such as the Canadian CanMEDS roles (Frank & Danoff, 2007), the competencies framework of the Accreditation Council for Graduate Medical Education (ACGME) in the United States (Batalden, Leach, Swing, Dreyfus, & Dreyfus, 2002) or the General Medical Council's Good Medical Practice domains in the United Kingdom (General Medical Council, 2013). Every individual assessment provides information in relation to this overarching framework, and assessment activities are planned in such a way that there is alignment between methods of assessment and the overarching framework.

Programmatic assessment has a number of rules (Box 16.1).

> ## Box 16.1 Guidelines for Programmatic Assessments
>
> 1. Pass/fail decisions are not based on a single data point (assessment event).
> 2. The program includes a deliberate mix of assessment methods.
> 3. Feedback use and self-directed learning are promoted through a continuous dialogue with the learner.
> 4. The number of data points needed is proportionally related to the stakes of the assessment decision.
> 5. High-stakes decisions are professional judgments made by a committee of assessors.

1. Pass/Fail Decisions Are Not Based on a Single Data Point

An individual assessment event, such as a multiple-choice question test or an observed patient encounter, is considered to be one data point in programmatic assessment. For a single data point, no compromises are made on learning goals. A single data point should provide meaningful information to the learner. It is feedback oriented, not decision oriented, since there is too little information in a single data point to make a high-stakes decision. Metaphorically, an individual data point can be compared to a pixel in a photograph. With a single pixel, we cannot see the image in the photograph. Feedback from a single data point can be of quantitative or qualitative nature. Standardized tests usually provide quantitative information and comparative information regarding where the learners stand in relation to peers. Non-standardized (e.g., workplace-based) assessments may also report scores, but should also include rich narrative information. The information from the assessment should inform the overarching framework; this means that instruments are structured to be consistent with the overarching framework. For example, a mini-CEX form (see Chapter 10) provides ratings and narrative information on all (relevant) competencies such as communication. A multi-source feedback form is structured in the same way, allowing information on communication skills to be aggregated across instruments. In sum, a single data point is optimized for learning, not for decision-making on passing or failing.

2. The Program Includes a Deliberate Mix of Different Assessment Methods

Methods of assessment are chosen based on their alignment with the educational objectives. Choices are made deliberately. For example, if one wants to assess critical appraisal skills, a series of assessments may require learners to write, to verbalize, to synthesize and to act and be directly observed. Any method may be useful, objective or subjective, quantitative or qualitative. There is no particular need for a single method to be highly reliable. The utility of a method comprising a single data point fully lies in the educational justification for using that method in that moment in time in the learning program.

Traditionally, most assessment is modular. However, to monitor the development of learners, some of the assessment should be longitudinal in nature, evaluating a learner in relation to the endpoint of learning. This can be done by formulating standards in a longitudinal or developmental way, as do the ACGME milestones (Holmboe, Edgar, & Hamstra, 2016). An example of longitudinal assessment in the cognitive domain is progress testing (Wrigley, van der Vleuten, Freeman, & Muijtjens, 2012; Heeneman, Schut, Donkers, van der Vleuten, & Muijtjens, 2017). A progress test is a comprehensive test consisting of multiple-choice items representing the end objectives of a training program. Progress tests are administered to all students in the program multiple times each year, and the development of knowledge is monitored. Maximum alignment with the goals of the training program is achieved through a mix of assessment methods.

Assessment optimization is strongly influenced by educational goals, with the deliberate intent to have assessment drive learning in a desired way.

3. Feedback Use and Self-Directed Learning Are Promoted Through a Continuous Dialogue With the Learner

The provision of feedback does not guarantee the use of feedback (Hattie & Timperley, 2007). This is particularly true in summative assessment programs where learners are inclined to ignore feedback (Harrison et al., 2015), and this is particularly true for learners who need the feedback most (Harrison et al., 2016). A summative approach seems to hinder the formative use of assessment. The use of feedback should therefore be educationally scaffolded through creating a dialogue around feedback. One approach is to coach students by means of a mentoring program (Driessen & Overeem, 2013); reflection and feedback use is promoted by creating a relationship with a trusted person (Watling, Driessen, van der Vleuten, Vanstone, & Lingard, 2013; Telio, Ajjawi, & Regehr, 2015). The mentor has access to all assessment information (and other learning data) and periodically discusses this with the learner. The learner is stimulated to reflect on the assessment feedback and to plan study actions accordingly.

4. The Number of Data Points Needed Is Proportionally Related to the Stakes of the Assessment Decision

At some point in time, pass/fail or promotion decisions need to be made. In programmatic assessment, the conventional summative and formative distinction (Lau, 2016) is replaced by a continuum of stakes. A single data point is low stakes since no pass/fail consequences are connected to it. It is not of 'no stakes', since the information from the assessment may feed into higher-stakes decisions at a later moment of time. In general, the higher the stakes of the decision-making involved, the more data points are needed. In the pixel metaphor, one needs many pixels to see the image. In most training programs, high-stakes decisions are often connected to promotion to the next year or to graduation. It is wise to also have one or more intermediate decisions throughout the year. The outcome of a high-stakes decision should never come as a surprise to the learner. The intermediate decision provides both feedback and feedforward information and can be used in the mentoring program to tailor remediation activities.

In general, decision-making in programmatic assessment is optimized by using sufficient data to make such a decision.

5. High-Stakes Decisions Are Professional Judgments Made by a Committee of Assessors

Given the quantitative and qualitative nature of the assessment information, high(er)-stakes decision-making regarding passing or failing cannot be a statistical algorithm. The decision requires a professional judgement, usually within a group such as a clinical competency committee (Hauer et al., 2016). All assessment (and other learning) information, usually in the form of an electronic portfolio, is held against performance standards relevant to the phase of training and a decision is made. The decision may be pass or fail and may include a distinction such as 'honors'. Sometimes a letter grade is given (Bok et al., 2013). A decision is usually made separately for each element of the overarching framework, followed by a final overall decision. The committee may also recommend remediation activities.

To return to the example of communication, all quantitative and qualitative (narrative) information on all instruments that have informed this competency are taken together and a judgment is made as to whether the performance constitutes a pass or fail (or distinction). All the information in the portfolio is aggregated using the overarching framework. This is fundamentally different from the traditional approach in assessment, in which we aggregate *within a method* to arrive at a decision. In programmatic assessment, information is aggregated *across instruments and across time* towards meaningful constructs that stem from the overarching framework.

A number of measures can be taken to further enhance the trustworthiness of the decision (Driessen, van der Vleuten, Schuwirth, Van Tartwijk, & Vermunt, 2005):

- Independence of the committee in relation to the learner increases the credibility of the judgment, because bias will not be introduced due to direct social relationships. However, it also brings a dilemma. The mentor is the person who knows the learner best; the mentor should therefore be in the best position to make a judgment. However, allowing a mentor to make pass/fail judgments can jeopardize the trusting relationship between learner and mentor. In practice, compromise solutions may be created. For example, the mentor may provide a recommendation, but the final decisions are made by other people.
- The size of the committee and the level of preparation of the assessors contributes to the credibility of the judgment, with larger committees making better judgments (Bok et al., 2013).
- The amount of deliberation in the committee and the justification of the judgment contributes to the credibility of the decision.
- Finally, prior intermediate decisions will increase the credibility of the final decision.

All of these due process measures will raise the trustworthiness of decision-making in competency committees.

Committee meetings can be efficiently planned to save time and resources. For most learners, decision-making will be quite straightforward and will not require the full committee's attention. Committee meetings can be planned in such a way that a discussion only takes place for learners who need discussion; basically, one titrates committee or assessor involvement based on the clarity of the information on the learner.

High-stakes decisions in assessment are optimized by having many data points that are judged by experts in groups. The judgment process is anchored by due process procedural measures that support the trustworthiness of the decision. It should be noted that trustworthiness is a term used in qualitative research methodology. The above measures to build rigor in decision-making are inspired by qualitative research strategies (van der Vleuten et al., 2010; Frambach, van der Vleuten, & Durning, 2013). Table 16.1 provides a set of assessment strategies related to qualitative rigor.

Programmatic assessment is an integral approach to assessment that contrasts strongly with the traditional approach to assessment. Table 16.2 provides some contrasting characteristics of both approaches. Box 16.2 describes an example of a programmatic assessment implementation.

Table 16.1 Assessment Strategies Related to Qualitative Research Methodologies for Building Rigor in Assessment Decisions

Strategies to Establish Trustworthiness	Criteria	Assessment Strategy
Credibility	Prolonged engagement	Training of assessors. The persons who know the student the best (a coach, peers) provide information for the assessment. Incorporate in the procedure intermittent feedback cycles.
	Triangulation	Many assessors should be involved and different credible groups should be included. Use multiple sources of assessment within or across methods. Organize a sequential judgment procedure in which conflicting information necessitates the gathering of more information.

(Continued)

Table 16.1 (continued)

Strategies to Establish Trustworthiness	Criteria	Assessment Strategy
	Peer examination (sometimes called peer debriefing)	Organize discussion between assessors (before and intermediate) for benchmarking and discussion of the process and the results. Separate multiple roles of the assessors by removing the summative assessment decisions from the coaching role.
	Member checking	Incorporate the learner's point of view in the assessment procedure. Incorporate in the procedure intermittent feedback cycles.
	Structural coherence	Organize assessment committee to discuss inconsistencies in the assessment data.
Transferability	Time sampling	Sample broadly over different contexts and patients.
	Thick description (or dense description)	Incorporate in the assessment instruments possibilities to give qualitative, narrative information. Give narrative information a lot of weight in the assessment procedure.
Dependability	Stepwise replication	Sample broadly over different assessors.
Dependability/ Confirmability	Audit	Document the different steps in the assessment process (a formal assessment plan approved by an examination board; overviews of the results per phase). Organize quality assessment procedures with external auditor. Give learners the possibility to appeal to the assessment decision.

Source: Reprinted from van der Vleuten, C., Schuwirth, L., Scheele, F., Driessen, E., & Hodges, B. (2010). The Assessment of Professional Competence: Building Blocks for Theory Development. *Best Practice & Research Clinical Obstetrics & Gynaecology*, *24*(6), 703–719; with permission from Elsevier, www.journals.elsevier.com/best-practice-and-research-clinical-obstetrics-and-gynaecology

Table 16.2 Overview of the Salient Differences Between a Traditional and a Programmatic Approach to the Assessment of Competence

Feature	Traditional Summative Assessment Approach	Programmatic Assessment Approach
Education philosophy	Behaviouristic	Constructivist
Use of single data points	Pass/fail decision oriented	Feedback oriented
Performance information	Grades	Profile scores, narrative information, information-rich data
Performance orientation	Modular	Longitudinal, developmental
Remediation	Resits	Personalized ongoing remediation activities
Use of methods	Restricted to reliable methods	Eclectic, depending on the educational justification
Aggregation of information	Across skills/content areas within methods	Across methods to skills/content areas
Learner support	Unstructured	Mentoring
Progress decisions	Algorithmic	Professional judgment (in committees)

Box 16.2 Case Study: A Programmatic Assessment Approach

The graduate entry program in medicine at the University of Maastricht is a four-year program with a strong emphasis on clinical research; in addition to the MD degree, an MSc is awarded for research. The first year is comprised of a classical problem-based learning curriculum. In the second year, real patients are seen and serve as starting point for learning. The third year consists of clinical rotations, and the final year is comprised of 18 weeks of research and 18 weeks of clinical work in a specialty of the learner's choice. The CanMEDS framework (Frank & Danoff, 2007, p. 21) is used on a national basis. There is no national licensing exam in The Netherlands.

The assessment program in the first two years has block-related elements with variable assessment formats. Classic multiple-choice tests are used to assess the "medical expert" (medical knowledge) role. Some of the units use other written formats or have smaller tests spread out through the block. In the first year, learners see simulated patients, and in the second year, real patients. Patient encounters are evaluated with mini-CEX-like forms (see Chapter 10) that assess the different competencies from the CanMEDS framework; forms are completed by faculty or peers. In years 3 and 4, an elaborate work-based assessment system is implemented using field notes, mini-CEXs and multisource feedback rounds. Longitudinal assessment is done in the form of progress testing for the medical expert role: all students in all years are assessed with a comprehensive written test four times a year. Growth of knowledge is monitored across time (and in collaboration with six of the eight medical schools in the country). All other competencies are assessed through periodic self, peer, and tutor or clinical supervisor assessment. The purpose of these assessments is to provide feedback, not to pass or fail the learner. There is elaborate (online) profile scoring on standardized (written) tests and both online and verbal feedback from observational instruments such as the mini-CEX. All information is stored in an electronic portfolio.

All learners have a mentor who follows the learner throughout all four years. Each mentor has about ten learners. Learners and mentors have regular meetings that are prepared by learners, who have to self-analyse their feedback and develop a plan for further study. The mentor has access to the e-portfolio and all the information in it, including graphical performance overviews and aggregations of narrative information. It is easy to navigate and to quickly get an overview of the learner's progress.

Halfway through the year is an intermediate assessment by another mentor (not the student's mentor), and at the end of the year a high-stakes decision is made by a committee. The committee consists of mentors, but a mentor has no say in decisions regarding their own students. The judgment is either pass, fail or distinction. The meetings are prepared by the chair of the committee. Hardly any committee time is spent on clear-cut decisions; on the other hand, there is ample discussion of borderline learners, during which arguments are exchanged and intense deliberation conducted until consensus is achieved. A justification or rationale is provided to learners who fail. The committee may also provide recommendations for remediation.

EVALUATION OF PROGRAMMATIC ASSESSMENT

Although programmatic assessment is based on assessment research insights (van der Vleuten, 2016) and resonates with similar calls for assessment at the program level (Knight, 2000; Fielding & Regehr, 2017; Eva et al., 2016; Bowe & Armstrong, 2017; Gibbs & Dunbar-Goddet, 2009;

Harris et al., 2017; Konopasek, Norcini, & Krupat, 2016), research on programmatic assessment is in its infancy. The literature on programmatic assessment implementations is rapidly growing, at both the undergraduate (Dannefer & Henson, 2007; Bok et al., 2013; Heeneman, Oudkerk Pool, Schuwirth, van der Vleuten, & Driessen, 2015; Jamieson, Jenkins, Beatty, & Palermo, 2017; Schut, Driessen, van Tartwijk, van der Vleuten, & Heeneman, 2018) and the postgraduate levels (Chan & Sherbino, 2015; Li, Sherbino, & Chan, 2017; Schuwirth, Valentine, & Dilena, 2017; McEwen, Griffiths, & Schultz, 2015; Perry et al., 2018). These descriptions generally report successful and satisfying implementations as proof of concept. However, much further research needs to be done. We will summarize some of the research done so far and some of our experiences with programmatic assessment implementations.

One of the critical features of programmatic assessment is the blurred distinction between formative and summative elements of assessment. A few studies have shown that a low-stakes assessment may be perceived by students as a high-stakes assessment (Bok et al., 2013; Heeneman et al., 2015). A recent study investigated how stakes are perceived by learners and what influences these perceptions (Schut et al., 2018). A central finding was that stakes are mediated by perceived learner agency: when more learner control was perceived by the learners, the stakes were perceived as lower. Several design factors and cultural/relational factors were mediating perceived agency and stakes. These included the opportunity to influence assessment outcomes (for example, the ability to interact with an assessor in an oral assessment), the freedom of the learner to gather and select evidence for performance monitoring, and opportunities for remediation within the program. The stakes were also strongly mediated by the relationship between learner and assessor. When this relationship was safe and learners felt supported, the stakes were perceived to be low.

The importance of the assessment culture was also found in a study on different assessment approaches (summative vs. programmatic) (Harrison et al., 2017). Receptivity to feedback was increased when students had control over the assessment, when the assessment was authentic and relevant, and when support was provided in the interpretation of feedback. The provision of grades or ranking information provided helpful external reference information but hindered the promotion of excellence. Not providing grades led to initial uncertainty but later promoted an aspiration to excellence. Another study (Perry et al., 2018) confirmed that learners in a programmatic assessment system engaged more with feedback than learners in a summative system.

After implementing programmatic assessment in an undergraduate medical training program in New Zealand, earlier detection of failing students was reported with fewer "failures to fail" (Wilkinson et al., 2011). The system also helped detect learners in difficulty in challenging-to-assess areas such as professionalism.

Finally, a study on mentoring in a programmatic approach to assessment showed that the quality and skills of the mentor influenced the quality of self-directed learning (Heeneman & de Grave, 2017). More longitudinal mentoring helps build the expertise of the mentor and promotes the creation of a mentoring community in which experiences may be shared.

From our own experience with programmatic assessment, which has been implemented in several of our training programs, and from our involvement in a number of other implementations, we can conclude a number of things. First, the quality of implementation determines the success of programmatic assessment. Moving a traditional summative-approach program to programmatic assessment is a major operation that necessitates change management. Programmatic assessment demands a different mind-set from teachers and learners in order to achieve a learning and feedback culture. Successful participatory design in which staff development and design of the program went hand in hand has been reported (Jamieson et al., 2017), but it can be very difficult for teachers and learners to think outside the summative paradigm (Harrison et al., 2017). The magnitude of the needed change can be compared to moving a school from a didactic learning approach to problem-based learning (PBL). Similar to PBL, implementation may fail due to insufficient buy-in from the teaching faculty. Just as in PBL, 'hybrid' programmatic assessment approaches will appear as a result of compromises on the original intended model, but just as in PBL (Frambach, Driessen, Chan, & van der Vleuten, 2012), they will probably achieve only 'hybrid' success.

A second lesson is that obtaining high-quality feedback from assessments is a challenge. Giving good feedback requires time and effort from faculty. Narrative feedback can be more informative than quantitative feedback, particularly for complex and behavioural skills, but is more time consuming and thus harder to get. Programmatic assessment relies on the richness of assessment data to monitor progress and to arrive at trustworthy decisions. Faculty development regarding feedback is important, as is the articulation of the role of the learner in eliciting good feedback.

A third lesson resonates with the above study on mentoring (Heeneman & de Grave, 2017). High-quality mentoring is crucial for reflection and feedback utilization. Self-directed learning is strongly promoted when guided through a relationship with a trusted person. Mentors find the mentoring role engaging, due to the personal contact with learners.

A fourth lesson is that decision-making regarding learner progress is generally a smooth process that only rarely leads to complications or appeals by learners. When organized well, consensus is relatively easily reached despite differences between assessors (Pool, Govaerts, Jaarsma, & Driessen, 2018).

A final lesson is that an electronic portfolio greatly facilitates the process. Essential features of an electronic portfolio include the ability to collect assessment data (e.g., from multisource feedback), the capacity to aggregate the information in quantitative or qualitative overviews and summaries, and ease of access and navigation.

Programmatic assessment can improve content validity by ensuring that many data points within and across content areas are obtained. The blueprint, however, has moved from the test level to the program level, and content validity will depend on mapping data points in relation to the overarching competency framework. Construct-irrelevant variance is reduced by assessing across time, methods and raters. When properly implemented, programmatic assessment can improve consequential validity since there is a strong focus on providing feedback, on educational scaffolding of the feedback and on creating a safe culture of feedback and reflection. Naturally, all these benefits from validity evidence need further empirical verification.

CONCLUSION

Programmatic assessment provides a new framework for assessment. The approach carefully optimizes assessment design choices based on the purpose of the assessment and improves the decision-making process. To a large extent, it disconnects *data gathering* in assessment from *decision-making* in assessment, two functions that are traditionally fully mixed. Programmatic assessment has the potential to promote more constructivist education in health professions education, at both the undergraduate and the postgraduate levels. With more programs adopting programmatic assessment and through more research, we will learn if and how it can transform educational practice.

Note: Additional material and resources may be available at the UIC AHPE website: https://go.uic.edu/AHPE

REFERENCES

Baartman, L.K., Bastiaens, T.J., Kirschner, P.A., & van der Vleuten, C.P. (2006). The wheel of competency assessment: Presenting quality criteria for competency assessment programs. *Studies in Educational Evaluation*, 32(2), 153–170.

Batalden, P., Leach, D., Swing, S., Dreyfus, H., & Dreyfus, S. (2002). General competencies and accreditation in graduate medical education. *Health Affairs, 21*(5), 103–111.

Berkhout, J.J., Helmich, E., Teunissen, P.W., van der Vleuten, C.P., & Jaarsma, A.D.C. (2018). Context matters when striving to promote active and lifelong learning in medical education. *Medical Education, 52*(1), 34–44.

Bok, H.G., Teunissen, P.W., Favier, R.P., Rietbroek, N.J., Theyse, L.F., Brommer, H., . . . Jaarsma, D.A. (2013). Programmatic assessment of competency-based workplace learning: When theory meets practice. *BMC Medical Education, 13*(1), 123.

Bowe, C.M., & Armstrong, E. (2017). Assessment for systems learning: A holistic assessment framework to support decision making across the medical education continuum. *Academic Medicine, 92*(5), 585–592.

Chan, T., & Sherbino, J. (2015). The McMaster modular assessment program (McMAP): A theoretically grounded work-based assessment system for an emergency medicine residency program. *Academic Medicine, 90*(7), 900–905.

Cilliers, F.J., Schuwirth, L.W., Adendorff, H.J., Herman, N., & van der Vleuten, C.P. (2010). The mechanism of impact of summative assessment on medical students' learning. *Advances in Health Sciences Education, 15*(5), 695–715.

Dannefer, E.F., & Henson, L.C. (2007). The portfolio approach to competency-based assessment at the Cleveland Clinic Lerner College of Medicine. *Academic Medicine, 82*(5), 493–502.

Dijkstra, J., Galbraith, R., Hodges, B.D., McAvoy, P.A., McCrorie, P., Southgate, L.J., . . . Schuwirth, L.W. (2012). Expert validation of fit-for-purpose guidelines for designing programmes of assessment. *BMC Medical Education, 12*(1), 20.

Dijkstra, J., van der Vleuten, C., & Schuwirth, L. (2010). A new framework for designing programmes of assessment. *Advances in Health Sciences Education, 15*(3), 379–393.

Driessen, E.W., & Overeem, K. (2013). Mentoring. In K. Walsh (Ed.), *Oxford Textbook of medical education*. Oxford: Oxford University Press.

Driessen, E., van der Vleuten, C., Schuwirth, L., Van Tartwijk, J., & Vermunt, J. (2005). The use of qualitative research criteria for portfolio assessment as an alternative to reliability evaluation: A case study. *Medical Education, 39*(2), 214–220.

Eva, K.W., Bordage, G., Campbell, C., Galbraith, R., Ginsburg, S., Holmboe, E., & Regehr, G. (2016). Towards a program of assessment for health professionals: From training into practice. *Advances in Health Sciences Education, 21*(4), 897–913.

Fielding, D.W., & Regehr, G. (2017). A call for an integrated program of assessment. *American Journal of Pharmaceutical Education, 81*(4), 77.

Frambach, J.M., Driessen, E.W., Chan, L.C., & van der Vleuten, C.P. (2012). Rethinking the globalisation of problem-based learning: How culture challenges self-directed learning. *Medical Education, 46*(8), 738–747.

Frambach, J.M., van der Vleuten, C.P., & Durning, S.J. (2013). AM last page: Quality criteria in qualitative and quantitative research. *Academic Medicine, 88*(4), 552.

Frank, J.R., & Danoff, D. (2007). The CanMEDS initiative: Implementing an outcomes-based framework of physician competencies. *Medical Teacher, 29*(7), 642–647.

General Medical Council: Good medical practice: Working with doctors for patients. (2013). Retrieved from www.gmc-uk.org/guidance.

Gibbs, G., & Dunbar-Goddet, H. (2009). Characterising programme-level assessment environments that support learning. *Assessment & Evaluation in Higher Education, 34*(4), 481–489.

Ginsburg, S., Eva, K., & Regehr, G. (2013). Do in-training evaluation reports deserve their bad reputations? A study of the reliability and predictive ability of ITER scores and narrative comments. *Academic Medicine, 88*(10), 1539–1544.

Ginsburg, S., van der Vleuten, C.P., & Eva, K.W. (2017). The hidden value of narrative comments for assessment: A quantitative reliability analysis of qualitative data. *Academic Medicine, 92*(11), 1617–1621.

Govaerts, M., & van der Vleuten, C.P. (2013). Validity in work-based assessment: Expanding our horizons. *Medical Education, 47*(12), 1164–1174.

Harris, P., Bhanji, F., Topps, M., Ross, S., Lieberman, S., Frank, J.R., . . . Collaborators, I. (2017). Evolving concepts of assessment in a competency-based world. *Medical Teacher, 39*(6), 603–608.

Harrison, C.J., Könings, K.D., Dannefer, E.F., Schuwirth, L.W., Wass, V., & van der Vleuten, C.P. (2016). Factors influencing students' receptivity to formative feedback emerging from different assessment cultures. *Perspectives on Medical Education, 5*(5), 276–284.

Harrison, C.J., Könings, K.D., Schuwirth, L., Wass, V., & van der Vleuten, C. (2015). Barriers to the uptake and use of feedback in the context of summative assessment. *Advances in Health Sciences Education, 20*(1), 229–245.

Harrison, C.J., Könings, K.D., Schuwirth, L.W., Wass, V., & van der Vleuten, C.P. (2017). Changing the culture of assessment: The dominance of the summative assessment paradigm. *BMC Medical Education, 17*(1), 73.

Hattie, J., & Timperley, H. (2007). The power of feedback. *Review of Educational Research, 77*(1), 81–112.

Hauer, K.E., Cate, O.t., Boscardin, C.K., Iobst, W., Holmboe, E.S., Chesluk, B., . . . O'Sullivan, P.S. (2016). Ensuring resident competence: A narrative review of the literature on group decision making to inform the work of clinical competency committees. *Journal of Graduate Medical Education, 8*(2), 156–164.

Heeneman, S., & de Grave, W. (2017). Tensions in mentoring medical students toward self-directed and reflective learning in a longitudinal portfolio-based mentoring system—An activity theory analysis. *Medical Teacher, 39*(4), 368–376.

Heeneman, S., Oudkerk Pool, A., Schuwirth, L.W., van der Vleuten, C.P., & Driessen, E.W. (2015). The impact of programmatic assessment on student learning: Theory versus practice. *Medical Education, 49*(5), 487–498.

Heeneman, S., Schut, S., Donkers, J., van der Vleuten, C., & Muijtjens, A. (2017). Embedding of the progress test in an assessment program designed according to the principles of programmatic assessment. *Medical Teacher, 39*(1), 44–52.

Holmboe, E.S., Edgar, L., & Hamstra, S. (2016). *The milestones guidebook*. Chicago, IL: American Council for Graduate Medical Education.

Jamieson, J., Jenkins, G., Beatty, S., & Palermo, C. (2017). Designing programmes of assessment: A participatory approach. *Medical Teacher, 39*(11), 1182–1188.

Knight, P.T. (2000). The value of a programme-wide approach to assessment. *Assessment & Evaluation in Higher Education, 25*(3), 237–251.

Kogan, J.R., Hatala, R., Hauer, K.E., & Holmboe, E. (2017). Guidelines: The do's, don'ts and don't knows of direct observation of clinical skills in medical education. *Perspectives on Medical Education, 6*(5), 286–305.

Kogan, J.R., Holmboe, E.S., & Hauer, K.E. (2009). Tools for direct observation and assessment of clinical skills of medical trainees: A systematic review. *Jama, 302*(12), 1316–1326.

Konopasek, L., Norcini, J., & Krupat, E. (2016). Focusing on the formative: Building an assessment system aimed at student growth and development. *Academic Medicine, 91*(11), 1492–1497.

Lau, A.M.S. (2016). "Formative good, summative bad?"—A review of the dichotomy in assessment literature. *Journal of Further and Higher Education, 40*(4), 509–525.

Li, S.A., Sherbino, J., & Chan, T.M. (2017). McMaster Modular Assessment Program (McMAP) Through the years: Residents' experience with an evolving feedback culture over a 3-year period. *AEM Education and Training, 1*(1), 5–14.

McEwen, L.A., Griffiths, J., & Schultz, K. (2015). Developing and successfully implementing a competency-based portfolio assessment system in a postgraduate family medicine residency program. *Academic Medicine, 90*(11), 1515–1526.

Norcini, J., Anderson, B., Bollela, V., Burch, V., Costa, M.J., Duvivier, R., . . . Perrott, V. (2011). Criteria for good assessment: Consensus statement and recommendations from the Ottawa 2010 Conference. *Medical Teacher, 33*(3), 206–214.

Perry, M., Linn, A., Munzer, B.W., Hopson, L., Amlong, A., Cole, M., & Santen, S.A. (2018). Programmatic assessment in emergency medicine: Implementation of best practices. *Journal of Graduate Medical Education, 10*(1), 84–90.

Pool, A.O., Govaerts, M.J., Jaarsma, D.A., & Driessen, E.W. (2018). From aggregation to interpretation: How assessors judge complex data in a competency-based portfolio. *Advances in Health Sciences Education, 23*(2), 275–287.

Schut, S., Driessen, E., van Tartwijk, J., van der Vleuten, C., & Heeneman, S. (2018). Stakes in the eye of the beholder: An international study of learners' perceptions within programmatic assessment. *Medical Education, 52*(6), 654–663.

Schuwirth, L., Valentine, N., & Dilena, P. (2017). An application of programmatic assessment for learning (PAL) system for general practice training. *GMS Journal for Medical Education, 34*(5).

Schuwirth, L.W., & van der Vleuten, C.P. (2011). Programmatic assessment: From assessment of learning to assessment for learning. *Medical Teacher, 33*(6), 478–485.

Shute, V.J. (2008). Focus on formative feedback. *Review of Educational Research, 78*(1), 153–189.

Telio, S., Ajjawi, R., & Regehr, G. (2015). The "educational alliance" as a framework for reconceptualizing feedback in medical education. *Academic Medicine, 90*(5), 609–614.

Van den Eertwegh, V., van Dalen, J., van Dulmen, S., van der Vleuten, C., & Scherpbier, A. (2014). Residents' perceived barriers to communication skills learning: Comparing two medical working contexts in postgraduate training. *Patient Education and Counseling, 95*(1), 91–97.

van der Vleuten, C.P. (1996). The assessment of professional competence: Developments, research and practical implications. *Advances in Health Sciences Education, 1*(1), 41–67.

van der Vleuten, C.P. (2016). Revisiting "Assessing professional competence: From methods to programmes". *Medical Education, 50*(9), 885–888.

van Der Vleuten, C.P., & Schuwirth, L.W. (2005). Assessing professional competence: From methods to programmes. *Medical Education, 39*(3), 309–317.

van der Vleuten, C.P., Schuwirth, L., Driessen, E., Dijkstra, J., Tigelaar, D., Baartman, L., & van Tartwijk, J. (2012). A model for programmatic assessment fit for purpose. *Medical Teacher, 34*(3), 205–214.

van der Vleuten, C., Schuwirth, L., Scheele, F., Driessen, E., & Hodges, B. (2010). The assessment of professional competence: Building blocks for theory development. *Best Practice & Research Clinical Obstetrics & Gynaecology, 24*(6), 703–719.

Watling, C., Driessen, E., van der Vleuten, C.P., Vanstone, M., & Lingard, L. (2013). Music lessons: Revealing medicine's learning culture through a comparison with that of music. *Medical Education, 47*(8), 842–850.

Wilkinson, T.J., Tweed, M.J., Egan, T.G., Ali, A.N., McKenzie, J.M., Moore, M., & Rudland, J.R. (2011). Joining the dots: Conditional pass and programmatic assessment enhances recognition of problems with professionalism and factors hampering student progress. *BMC Medical Education, 11*(1), 29.

Wrigley, W., van der Vleuten, C.P., Freeman, A., & Muijtjens, A. (2012). A systemic framework for the progress test: Strengths, constraints and issues: AMEE guide no. 71. *Medical Teacher, 34*(9), 683–697.

17

ASSESSMENT AFFECTING LEARNING

Matthew Lineberry

This chapter approaches assessment from a quite different perspective, focusing not on how an assessment *measures* learning processes and outcomes, but on how it *affects* them. That perspective may seem like a suitable afterthought: interesting, but secondary to measurement goals. However, the theory and evidence outlined here suggest that an assessment's effects can be as important as its measurement properties or more so. Assessment may also be among the most powerful methods for fostering learning, superior even to many sophisticated educational methods.

This is written with an eye to a future when assessment *affecting* learning (AAL) is a perspective as well studied and refined as our thinking about assessment *of* learning (AOL). First, I will explore current assessment terminology and suggest how an AAL perspective might lead us to think differently about such terms. Second, I will draw together research on how assessment can affect learning during four phases of education: course development, anticipation of an assessment event, the assessment event itself, and post-assessment reflection and improvement. At the end of the chapter, we won't yet arrive at a prescriptive set of AAL design guidelines; rather, I hope this serves as a map of the terrain, for the field to see opportunities for exploration and early application.

Before continuing, I invite you to take a "pop quiz"! This should give you direct experience with concepts in this chapter, and could reinforce what you've learned about assessment. I will share two questions about content from Chapter 2, "Validity and Quality." If you would, please physically write down answers—perhaps on a sheet of paper, if you don't want to mark up this book. While answering, please pay attention to thoughts or emotions that arise for you. When you are done, you can check your answers using the answer key at the end of this chapter.

Question 1:

Michael Kane's framework for assessment validity lists four main inferences (or "assumptions") involved when we interpret and use assessment scores. What are they? Give both the one-word term for each, plus a short definition.

	Kane inference (one word)	Short definition
1		
2		
3		
4		

Question 2:

What are two validity threats that could lead to *construct-irrelevant variance* during a multiple-choice test of pathophysiology knowledge (or any other content area you prefer)?

1	
2	

Once you are done: Thank you for participating! Now, please reflect on the thoughts and emotions you had while answering those questions and reviewing the answer key:

- What is the most salient thought you had during this?
  What was the most noticeable emotion?
- How do you suppose your thoughts and emotions might have differed if I used a different response format, such as multiple choice rather than free response?
- Does answering such questions feel natural—perhaps you typically test yourself after reading—or, is answering questions not the normal way you engage with material like this?

Hold on to those self-reflections as you read through the chapter—which I promise includes no further pop quizzes!—and see if any of them are reflected in the key theories and findings about AAL.

RECONSIDERING KEY CONCEPTS AND TERMS

For this chapter, when I say "assessment," I mean a whole social and technical *system* that challenges a person or persons to perform a task, and then collects and interprets data on whether their performance demonstrates knowledge, skill, ability, or other characteristics (KSAOs) of interest against a scoring key. Assessments aren't just about our test formats or their content; a certification examination isn't just "a lot of questions on a sheaf of papers." Rather, assessments function as a system of *people* participating, such as learners, educators, administrators, and test developers; *social structures*, such as power dynamics and interpersonal relationships between and among learners and educators; *tasks*, such as developing the assessment, preparing for it, running the event (and associated communications, logistics, etc.), completing the assessment, and reflecting and acting on it; and *technologies* both physical and conceptual, such as assessment methods, data collection equipment, scoring processes, and report formats (Figure 17.1). The "system-ness" of assessment will be a key consideration as we explore ways assessments can affect learning—recognizing, for instance, that while assessment techniques matter, so too do the social dynamics among and between examinees and educators.

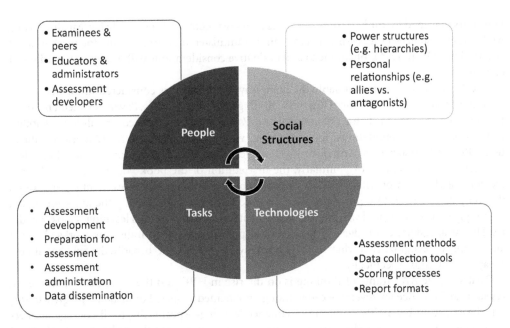

Figure 17.1 Assessments as sociotechnical systems

Also, per the definition above, I consider many activities to count as assessments—not just "formal examinations administered by educators." For instance, if several learners complete a simulated patient case and then review with an educator whether the actions they took adhered to key clinical practice guidelines, even if no "grade" is recorded, that's an assessment, for present purposes at least.

In HPE, we often refer to two types of assessment. "Summative" assessments involve decision-making and assignment of important labels or outcomes, such as grades or admission to a subsequent opportunity. Meanwhile, "formative" assessments lack such decision-making and are meant to support learning. These terms have also come to be closely related to the concept of "stakes," where summative assessments are often described as "high-stakes," meaning they influence major consequences for examinees, while formative assessments are labeled "low-stakes." These terms are reasonable but can be limiting. First, their use implies a dichotomy of judgment versus learning, when in fact every assessment involves some judgment, *and* every assessment is likely to affect learning in appreciable ways. Second, those terms focus on what educators *intend* but may not reflect how assessments are experienced. Even when educators think an assessment is low-stakes, learners can consider it high-stakes (Bok et al., 2013; Heeneman, Oudkerk Pool, Schuwirth, van der Vleuten, & Driessen, 2015; Schut, Driessen, van Tartwijk, van der Vleuten, & Heeneman, 2018; Watling & Ginsburg, 2019), and even summative assessments, such as national licensing examinations, can have dramatic effects on learning behaviors (London et al., 2016; Mehta, Hull, & Young, 2016; Prober, Kolars, First, & Melnick, 2016). Recent literature has promoted two new terms: "assessment of learning" (AOL) and "assessment for learning" (AFL; Dannefer, 2013). However, these terms might perpetuate the conflation of intents with effects, as much as saying a thing is "for" some purpose implies intent. These terms may also continue to imply a false dichotomy, especially if they are used to label different assessment activities, such as to say "our third-year students complete two assessments for learning before they complete the final assessment of learning."

I propose we recognize that all assessments have two important dimensions: their quality as assessments of learning and their effects on learning processes and outcomes, i.e., AOL *and* AAL.

Educators may tend to think of some instances of assessments as being mainly for learning (AFL), while other instances of assessments are mainly administered as assessments for measurement (AFM), but AOL and AAL phenomena and evaluative considerations will be at play regardless of educator intent.

The AOL frame is understandably the main way "assessment" is considered in formal assessment theory and design guidance (Harrison, Könings, Schuwirth, Wass, & van der Vleuten, 2017). For instance, the Standards for Educational and Psychological Testing cover validity, reliability, and fairness as the "foundations" for assessment, without considering AAL (American Educational Research Association, American Psychological Association, & National Council on Measurement in Education, 2014). Similarly, the first edition of the book you are reading did not include this chapter. Consistent with this, a review of simulation-based assessment reports found that only 20 of 217 (9%) reports considered the consequences of applying the assessment, and seemingly none investigated whether the assessment fostered or inhibited learning (Cook, Zendejas, Hamstra, Hatala, & Brydges, 2014). I do not point these out to indict the works above at all—simply to recognize that when we have been saying "assessment" broadly, the field has almost always meant "AOL" specifically.

That said, the AAL frame of thinking is on the rise in HPE, and there has been AAL theory, research, and practice for several decades, though not named as such. For instance, *progress testing* was developed in the 1970s primarily to enhance learning—specifically, to discourage learners from "cramming" by repeatedly giving comprehensive examinations throughout medical school (Albanese & Case, 2015; Norman, Neville, Blake, & Mueller, 2010). Similarly, *mastery learning* is an instructional design approach primarily concerned with supporting effective learning trajectories through assessment (Lineberry, Park, Cook, & Yudkowsky, 2015; McGaghie, 2015). The broader push toward competency-based medical education in many countries currently is also couched as an effort to use assessment to better support learning and development (Holmboe et al., 2017; Holmboe et al., 2015; Nasca, Philibert, Brigham, & Flynn, 2012).

AAL concepts are also beginning to appear in formal assessment theory and standards. An influential assessment model by Cees van der Vleuten pointed to assessment *utility* as the key criterion of interest in deciding how to apply assessments, noting that it involves a trade-off among five facets: validity, reliability, educational impact, acceptability, and cost (van der Vleuten, 1996). While all facets are important for effective assessment, van der Vleuten specifically called out educational impact as one that should rarely be compromised. Similarly, the 2018 Ottawa Consensus Framework for Good Assessment still lists "Validity" and "Reliability" as the first criteria, but then includes five other criteria for individual assessments, including "Educational Effect: That the assessment motivates those who take it to prepare in a fashion that has educational benefit" and "Catalytic Effect: That the assessment provides results and feedback in a fashion that motivates all stakeholders to create, enhance, and support education; it drives future learning forward and improves overall program quality" (Norcini et al., 2018). Thus, there is significant movement in the field toward seeing assessments as having important effects on learning.

MECHANISMS OF ACTION IN ASSESSMENT FOR LEARNING

Understanding *how* assessments affect learning can help us better design, use, and evaluate them. I see four main mechanisms of AAL, ordered as "phases" in assessment development and use (Box 17.1).

MECHANISM OF ACTION #1: COURSE DEVELOPMENT

A good educational program starts with effective design of educational experiences, and any sensible framework for curriculum design will recommend setting learning objectives and then using

Box 17.1 Assessment Affecting Learning: Mechanisms of Action at Each Stage of Assessment Design and Use

Stage	Mechanisms of action (under ideal design and use)
Course Development	Greater clarification of course objectives, *which should promote:* tighter linking of learning activities with achievement of objectives
Pre-Assessment Anticipation and Preparation	Clear and compelling communication of learning objectives, *which should promote:* learners and educators devoting sufficient effort and persistence, in directions that support achievement of objectives
Assessment Completion	Challenging and real-world-applicable exercise of targeted learner attributes (e.g., knowledge or skill), *which should promote:* deeply encoded, transfer-ready learning
Post-Assessment Reflection and Correction	Clear identification of performance gaps and underlying reasons, *which should promote:* effective adjustments toward improved learning and performance

those to guide educational activity design. However, even well-written learning objectives are not fully detailed specifications, but rather are moderately broad collections of targeted KSAOs. Consider, for instance, the learning objectives defined in the American Physiology Society's Medical Curriculum Objectives Project (Carroll, Navar, & Blaustein, 2012), such as that students should be able to "describe the organization of the circulatory system and explain how the systemic and pulmonary circulations are linked physically and physiologically." This leaves room for interpretation: for instance, what aspects of the organization of the circulatory system must be described? Is it acceptable if students can describe that organization in the abstract, but fail to apply understanding when diagnosing cardiac pathology?

Several curriculum design frameworks advocate that, beyond defining learning objectives, educators should select or develop assessments sensitive to the desired end state for learning, and then work backwards to develop learning activities that foster achievement of that end state. Such frameworks include backwards design (Wiggins & McTighe, 2005), mastery learning (McGaghie, 2015), and four-component instructional design (van Merriënboer & Kirschner, 2012). Augmenting learning objectives with assessment helps operationalize abstract ideas about desired KSAOs into concrete, observable learner behaviors. This is likely to prompt deliberative conversations that help education developers clarify their focus and then align learning activities with that intent. Assessment development processes have revealed that even experts who might be expected to "naturally" know and agree upon the important aspects of a learning objective may have many unstated, divergent notions of what that objective entails. For instance, one study found that expert cardiothoracic surgeons' opinions about the mandatory behaviors for a coronary artery bypass anastomosis (a basic surgical technique) were widely divergent; only 25% of each expert's initial "mandatory" steps were agreed to be mandatory after an assessment development exercise (Vaporciyan, Fikfak, Lineberry, Park, & Tekian, 2017). Another study observed experts teaching what they believed to be the key aspects of performing a cricothyrotomy; the authors found that experts omitted between 51% to 73% of the key aspects of the procedure, as defined within a gold-standard assessment (Sullivan, Yates, Inaba, Lam, & Clark, 2014). Of course, the core AOL principle that one should thoroughly sample the construct being assessed warns us against designing courses around any assessments with considerable construct underrepresentation. For instance, if only a limited number of multiple-choice questions were used to assess a quite broad construct, that may lead to problematic "teaching to the test."

MECHANISM OF ACTION #2: ANTICIPATION OF AN ASSESSMENT EVENT

Just as assessment items operationalize learning objectives for curriculum designers, they should be similarly clear and useful to learners and educators. Ideally, assessments also motivate learners and educators to strive toward the targeted learning. Motivation has three components: (1) *intensity*, e.g., how intently an educator listens for hints of a learner's underlying frame of thinking; (2) *persistence*, e.g., how long a learner spends in studying some content; and (3) *direction* of effort, e.g., which content an educator focuses their teaching on. Optimal learning should occur when learners and educators engage effortfully, for sufficient amounts of time, with high-quality learning content and approaches.

Assessments exemplify what is broadly known about goal setting and striving: that goals can create powerful motivation for behavior (Austin & Vancouver, 1996; Locke & Latham, 2002). Even miniscule assignment of formal grades in assessments seems to matter. In one study, associating just 1% of a course's grade with a learning module led to learners being four times more likely to devote extra study time to it (Raupach, Brown, Anders, Hasenfuss, & Harendza, 2013). Similar tight "coupling" between the assignment of grades and learner motivation has been found in other studies (Buss et al., 2012; Wormald, Schoeman, Somasunderam, & Penn, 2009). When assessments are used for licensing, selection, or credentialing, they can elicit especially strong motivation. In US medical education, for instance, medical students are so concerned with scoring well on the United States Medical Licensing Examination (USMLE) Step 1 examination that they preferentially study for that, skipping large parts of their schools' formal curricula (Burk-Rafel, Santen, & Purkiss, 2017; Chen et al., 2019; Schwartz, Lineberry, Park, Kamin, & Hyderi, 2018). Certain assessments may thus lead to great *intensity* and *persistence* of effort, but perhaps not in the *direction* desired by educators or learners, hence the controversy over whether examinations like the USMLE Step 1 are influencing motivation and learning appropriately (Katsufrakis & Chaudhry, 2019; London et al., 2016; Mehta et al., 2016; Prober et al., 2016).

Learners can be quite sophisticated in planning their studying for assessments. Cilliers, Schuwirth, Herman, Adendorff, and van der Vleuten (2012) interviewed medical students about how they prepared for assessments in end-of-course modules, finding that as assessments became imminent, the perceived workload of preparation became overwhelming. As such, even students who preferred to deeply master material switched to superficial "rote" memorization. Students also predicted the types of questions assessments would likely feature, based on prior assessments, peer guidance, and past educator behavior, along with sophisticated reasoning about practical limits of specific assessments. For instance, one learner realized,

> they can't just ask 20 [points' worth of questions] about one disease's pathophysiology . . . [they will] cover stuff as widely as possible . . . so, at the end of the day, you leave pretty important stuff out for now to learn ridiculous lists of thingeys.
>
> (Cilliers et al., 2012, p. 49)

The authors concluded that assessment affected learning substantially—but not as educators intended, consistent with the supposition that educational effects of assessments are often not what educators predict them to be (van der Vleuten, 1996).

Among other things, assessments are likely not only energizing learners toward a goal but also influencing the *goal orientations* they adopt, that is, the *types* of learning goals they are seeking

(DeShon & Gillespie, 2005; Dweck, 1986). There are three main orientations learners adopt to varying degrees: *mastery* or *learning* orientation, which is marked by seeking deep understanding for its own sake; *performance-prove* orientation, characterized by trying to demonstrate one's proficiency; and relatedly, *performance-avoid* orientation, which reflects trying to *not* show a *lack* of proficiency. It seems suitable for educators to encourage mastery orientation as much as possible, to hopefully foster life-long learners; additionally, some performance-prove orientation can also be functional for learning and performance (Harackiewicz, Barron, Carter, Lehto, & Elliot, 1997; Payne, Youngcourt, & Beaubien, 2007). Goal orientations have been found to predict the emotions that learners have as they anticipate assessments. For instance, those with dominant mastery orientations report more enjoyment, pride, and hope just prior to a test, while those with dominant performance-avoid orientations report anger, anxiety, hopelessness, and shame (Pekrun, Elliot, & Maier, 2009). These goal orientations and emotional responses represent important learning *processes* that assessments may affect, such that all else being equal, we should likely prefer assessment designs that foster deep, inquisitive learning behaviors and healthy emotion regulation.

Recognizing that learners will schedule and orient their learning and study behaviors according to how educators schedule and assign grades to assessments, a significant movement in health professions education is pushing for *programmatic assessment*, which among other things calls for more frequent, brief, "low-stakes" assessments and de-emphasis of large "high-stakes" assessments (Schuwirth & van der Vleuten, 2011) (see Chapter 16). On principle, this approach would seem to encourage more mastery orientation and more evenly spaced study behaviors among learners. However, the frequent and supposedly low-stakes assessments are not *zero* stakes; in fact, they are summed over time to facilitate decisions and lead to important consequences. Therefore, learners see and respond to the frequent small assessments much the same as more traditional "summative" assessments (Bok et al., 2013; Heeneman et al., 2015; Schut et al., 2018; Watling & Ginsburg, 2019). All the same, distributing assessments across multiple time points does seem to lead learners to space out their studying more broadly (Kerdijk, Cohen-Schotanus, Mulder, Muntinghe, & Tio, 2015); since spacing out learning over time has powerful positive effects for learning (Cepeda, Pashler, Vul, Wixted, & Rohrer, 2006), this seems like a very desirable result.

Just as learners are motivated by assessments, so too might educators feel at least partly responsible for their learners' assessment performance. This potentially leads to a familiar phenomenon: "teaching to the test." That often is a pejorative, for instance, to decry educators emphasizing rote memorization rather than facilitating learners' development of critical thinking. However, the root problem in such instances is not the teaching to the test, but rather the *test itself*, which may be misaligned with educational objectives. When assessments requiring higher-order cognitive processing are administered, learners tend to better develop the requisite thinking processes (Jensen, McDaniel, Woodard, & Kummer, 2014). Relatedly, van der Vleuten suggests that we may be unduly biased against certain *response formats*, like multiple-choice question-based tests, when really what we should be concerned with is *stimulus formats*, i.e., the *content* of items. That is, an excellent multiple-choice test can feature cases and choices that stimulate rich critical thinking, just as an essay-format test might only require rote recitation of simple concepts (van der Vleuten, 1996). One example of an AAL perspective on assessment content selection is the research and practice in *hypothesis-driven physical examination* education. Rather than assessing (and thus promoting) learners' relatively unthinking performance of an exhaustive set of "head to toe" physical examination maneuvers, one may assess whether learners can anticipate what maneuvers would be clinically discriminating in the context of a given patient case (Yudkowsky et al., 2009). Similar focus on learners' critical thinking during both physical examination and history taking has been explored as well, again in an effort to promote thoughtful and efficient data collection rather than thorough "regurgitation" without strategy or reflection (Yudkowsky, Park, Riddle, Palladino, & Bordage, 2014). Discomfort with "teaching to the test" may often be warranted, though it should arguably motivate better alignment of assessment practices with desired learning processes and outcomes, not abandonment of assessment entirely.

MECHANISM OF ACTION #3: THE ASSESSMENT EVENT ITSELF

The direct learning benefit of completing an assessment—what we could call assessment *as learning*—has proven to be remarkably strong and robust, a phenomenon referred to as the *testing effect* or *test-enhanced learning*. A large-scale review of common learning strategies found that assessment as learning is one of the two highest-utility strategies for fostering long-term learning, the second strategy being to study or practice learned material repeatedly with time in between, known as the *spacing effect* (Dunlosky, Rawson, Marsh, Nathan, & Willingham, 2013).

Several studies illustrate how strong and generalizable the testing effect is. For instance, Karpicke and Blunt (2011) found that testing was dramatically more effective than content mapping as a strategy to facilitate performance on a delayed science assessment ($d = 1.50$), even though concept mapping is generally thought to be a highly active and effective strategy, and in spite of the fact that the final assessment required relatively complex reasoning. Raupach and colleagues found that among fourth-year medical students learning clinical reasoning, brief key-features-style practice questions led to greater learning than a case-based learning approach, even after a six-month delay ($d = .29$) (Raupach et al., 2016). Meanwhile, Larsen, Butler, Lawson, and Roediger (2012) found that, for first-year medical students, the use of standardized patient-based practice testing of history and physical examination skills led to greater learning than both written practice testing ($d = .55$) and typical studying ($d = .84$). Similarly, a comparison of testing vs. typical study of physiology content found that testing supported better recall of learning after a delay ($d = .62–.82$) and greater ability to critique scientific articles relevant to the learned content ($d = .65–.81$) (Dobson, Linderholm, & Perez, 2018). A recent meta-analysis showed that testing also enhances learning of unstudied related material in the future ($g = .75$) (Chan, Meissner, & Davis, 2018), akin to the recent call to foster learners' *preparation for future learning* (Mylopoulos, Brydges, Woods, Manzone, & Schwartz, 2016). The mechanisms of this enhancement of future learning are under investigation; one theory is that testing causes learners to shift to more effective memory encoding strategies in general, not just for the learned content (Wissman, Rawson, & Pyc, 2011).

While several mechanisms are being investigated as to why assessment as learning has such strong effects, two simple mechanisms may explain much of the phenomenon. First, assessment as learning is *hard*—it requires effortful mental processing—which signals the brain to form new or stronger connections, making it what education scholar Robert Bjork calls a "desirable difficulty" (Bjork, 1994). This is the "no pain, no gain" theory of the testing effect. Second, when designed well, assessment as learning challenges learners in ways that are similar to how they will be challenged when they try to apply learning in the future, i.e., it requires "transfer-appropriate processing" (Kulasegaram & McConnell, 2016). These two mechanisms help explain why certain assessment design features can make the testing effect especially strong. For instance, constructed-response assessments, such as short answer or essay-based tests, lead to greater learning than selected-response assessments, like multiple-choice tests (Kang, McDermott, & Roediger, 2007; McDaniel, Roediger, & McDermott, 2007). The former response format requires that examinees *retrieve* the tested concepts from memory and then *produce* a response, whereas the latter only requires *recognizing* a correct answer from a list of options. The former is a more challenging mental task and is also more like real life, in which learning usually must be applied without the benefit of strong reminders of correct responses. (Reflecting on your experience of the pop quiz in this chapter: I wonder if you found it difficult to complete the short-answer format questions! I am also curious: did answering those questions change how well you believed you had learned the content?

I myself struggle at least a little—sometimes a lot—to answer questions like those, even about content I am relatively expert in. That struggle is beneficial!)

One drawback of constructed-response item formatting is that scoring can be time-consuming. A way to balance educational effect and ease of scoring is to use *sequentially-presented answer options* in multiple-choice testing: rather than examinees seeing all options and being asked to choose the correct one, they are shown one option at a time and must decide if each is correct or not (Willing, Ostapczuk, & Musch, 2014). Research and development is also in progress to allow for more computer-automated scoring of short answer responses (Waters, Grimaldi, Lan, & Baraniuk, 2017).

Despite its strength, assessment as learning seems deeply misunderstood and underutilized by learners and educators. Learners infrequently use assessment as learning during study, underestimate how effective it is, and tend to think of it mainly as a *diagnostic* tool rather than as a form of deliberate practice or study (Karpicke, Butler, & Roediger, 2009; Karpicke & Roediger, 2008; Kornell & Bjork, 2007, 2008; McCabe, 2011; Wissman, Rawson, & Pyc, 2012). This may be due partly to the high level of mental exertion needed in assessment as learning; learners with limited spare energy may opt for more passive forms of study. Assessment as learning also feels ineffective in the short-term—and in fact, it *is* less effective for stimulating very short-term learning, compared to more passive study activities (Mulligan & Peterson, 2014). This suggests a "blind spot" in our understanding of our own learning: ineffective strategies feel effective in the moment, help us feel competent, and require little energy, so we use them, even though they are ineffective in the long run. Kornell and Bjork (2007) put it well, that "becoming a meta-cognitively sophisticated learner is far from simple; it requires going against certain intuitions and standard practices, having a reasonably accurate model of how learning works, and not being misled by short-term performance." So, if you found it strange to answer quiz questions at the beginning of this chapter, know that that is normal—but that you might consider doing it more often! I find that I appreciate such questions when they are available, though it is uncommon for learning materials to be accompanied by good practice questions.

MECHANISM OF ACTION #4: POST-ASSESSMENT REFLECTION AND IMPROVEMENT

Assessment data can be analyzed and shared with learners and educators to guide future learning. However, skepticism is in order as to whether typical assessment practices are well designed to facilitate learning from feedback. For instance, Humphrey-Murto et al. (2016) found that residents who completed an OSCE remembered very little of the feedback they had been given after each station, either immediately after the OSCE or one month later. Harrison et al. (2013) found that for post-OSCE feedback available online, high-performing students viewed feedback the most; those who had just barely passed the OSCE, and presumably needed considerable improvement, viewed feedback the least. A classic synthesis of feedback research by Kluger and DeNisi (1996) found that a surprising proportion of feedback interventions were in fact ineffective, and roughly one-third of feedback interventions actually caused performance to *decrease*. Learning from feedback is a very large topic in education, so here, we will share only a broad model of the process and consider a few key considerations from an AAL perspective.

Identifying Performance Gaps

Learning from feedback might break down at the very beginning of the learning cycle if a learner is unable or unwilling to notice important information in feedback and engage with it cognitively and emotionally. Educators should thus ask, Is my assessment's feedback designed to be easy to meaningfully interpret toward learning, and are learners emotionally prepared to receive it? Cognitive load theory (Van Merrienboer & Sweller, 2010) and related theories of learning from multimedia (Mayer, 2014) offer many principles to enhance the cognitive interpretability of feedback. For instance, making feedback *contiguous* with learners' responses—such as by presenting feedback in an online assessment right next to each question, rather than in a separate feedback report—helps learners process feedback without having to split their attention. When assessments require expert judgment for scoring, providing feedback promptly can be a challenge, illustrating how AOL and AAL priorities can sometimes require trade-offs. For instance, experienced clinicians' expertise often makes them desirable as raters, but such clinicians are often profoundly busy, making it difficult to collect ratings promptly. One study simulating the process of using medical faculty to rate student OSCE videos found that it took as long as 16 days to collect ratings for just six learners from four faculty members (Grichanik, 2017). In that same study, recruiting laypersons as raters resulted in similar validity and reliability and was also much faster; 20 laypersons' ratings could be collected in just over five hours. Similar speed differences between laypersons and faculty have been found in a study of patient note scoring (Yudkowsky et al., 2019). In such situations, educators might trade some validity to improve speed of feedback and thus learning.

Helping learners be emotionally prepared for feedback can be challenging, especially in assessments, to which many learners tend to have strong emotional reactions. The core finding of Kluger and DeNisi's (1996) research was that when feedback draws learners' attention to the task or task strategies, it is more likely to be effective, whereas it is ineffective or even harmful when it draws learners' attention to their self-concept or sense of self-worth. While we tend to think of cognitions and emotions as separate processes, they both compete for limited attention and energy. If feedback targets the learners' self and triggers either intense pride (as might occur if we say, "Wow, you are remarkably skilled!"), shame ("Hmm . . . you are really not at the level of your peers"), or any other strong self-relevant emotions, cognitive load theory predicts the learner would have less spare attentional capacity for learning-focused processing to occur. With this in mind, learning theorists have emphasized several related principles: the importance of creating an environment of *psychological safety* for learners (Edmondson, 1999; Rudolph, Raemer, & Simon, 2014) and of establishing an *educational alliance* between learners and educators (Telio, Ajjawi, & Regehr, 2015). That is, while much of the popular guidance around feedback treats it like a thing that is "delivered" to learners, feedback is part of a *relationship* that may be more or less conducive to trust, positive expectations, and calm emotions.

Generating New Approaches

If a learner successfully attends to important feedback about a gap in performance, they must then generate an appropriate strategy to improve. Educators may assist by helping learners understand the underlying causes for performance gaps. For instance, learners benefit from seeing *rationales* for multiple-choice answers being correct vs. incorrect, rather than just being told which answers are correct (Levant, Zückert, & Paolo, 2018; Wojcikowski & Kirk, 2013). In debriefing of performance after simulated or actual patient care episodes, Rudolph, Simon, Raemer, and Eppich (2008) suggest that debrief facilitators should act as "cognitive detectives," eliciting learners' thoughts to discover the underlying frames of thinking that may explain learners' current performance, then helping them to generate new strategies for future performance.

An AAL perspective can help us think differently about how assessment formats might influence feedback and learning. There has been debate as to how useful checklist vs. global rating scale formats are for observational assessments, a debate historically focused on the measurement properties of each format (Ilgen, Ma, Hatala, & Cook, 2015). In either format, one should wonder not only whether the scores are valid and reliable, but also whether corrective actions are readily apparent when performance gaps are identified. For instance, a certain learner's global "Professionalism" rating might be reliably and validly scored as a "3" on a five-point scale, perhaps anchored as "Acceptable." It is not clear, however, what the learner is supposed to make of that;

should they behave differently, and if so, how? Checklists and behaviorally anchored rating scales (BARS) (see Chapter 9), being inherently more concrete, seem likely to have clearer implications for learning in many cases. That said, even checklists and BARS would benefit from careful attention to ensure correct vs. incorrect scores are tied to clear behaviors that can be improved. For example, it would be useful for a learner receiving feedback on a procedure they performed to know that their technique was deemed "incorrect" for some step of a procedure, such as "secure the patient's informed consent." However, it would be even more useful for them to know that their informed consent was specifically incorrect due to failure to "explain the procedure in clear, non-technical language"; that is, something they can readily improve.

Applying and Reinforcing New Approaches

Finally, learners must reinforce new ways of thinking and behaving strongly enough that they will recognize and take advantage of later opportunities to apply their learning. It should perhaps not be so surprising if learners are often disinterested in post-assessment feedback and performance improvement, because particularly after challenging assessments, they just "survived" what can often seem like the only time they will need to perform in that way for a long time. Just as a marathon runner will stop running once they cross the finish line, learners' engagement in learning may plummet after a major assessment (Pugh & Regehr, 2016). One way to help reinforce learners' motivation enough to ensure they reflect, practice, and solidify performance improvements after assessments is to stop administering "one-off" assessments, instead providing multiple opportunities for learners to perform (see Chapter 16). For instance, mastery learning-based instructional designs accomplish this by administering assessments two or more times: if learners can perform well enough on an assessment before an educational module, they can skip the module entirely; conversely, if they still struggle to perform on the assessment after the module, then they must restudy and retake the assessment as many times as needed until they can demonstrate sufficiently strong performance (Lineberry et al., 2015). Similarly, assessment experiences should be timed within a curriculum so that they are promptly followed by real-life practice and assessment opportunities; for instance, assessing catheter insertion just before learners are likely to begin observing or placing catheters in the clinical environment.

SUMMARY AND NEXT STEPS

Given the theory and findings above, I posit that assessments, approached with an assessment affecting learning (AAL) frame of thinking and design, along with more traditional assessment of learning (AOL) thinking and design, should be a primary method for fostering learning and performance in education. The AAL frame can promote focused and insightful deliberation in course design, clarity and motivation for learning and teaching, desirably difficult exercise of targeted learner KSAOs, and facilitation of reflection and growth.

That said, we also note that challenges in applying AAL are many and varied. To realize the educational program-level potential of AFL will be a major undertaking, and we may tend to underestimate how difficult it would be to change an educational system and culture to adopt it (Harrison et al., 2017). While AAL is becoming more popular in HPE, it is still an uncommon area in faculty development and formal education degree programs. Even professionals with advanced degrees in educational assessment are likely to have little to no training in it, since those degrees are generally focused only on AOL. And as mentioned previously, AOL frames of thinking tend to be well established, and some AAL principles are outright counterintuitive.

However, AAL "micro-interventions" are quite feasible. Any course that currently features an assessment can evaluate that assessment from the AAL lens and redesign it incrementally to enhance learning. Similarly, any course that currently features little or no assessment can develop or borrow suitable assessments and incorporate them, even if only as practice questions interspersed within existing learning activities. Schools hoping to develop capacity for AAL might also look to aim existing faculty development offerings in that direction, such as through journal clubs, short workshops, and developmental grants. We look forward to the field continuing to study, innovate, and incorporate AAL considerations in education in the years to come.

POP QUIZ ANSWERS

Question 1:

For the one-word terms, knowing exact terms may be useful, but close synonyms probably suffice. For the short definitions, specific phrasing is of course unimportant, so long as your answer is conceptually equivalent to these:

- *Scoring:* the inference (or assumption) that assessment scores reflect what happened in the "microcosm" of the assessment environment.
- *Generalization:* the inference (or assumption) that assessment scores reflect the scores examinees would have gotten if they took the assessment many times, in all the different ways the assessment details might have trivially differed (e.g., over different days of the week, equally suitable items, different raters, etc.).
- *Extrapolation:* the inference (or assumption) that assessment scores reflect examinees' real-world performance of interest, that is, that they correspond to the "macrocosm."
- *Decisions (or "Consequences" or "Implications"):* that assessment score interpretations and uses lead to appropriate decisions and consequences for all those affected.

Question 2:

Here, there are many possible examples of construct-irrelevant variance; refer to Chapter 2, Table 2.3, for several examples, denoted with the abbreviation "CIV." To count as construct-irrelevant variance, each validity threat must be such that the test *is* measuring something, but *not* what you meant to measure. For instance, if some students score better because they stole the answer key, the test *is* measuring "answer key theft (yes vs. no)," and that's not what you hoped the scores were measuring. Similarly, if the multiple choices were such that correct answers tended to be shorter than the incorrect distractor answers, then you might say the test is inadvertently measuring "examinees' test-wiseness"—again, probably not what you meant to be measuring.

If either of your answers referred to the test *failing* to measure something important, that's *construct underrepresentation*, not construct-irrelevant variance. For instance, if the test covers pathophysiology of respiratory conditions but not cardiac conditions (and you meant to cover both), then the broader construct is under-represented by your test.

Note: Additional material and resources may be available at the UIC AHPE website: https://go.uic.edu/AHPE

REFERENCES

Albanese, M., & Case, S.M. (2015). Progress testing: Critical analysis and suggested practices. *Advances in Health Sciences Education, 21*(1), 221–234.

American Educational Research Association, American Psychological Association, & National Council on Measurement in Education. (2014). *Standards for educational and psychological testing.* Washington, DC: AERA.

Austin, J.T., & Vancouver, J.B. (1996). Goal constructs in psychology: Structure, process, and content. *Psychological Bulletin, 120*(3), 338–375.

Bjork, R.A. (1994). Memory and metamemory considerations in the training of human beings. In J. Metcalfe & A. Shimamura (Eds.), *Metacognition: Knowing about knowing* (pp. 185–205). Cambridge, MA: MIT Press.

Bok, H.G., Teunissen, P.W., Favier, R.P., Rietbroek, N.J., Theyse, L.F., Brommer, H., . . . Jaarsma, D.A. (2013). Programmatic assessment of competency-based workplace learning: when theory meets practice. *BMC Medical Education, 13*, 123.

Burk-Rafel, J., Santen, S.A., & Purkiss, J. (2017). Study behaviors and USMLE Step 1 performance: Implications of a student self-directed parallel curriculum. *Academic Medicine: Journal of the Association of American Medical Colleges, 92*(11S Association of American Medical Colleges Learn Serve Lead: Proceedings of the 56th Annual Research in Medical Education Sessions), S67–S74.

Buss, B., Krautter, M., Möltner, A., Weyrich, P., Werner, A., Jünger, J., & Nikendei, C. (2012). Can the "Assessment Drives Learning" effect be detected in clinical skills training?—Implications for curriculum design and resource planning. *GMS Zeitschrift Für Medizinische Ausbildung, 29*(5).

Carroll, R.G., Navar, L.G., & Blaustein, M.P. (2012). *APS/ACDP Medical Physiology Learning Objectives Project.* Bethesda, MD: American Physiology Society and Association of Chairs of Departments of Physiology.

Cepeda, N.J., Pashler, H., Vul, E., Wixted, J.T., & Rohrer, D. (2006). Distributed practice in verbal recall tasks: A review and quantitative synthesis. *Psychological Bulletin, 132*(3), 354–380.

Chan, J.C.K., Meissner, C.A., & Davis, S.D. (2018). Retrieval potentiates new learning: A theoretical and meta-analytic review. *Psychological Bulletin, 144*(11), 1111–1146.

Chen, D.R., Priest, K.C., Batten, J.N., Fragoso, L.E., Reinfield, B.I., & Laitman, B.M. (2019). Student perspectives on the "Step 1 Climate" in preclinical medical education. *Academic Medicine, 94*(3), 302–304.

Cilliers, F.J., Schuwirth, L.W.T., Herman, N., Adendorff, H.J., & van der Vleuten, C.P.M. (2012). A model of the pre-assessment learning effects of summative assessment in medical education. *Advances in Health Sciences Education: Theory and Practice, 17*(1), 39–53.

Cook, D.A., Zendejas, B., Hamstra, S.J., Hatala, R., & Brydges, R. (2014). What counts as validity evidence? Examples and prevalence in a systematic review of simulation-based assessment. *Advances in Health Sciences Education, 19*, 233–250.

Dannefer, E.F. (2013). Beyond assessment of learning toward assessment for learning: Educating tomorrow's physicians. *Medical Teacher, 35*(7), 560–563.

DeShon, R.P., & Gillespie, J.Z. (2005). A motivated action theory account of goal orientation. *Journal of Applied Psychology, 90*(6), 1096–1127.

Dobson, J., Linderholm, T., & Perez, J. (2018). Retrieval practice enhances the ability to evaluate complex physiology information. *Medical Education, 52*(5), 513–525.

Dunlosky, J., Rawson, K.A., Marsh, E.J., Nathan, M.J., & Willingham, D.T. (2013). Improving students' learning with effective learning techniques: Promising directions from cognitive and educational psychology. *Psychological Science in the Public Interest, 14*(1), 4–58.

Dweck, C.S. (1986). Motivational processes affecting learning. *American Psychologist, 41*(10), 1040–1048.

Edmondson, A. (1999). Psychological safety and learning behavior in work teams. *Administrative Science Quarterly, 44*(2), 350–383.

Grichanik, M. (2017). Many hands make light work: Crowdsourced ratings of medical student OSCE performance. *Unpublished Doctoral Dissertation, University of South Florida.* Retrieved from https://scholarcommons.usf.edu/etd/6706.

Harackiewicz, J.M., Barron, K.E., Carter, S.M., Lehto, A.T., & Elliot, A.J. (1997). Predictors and consequences of achievement goals in the college classroom: Maintaining interest and making the grade. *Journal of Personality and Social Psychology, 73*(6), 1284–1295.

Harrison, C.J., Könings, K.D., Molyneux, A., Schuwirth, L.W.T., Wass, V., & van der Vleuten, C.P.M. (2013). Web-based feedback after summative assessment: How do students engage? *Medical Education, 47*(7), 734–744.

Harrison, C.J., Könings, K.D., Schuwirth, L.W.T., Wass, V., & van der Vleuten, C.P.M. (2017). Changing the culture of assessment: The dominance of the summative assessment paradigm. *BMC Medical Education, 17*(1), 73.

Heeneman, S., Oudkerk Pool, A., Schuwirth, L.W.T., van der Vleuten, C.P.M., & Driessen, E.W. (2015). The impact of programmatic assessment on student learning: Theory versus practice. *Medical Education, 49*(5), 487–498.

Holmboe, E.S., Sherbino, J., Englander, R., Snell, L., Frank, J.R., & ICBME Collaborators. (2017). A call to action: The controversy of and rationale for competency-based medical education. *Medical Teacher, 39*(6), 574–581.

Holmboe, E.S., Yamazaki, K., Edgar, L., Conforti, L., Yaghmour, N., Miller, R.S., & Hamstra, S.J. (2015). Reflections on the first 2 years of milestone implementation. *Journal of Graduate Medical Education, 7*(3), 506–511.

Humphrey-Murto, S., Mihok, M., Pugh, D., Touchie, C., Halman, S., & Wood, T.J. (2016). Feedback in the OSCE: What do residents remember? *Teaching and Learning in Medicine, 28*(1), 52–60.

Ilgen, J.S., Ma, I.W.Y., Hatala, R., & Cook, D.A. (2015). A systematic review of validity evidence for checklists versus global rating scales in simulation-based assessment. *Medical Education, 49*(2), 161–173.

Jensen, J.L., McDaniel, M.A., Woodard, S.M., & Kummer, T.A. (2014). Teaching to the test . . . or testing to teach: Exams requiring higher order thinking skills encourage greater conceptual understanding. *Educational Psychology Review, 26*(2), 307–329.

Kang, S.H.K., McDermott, K.B., & Roediger III, H.L. (2007). Test format and corrective feedback modify the effect of testing on long-term retention. *European Journal of Cognitive Psychology*, *19*(4–5), 528–558.

Karpicke, J.D., & Blunt, J.R. (2011). Retrieval practice produces more learning than elaborative studying with concept mapping. *Science*, *331*(6018), 772–775.

Karpicke, J.D., Butler, A.C., & Roediger, H.L. (2009). Metacognitive strategies in student learning: Do students practise retrieval when they study on their own? *Memory*, *17*(4), 471–479.

Karpicke, J.D., & Roediger, H.L. (2008). The critical importance of retrieval for learning. *Science*, *319*(5865), 966–968.

Katsufrakis, P.J., & Chaudhry, H.J. (2019). Improving residency selection requires close study and better understanding of stakeholder needs. *Academic Medicine*, *94*(3), 305–308.

Kerdijk, W., Cohen-Schotanus, J., Mulder, B.F., Muntinghe, F.L.H., & Tio, R.A. (2015). Cumulative versus end-of-course assessment: Effects on self-study time and test performance. *Medical Education*, *49*(7), 709–716.

Kluger, A.N., & DeNisi, A. (1996). The effects of feedback interventions on performance: A historical review, a meta-analysis, and a preliminary feedback intervention theory. *Psychological Bulletin*, *119*(2), 254–284.

Kornell, N., & Bjork, R.A. (2007). The promise and perils of self-regulated study. *Psychonomic Bulletin & Review*, *14*(2), 219–224.

Kornell, N., & Bjork, R.A. (2008). Optimising self-regulated study: The benefits—and costs—of dropping flashcards. *Memory*, *16*(2), 125–136.

Kulasegaram, K.M., & McConnell, M. (2016). When I say . . . transfer-appropriate processing. *Medical Education*, *50*(5), 509–510.

Larsen, D.P., Butler, A.C., Lawson, A.L., & Roediger, H.L. (2012). The importance of seeing the patient: Test-enhanced learning with standardized patients and written tests improves clinical application of knowledge. *Advances in Health Sciences Education*, *18*(3), 409–425.

Levant, B., Zückert, W., & Paolo, A. (2018). Post-exam feedback with question rationales improves re-test performance of medical students on a multiple-choice exam. *Advances in Health Sciences Education: Theory and Practice*, *23*(5), 995–1003.

Lineberry, M., Soo Park, Y., Cook, D.A., & Yudkowsky, R. (2015). Making the case for mastery learning assessments: key issues in validation and justification. *Academic Medicine: Journal of the Association of American Medical Colleges*, *90*(11), 1445–1450.

Locke, E.A., & Latham, G.P. (2002). Building a practically useful theory of goal setting and task motivation: A 35-year odyssey. *American Psychologist*, *57*(9), 705–717.

London, D.A., Kwon, R., Atluru, A., Maurer, K., Ben-Ari, R., & Schaff, P.B. (2016). More on how USMLE Step 1 scores are challenging academic medicine. *Academic Medicine*, *91*(5), 609–610.

Mayer, R.E. (Ed.). (2014). *The Cambridge handbook of multimedia learning* (2nd ed.). New York: Cambridge University Press.

McCabe, J. (2011). Metacognitive awareness of learning strategies in undergraduates. *Memory & Cognition*, *39*(3), 462–476.

McDaniel, M.A., Roediger, H.L., & Mcdermott, K.B. (2007). Generalizing test-enhanced learning from the laboratory to the classroom. *Psychonomic Bulletin & Review*, *14*(2), 200–206.

McGaghie, W.C. (2015). Mastery learning: It is time for medical education to join the 21st century. *Academic Medicine: Journal of the Association of American Medical Colleges*, *90*(11), 1438–1441.

Mehta, N.B., Hull, A., & Young, J. (2016). More on how USMLE Step 1 scores are challenging academic medicine. *Academic Medicine*, *91*(5), 609.

Mulligan, N.W., & Peterson, D.J. (2014). The spacing effect and metacognitive control. *Journal of Experimental Psychology: Learning, Memory, and Cognition*, *40*(1), 306–311.

Mylopoulos, M., Brydges, R., Woods, N.N., Manzone, J., & Schwartz, D.L. (2016). Preparation for future learning: A missing competency in health professions education? *Medical Education*, *50*(1), 115–123.

Nasca, T.J., Philibert, I., Brigham, T., & Flynn, T.C. (2012). The Next GME Accreditation System—Rationale and benefits. *New England Journal of Medicine*, *366*(11), 1051–1056.

Norcini, J., Anderson, M.B., Bollela, V., Burch, V., Costa, M.J., Duvivier, R., . . . Swanson, D. (2018). 2018 Consensus framework for good assessment. *Medical Teacher*, Online ahead of print, October 9, 1–8.

Norman, G., Neville, A., Blake, J.M., & Mueller, B. (2010). Assessment steers learning down the right road: Impact of progress testing on licensing examination performance. *Medical Teacher*, *32*(6), 496–499.

Payne, S.C., Youngcourt, S.S., & Beaubien, J.M. (2007). A meta-analytic examination of the goal orientation nomological net. *Journal of Applied Psychology*, *92*(1), 128–150.

Pekrun, R., Elliot, A.J., & Maier, M.A. (2009). Achievement goals and achievement emotions: Testing a model of their joint relations with academic performance. *Journal of Educational Psychology*, *101*(1), 115–135.

Prober, C.G., Kolars, J.C., First, L.R., & Melnick, D.E. (2016). In reply to Mehta, et al. (2016) and to London, et al. (2016) *Academic Medicine*, *91*(5), 610.

Pugh, D., & Regehr, G. (2016). Taking the sting out of assessment: Is there a role for progress testing? *Medical Education*, *50*(7), 721–729.

Raupach, T., Andresen, J.C., Meyer, K., Strobel, L., Koziolek, M., Jung, W., . . . Anders, S. (2016). Test-enhanced learning of clinical reasoning: A crossover randomised trial. *Medical Education, 50*(7), 711–720.

Raupach, T., Brown, J., Anders, S., Hasenfuss, G., & Harendza, S. (2013). Summative assessments are more powerful drivers of student learning than resource intensive teaching formats. *BMC Medicine, 11*, 61.

Rudolph, J.W., Raemer, D.B., & Simon, R. (2014). Establishing a safe container for learning in simulation: the role of the presimulation briefing. *Simulation in Healthcare, 9*(6), 339.

Rudolph, J.W., Simon, R., Raemer, D.B., & Eppich, W.J. (2008). Debriefing as formative assessment: Closing performance gaps in medical education. *Academic Emergency Medicine, 15*(11), 1010–1016.

Schut, S., Driessen, E., van Tartwijk, J., van der Vleuten, C., & Heeneman, S. (2018). Stakes in the eye of the beholder: An international study of learners' perceptions within programmatic assessment. *Medical Education, 52*(6), 654–663.

Schuwirth, L.W.T., & van der Vleuten, C.P.M. (2011). Programmatic assessment: From assessment of learning to assessment for learning. *Medical Teacher, 33*(6), 478–485.

Schwartz, L.F., Lineberry, M., Park, Y.S., Kamin, C.S., & Hyderi, A.A. (2018). Development and evaluation of a student-initiated test preparation program for the USMLE Step 1 examination. *Teaching and Learning in Medicine, 30*(2), 193–201.

Sullivan, M.E., Yates, K.A., Inaba, K., Lam, L., & Clark, R.E. (2014). The use of cognitive task analysis to reveal the instructional limitations of experts in the teaching of procedural skills. *Academic Medicine, 89*(5), 811–816.

Telio, S., Ajjawi, R., & Regehr, G. (2015). The "educational alliance" as a framework for reconceptualizing feedback in medical education. *Academic Medicine, 90*(5), 609.

van der Vleuten, C.P.M. (1996). The assessment of professional competence: Developments, research and practical implications. *Advances in Health Sciences Education, 1*(1), 41–67.

van Merriënboer, J.J.G., & Kirschner, P.A. (2012). *Ten steps to complex learning: A systematic approach to four-component instructional design* (2nd ed.). New York: Routledge.

van Merrienboer, J.J.G., & Sweller, J. (2010). Cognitive load theory in health professional education: Design principles and strategies. *Medical Education, 44*(1), 85–93.

Vaporciyan, A.A., Fikfak, V., Lineberry, M.C., Park, Y.S., & Tekian, A. (2017). Consensus-derived coronary anastomotic checklist reveals significant variability among experts. *The Annals of Thoracic Surgery, 104*(6), 2087–2092.

Waters, A., Grimaldi, P., Lan, A., & Baraniuk, R. (2017). Short-answer responses to STEM questions: measuring response validity and its impact on learning. In *Proceedings of the 10th International Conference on Data Mining* (pp. 374–375). Wuhan, China.

Watling, C.J., & Ginsburg, S. (2019). Assessment, feedback and the alchemy of learning. *Medical Education, 53*(1), 76–85.

Wiggins, G., & McTighe, J. (2005). *Understanding by design* (2nd Expanded ed.). Alexandria, VA: Association for Supervision & Curriculum Development.

Willing, S., Ostapczuk, M., & Musch, J. (2014). Do sequentially-presented answer options prevent the use of test-wiseness cues on continuing medical education tests? *Advances in Health Sciences Education, 20*(1), 247–263.

Wissman, K.T., Rawson, K.A., & Pyc, M.A. (2011). The interim test effect: Testing prior material can facilitate the learning of new material. *Psychonomic Bulletin & Review, 18*(6), 1140–1147.

Wissman, K.T., Rawson, K.A., & Pyc, M.A. (2012). How and when do students use flashcards? *Memory, 20*(6), 568–579.

Wojcikowski, K., & Kirk, L. (2013). Immediate detailed feedback to test-enhanced learning: An effective online educational tool. *Medical Teacher, 35*(11), 915–919.

Wormald, B.W., Schoeman, S., Somasunderam, A., & Penn, M. (2009). Assessment drives learning: An unavoidable truth? *Anatomical Sciences Education, 2*(5), 199–204.

Yudkowsky, R., Hyderi, A., Holden, J., Kiser, R., Stringham, R., Gangopadhyaya, A., . . . Park, Y.S. (2019). Can non-clinician raters be trained to assess clinical reasoning in post-encounter patient notes? *Academic Medicine,* October Supplement.

Yudkowsky, R., Otaki, J., Lowenstein, T., Riddle, J., Nishigori, H., & Bordage, G. (2009). A hypothesis-driven physical examination learning and assessment procedure for medical students: Initial validity evidence. *Medical Education, 43*(8), 729–740.

Yudkowsky, R., Park, Y.S., Riddle, J., Palladino, C., & Bordage, G. (2014). Clinically discriminating checklists versus thoroughness checklists: Improving the validity of performance test scores. *Academic Medicine, 89*(7), 1057–1062.

18

ASSESSMENT IN MASTERY LEARNING SETTINGS

Matthew Lineberry, Rachel Yudkowsky, Yoon Soo Park,
David Cook, E. Matthew Ritter, and Aaron Knox

Mastery learning is an instructional approach in which educational progress is based on demonstrated performance rather than curricular time (Block, 1971; McGaghie, 1978, 2015). Learners are provided with clear terminal objectives and performance metrics, opportunities for study and practice, and repeated formative testing with feedback about their progress towards performance goals. Learners cannot advance to the next curricular module, stage of training, or level of practice until the predetermined performance levels are achieved. A key characteristic of mastery testing is the ability to retest on multiple occasions to reach a designated "mastery" level; the final level of achievement is the same for all learners, though some learners may require more time for study and practice and more test attempts than others do. Given the emphasis on demonstrated performance over fixed curricular time, mastery learning and testing can be important elements of a competency-based curriculum (McGaghie, 2015) and are integral to the achievement and assessment of core entrustable professional activities (EPAs) for entering residency in undergraduate medical education (Association of American Medical Colleges, 2014) and of milestones (Holmboe, Edgar, & Hamstra, 2016) during residency.

Sound assessment is the cornerstone of mastery learning systems. Inaccurate assessment of learners' mastery or poor use of such assessments for decision-making would lead learners to be prematurely advanced or unnecessarily held back. Our aim in this chapter is to outline key issues in the validation and justification of mastery learning assessments (see Chapter 2 for a full discussion of assessment validity). Where possible, we suggest solutions to key challenges, and in all cases we focus on clearly identifying those challenges, which are summarized in Box 18.1.

INTERPRETATIONS OF AND USES FOR MASTERY LEARNING ASSESSMENTS

What does "mastery" mean? Colloquially, it suggests a high level of expertise. However, for mastery learning it only means readiness to proceed to the next phase of instruction. A medical student who understands mutagenesis enough to learn about genetic transmission has almost certainly not "mastered" mutagenesis in the lay sense but may have mastered it sufficiently to advance. The concept of "mastery" is also different from "borderline" or "minimally competent" performance

---

Box 18.1 Key Considerations for Validation and Justification of Mastery Learning Assessments

Interpretation and Use

- Specify what degree of achievement or readiness to progress is meant by mastery
- Specify how long mastery is intended to be retained
- Specify how complete mastery must be within a particular content area (*compensatory vs. non-compensatory scoring*)
- Specify how scores will be used to make decisions and actions about learners

Content Evidence

- Develop sufficient assessment content to allow for high-volume retesting as needed
- Use best practices for generating multiple equivalent retests
- When appropriate, assess aspects of performance beyond achievement of content, e.g., automaticity of performance

Response Process Evidence

- Examine whether learners' response processes on retests are consistent with true mastery, rather than memorization of particulars of the assessment content

Internal Structure and Reliability Evidence

- Use adjusted reliability estimates for the mastery vs. non-mastery distinction
- Carefully consider how to derive estimates of reliability and internal structure for mastery post-tests, when learner performance is likely to be restricted in range; consider using baseline scores, which will likely show greater variance
- If non-compensatory scoring is used, adjust reliability estimates accordingly

Relationships to Other Variables Evidence

- Carefully consider how to derive estimates of relationships to other variables for mastery post-tests, when learner performance is likely to be restricted in range
- Collect evidence as to whether a given mastery assessment relates to satisfactory vs. unsatisfactory progress in later educational units and/or subsequent patient care

Consequences of Assessment Use

- Examine potential positive *and* negative, and intended and unintended, effects of mastery assessment for individual learners, the education system, patient outcomes, and society

---

in standard setting (see Chapter 6); mastery connotes being *well prepared* to succeed in the next stage. Similarly, a resident who has "mastered" central venous catheter insertion in a simulation lab might be ready for supervised performance on patients, but will of course still have much to learn. This terminological confusion could lead to problems. Learners who advance through a unit may believe they have "mastered" its content in the lay sense when they have not. Conversely, educators asked to set mastery standards may set unnecessarily high standards, letting the lay connotation of "mastery" color their judgments.

How long is "mastery" expected to last? In mastery-learning-based courses, achievement is often assessed immediately after the completion of training. Yet most learning units in health professions education are connected to many later units, and achievement often decays rapidly following training (Arthur, Bennett, Stanush, & McNelly, 1998). Moreover, many of the learning activities that maximize short-term mastery are precisely the opposite of those that support long-term retention and generalization of mastery (Rohrer & Pashler, 2010). Although rigorous delayed testing is logistically challenging, particularly as learners rotate through different educational sites and assume time-consuming clinical commitments, limiting mastery assessment to the period immediately following training could subvert the intent of the mastery system, which is to ensure uniform, *enduring* competence (Norman, Norcini, & Bordage, 2014).

Mastery also may connote a *completeness* of knowledge or skill. In some contexts, mastery means that a learner has achieved sufficient competence in *all* the sub-units of a content area (e.g., a learner cannot master "genetic transmission" without understanding each of the modes of transmission), or that they are sufficiently competent at *all* aspects of a procedure. In such situations, for example, if a learner scores 90% on a procedural task, but the missed 10% reflect a serious error, designation of mastery would be inappropriate (Yudkowsky, Tumuluru, Casey, Herlich, & Ledonne, 2014). In such *non-compensatory* (aka *conjunctive*) scoring, performance on each sub-unit would be evaluated against a minimum standard and mastery would be achieved only when all sub-units are passed.

We usually want assessments to discriminate between examinees of a wide variety of ability levels. *However, the central inference in the mastery model is pass and advance or fail and repeat; there is no middle ground.* This implies that the passing mastery standard or cut score must be established with great rigor. This also has implications for how assessments are designed. Figure 18.1 depicts a hypothetical distribution of learners' true scores—their actual knowledge or skill levels—on a mastery assessment. For learners whose true scores are far below the mastery cut score, precision of measurement is not terribly important from a decision-making standpoint; the learner has clearly not mastered the content. For learners in this range, the assessment will be most useful if it generates specific feedback to help the learner make efficient progress to the standard. By contrast, for learners whose true scores are close to the mastery standard—perhaps within one standard error of measurement from the cut score—precise measurement becomes the priority. Assessment items that discriminate well in this range should be oversampled. Though identifying such items using classical test theory is possible, more robust techniques such as item response theory (IRT) can be especially helpful (see Chapter 19; Embretson & Reise, 2000). Such items may also need to be kept particularly secure from being released to learners, which runs counter to the goal of providing feedback. Finally, for learners whose true scores are well beyond the mastery standard, neither precision of measurement nor rich feedback are of much concern, so less effort could be spent on items that discriminate only in this range.

Along with the need to specify the inferences to be drawn from mastery assessment scores, the ways those scores are used to make decisions must be clearly specified. The most obvious use of such assessments is for deciding when to advance learners in the curriculum. Two key details related to that decision are (1) the resources and policies in place for learners who do not pass and (2) any special consequences for persistent failure to meet mastery standards. Less-obvious uses of mastery scores are possible and may have unintended consequences. For instance, if deans' letters to residency programs extol students who quickly mastered the curriculum, this

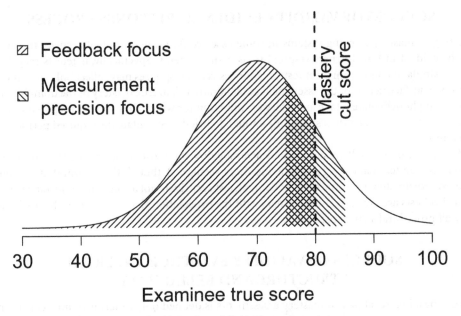

Figure 18.1 Assessment focus, by examinees' standing relative to the mastery cut score

Note: The location and shape of the examinee true score distribution, the location of the mastery cut score, and the width of the region of measurement focus are chosen only for illustration; these will vary for particular contexts.

inadvertently makes "time to mastery" a new achievement indicator, perhaps encouraging learners to rush through the curriculum rather than truly mastering it.

To summarize, adopting a mastery system requires clear specification about how assessment scores will be interpreted and used. For interpretation, it should be clear what level of achievement is meant by "mastery," how long it is expected to last, and how complete that achievement must be. Intended uses should be specified, with particular detail regarding remediation and retesting.

SOURCES OF VALIDITY EVIDENCE: CONTENT

One important source of validity evidence is the suitability of the assessment content. In mastery assessment programs, the number of items needed may be larger than in traditional settings, because many learners will take the mastery test more than once. Examinees who struggle will retest one or more times. Many mastery systems use pre-tests before initial instruction—a practice which may allow some learners to skip already-mastered educational units entirely, and which can enhance the effectiveness of initial instruction (Richland, Kornell, & Kao, 2009), but then requires at least one additional test for most learners. It is thus important to have a large enough bank of well-developed items and sound methods for generating multiple equivalent test forms (Crocker & Algina, 1986). Additionally, depending on one's definition of mastery, certain aspects of *how* examinees perform may be key criteria, beyond simply the products of their performance (e.g., correct answers or completed procedural tasks). For instance, if one defines "mastery" of suturing skill as the ability to suture automatically, with minimal to no conscious thought, a suitable assessment must detect when examinees can suture even while their attention is distracted (Stefanidis, Scerbo, Montero, Acker, & Smith, 2012).

SOURCES OF VALIDITY EVIDENCE: RESPONSE PROCESS

Retesting in mastery learning systems in some cases could create a content security threat that may be evident in how learners respond to assessment items. Specifically, if retests recycle the same or similar content from prior tests, examinees' retest responses may reflect only their memorization of surface details of the assessment content rather than true mastery of the domain. Savvy learners might deliberately take a mastery examination for which they weren't prepared in order to become "test-wise," and then study only enough to briefly regurgitate the required performance on a retest.

If retesting does result in superficial learning gains, the most straightforward solution is to build larger content banks (e.g., more items, more scenarios), though this is admittedly resource intensive. Fortunately, for some types of content, test security is not a concern; for instance, procedural checklists are given freely to learners with the expectation that they will be able to demonstrate all procedural steps satisfactorily.

SOURCES OF VALIDITY EVIDENCE: INTERNAL STRUCTURE AND RELIABILITY

Strictly speaking, reliability in mastery assessments is defined only in terms of how consistently the mastery vs. non-mastery distinction is made. Common reliability statistics such as coefficient alpha and test-retest correlations refer to the reliability of discriminations between examinees across the full range of examinee true scores. However, the reliability of a pass/fail decision at a particular cut score can be dramatically different from the overall score reliability. Generally, cut scores at or near the average examinee performance level will be the least reliable, whereas extremely high or low cut scores are often highly reliable (Brent Stansfield & Kreiter, 2007). Suitably modified reliability equations are available and should be used for mastery learning assessments, including the conditional error variance for absolute decisions generalizability coefficient (Webb, Shavelson, & Haertel, 2006) and decision-consistency reliability indices (Livingston & Lewis, 1995; Subkoviak, 1988). Both may be complex enough to require psychometric consultation to properly estimate and interpret.

Other unique aspects of mastery learning systems can also affect reliability estimates. If learners can choose when to take the mastery test, have a good sense of when they are sufficiently prepared to pass, and can retest as needed, the final test scores of all examinees will be very similar (i.e., everyone will be very near the passing score) (Figure 18.2). In situations of such reduced score variance (i.e., restriction in range), reliability estimates will be reduced. The very goal of mastery learning systems—uniform achievement from all learners—is thus at odds with classical reliability estimation. At the same time, remediation and retraining can affect item-level score variation and may actually increase reliability. Therefore, depending on the frequency of retesting, mastery assessments can show unstable reliability estimates. By extension, these issues may limit the ability to assess internal structure through methods such as factor analysis, which also requires a reasonable degree of variance between subjects and items. One solution is to use scores from the baseline, pre-instruction assessment—at which time examinees would still be expected to vary in ability—to estimate the reliability and factor structure of later mastery assessments.

Last, as with credentialing examinations generally, administrators may choose to score mastery assessments in a *non-compensatory* fashion, whereby learners must demonstrate mastery on many different sub-units before progressing (Norcini et al., 1993). While such scoring might be most consistent with a program's intended interpretation and use of scores, it is important to realize how the practice affects measurement reliability and associated psychometric inferences. In non-compensatory scoring, overall measurement error is an exponential function of the measurement error for each sub-unit and can thus "balloon" into very unreliable overall pass/fail decisions. For instance, if learners must pass all of five procedural skill stations that each have a

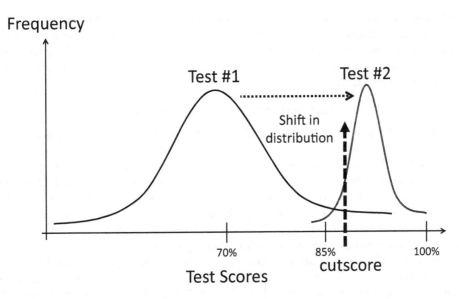

Figure 18.2 Learner performance distributions shift in a mastery setting as each round of practice and retesting increases learners' probability of mastery

pass/fail reliability of 0.8, overall non-compensatory pass/fail decision reliability would only be 0.8^5—an abysmally low 0.33 reliability coefficient (Hambleton & Slater, 1997).

SOURCES OF VALIDITY EVIDENCE: RELATIONSHIPS TO OTHER VARIABLES

Test scores should relate positively to measures of similar constructs and to outcomes they are meant to predict or measure concurrently ("convergent validity evidence") and should not correlate positively with conceptually dissimilar constructs ("discriminant validity evidence"). Many forms of convergent and discriminant validity evidence for mastery assessments will be similar to those for non-mastery assessments. However, a key important relationship to evaluate in a mastery system is whether assessment scores relate to examinees' success in their subsequent educational unit(s), including their eventual transition to practice on patients.

Just as it impairs estimation of reliability, restriction of range in mastery assessment scores makes it difficult to estimate relationships to other variables. However, it is possible to correlate relatively unrestricted assessment data obtained prior to implementing a mastery system with other variables. For instance, if residents were assessed on chest tube insertion using simulation, and then performed chest tubes on patients regardless of their assessment score, outcome data such as patient complication rates could be correlated with the assessment scores. Of course, in this example—where the consequences of allowing some failure in the criterion measure are dire—there is likely an ethical imperative *not* to allow low-scoring examinees to proceed to patient care in the first place (Ziv, Wolpe, Small, & Glick, 2003), thus disallowing estimation of this relationship.

SOURCES OF VALIDITY EVIDENCE: CONSEQUENCES OF ASSESSMENT USE

In contrast to validity evidence that focuses on the whether the assessment can support desired inferences, consequences evidence seeks to justify the uses or applications of scores by considering the intended and unintended consequences of the assessment and whether implementation of the assessment is reasonable and desirable (Kane, 2013; Cizek, 2012). Consequences evidence includes information about the process of setting standards and the impact of the assessment on the learning process, learning outcomes, and the practice of healthcare (Downing, 2003; Cook & Lineberry, 2016; Chapter 2).

Standard Setting in Mastery Settings

A thoughtful and rigorous approach to standard setting, establishing the performance levels and metrics that determine when a learner has demonstrated mastery, is essential to mastery learning. As described in Chapter 6, standards can be *normative* (an individual's performance relative to that of all learners, such as setting the pass score at a specified number of standard deviations below the mean examinee score), or *criterion-based* (also called "absolute"; for example, fixing the pass score at 80% correct) reflecting a specific performance standard. Normative standards, in which a learner's pass/fail status depends on the performance of other members of the group, have no place in competency-based curricula or mastery settings.

While criterion-based methods are appropriate for mastery settings, the central inference of mastery standards—that they predict success in subsequent training or practice—demands an evidence-based approach (AERA, APA, & NCME, 1985; O'Malley, Keng, & Miles, 2012). Thus, the information on which judgments are based should be focused on *predicting future performance*, a type of evidence only rarely used in traditional standard-setting exercises. Evidence can include the use of predictive past performance data, information about the consequences of different standards for future performance, the use of targeted reference groups, and consideration of patient safety in clinical settings.

Item-Based Standard-Setting Procedures: Predictive Performance Data

The item-based *Angoff method* (Angoff, 1971; Chapter 6) frequently used for written tests and performance checklists asks judges to predict the performance of the "borderline student," a student who is *just at the edge of minimal competence*. Judges indicate the probability that the borderline student would accomplish each item of a test or checklist correctly. In mastery settings, rather than predicting the behavior of a *minimally* competent student who is *just at the edge* of acceptable performance, judges will be modeling the performance of a student who is *well prepared to succeed* at the next stage of instruction or practice.

Data about past examinees' performance often is used to help judges calibrate item-based judgments (Cizek, 1996; Mee, Clauser, & Margolis, 2013). Judges frequently refer to percent-correct statistics from past administrations of each test or checklist item to help estimate item difficulty and the probability that a minimally competent examinee would accomplish that item. In traditional curricula, these statistics are based on a single test administration at the end of the learning unit, which most learners are expected to pass on the first attempt. In a mastery environment, on the other hand, the first test may have a very low pass rate. Learners may retake the exam a variable number of times—some will choose to retest early and often, others will wait until they've mastered most of the material. Eventually—after two, three, five, ten retests—they will reach the mastery level and move on. Which test results should be used to inform the judges?

When setting standards in the context of a mastery learning approach, item *difficulty* is less important than item *relevance* or *importance*. If a given item is important for learners to master prior to progressing to the next stage of learning or clinical practice, discovering that in the past only 50% of learners accomplished that item on first attempt does not make the item any less important. Such a finding should be interpreted as a gap in curriculum and instruction that needs to be closed, not as cause to lower the mastery standard.

An evidence-based approached to mastery standards implies that performance data are most valuable when they include information about past examinees' success or failure in *subsequent* learning experiences (O'Malley et al., 2012). Suppose a cohort of residents completed a basic laparoscopic skills assessment on a simulator, and then completed a number of basic laparoscopic procedures on patients. Analyses showing how scores on the simulation-based assessment predict examinees' performance on actual patients could be very useful to judges—for example, showing that "examinees with four or more instrument collisions on the simulation-based assessment have a significantly elevated risk of unsafe behaviors during patient care" would suggest that "fewer than four instrument collisions" be one of the criteria for advancement. Similarly, for pre-clinical written exams, predictive performance data might include the test performance of the subset of students who were subsequently successful in the pre-clinical curriculum overall.

As another example, Figure 18.3 shows a data display for a hypothetical simulation-based lumbar puncture (LP) training program. Figure 18.3a shows *past* performance data typically provided during standard-setting exercises; Figure 18.3b provides an example of *predictive* performance

Item	Residents Who Correctly Performed the Item No. (%)	Residents Who Omitted or Incorrectly Performed the Item No. (%)
Checked that all necessary equipment is available and ready to use.	181 (76)	48 (24)
Opened lumbar puncture kit carefully to maintain sterility.	170 (71)	69 (29)
Prepped insertion point with iodine swabs in concentric circles.	147 (61)	92 (39)
[Other checklist items, not shown here]	——	——
		Total Score Mean (SD): 65% (40%)

(a)

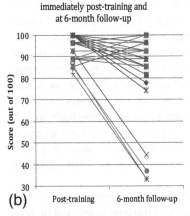

Trainee scores, immediately post-training and at 6-month follow-up

(b) Post-training   6-month follow-up

Correlation between post-training and 6-month follow-up: *r* = 0.44

If Post-Training Mastery Standard Is Set At:	Then at Six-Month Follow Up:	
	Minimum Score	Mean Score
100	74.07	88.10
95	74.07	89.95
90	44.44	88.74
85	33.33	86.20
80	33.33	86.20

Figure 18.3 Performance data examples for standard-setting judges in non-mastery and mastery contexts. The *top panel* (Figure 18.3a) presents a hypothetical past-performance data display for a traditional item-based standard-setting exercise for lumbar puncture, showing the number and percent of residents who did or did not accomplish each item; data based on performance of 239 residents. The *bottom panel* (Figure 18.3b) presents a hypothetical predictive performance data display for a mastery item-based standard-setting exercise for lumbar puncture; data based on performance of 34 residents

data. Suppose that all learners had to score at least 80% on an LP checklist at the end of training, and that learners were then certified to perform LPs into the indefinite future. By showing how participants' immediate post-training scores relate to the same learners' retest scores six months later (Figure 18.3b), this hypothetical example suggests that the mastery standard of 80% may have been too lenient, as a number of participants who scored below 95% on the post-training assessment earned extremely low scores at six-month follow-up. This type of data, clearly displayed, helps standard-setting judges estimate the levels of performance needed in early mastery learning modules in order to ensure safe and effective subsequent learning or patient care activities.

Examinee-Based Standard-Setting Procedures

Examinee-based procedures or methods such as *borderline group* or *contrasting groups* (Livingston & Zieky, 1982; Downing, Tekian, & Yudkowsky, 2006; Chapter 6) require judges or external criteria to categorize examinees into groups at contrasting levels of performance such as proficient vs. non-proficient or pass/marginal/fail. Group membership is defined by data other than scores on the test in question, for example by direct observation of performance or other relevant criteria. The standard for a particular exam is obtained by determining the test score that best discriminates between the two groups (contrasting groups method) or the median score of the marginal group (borderline group method) (see Chapter 6). Examinee-based methods are often used to set mastery standards for instrument-based metrics: measures obtained by a simulator, computer, or other measurement device during dynamic, real-time assessments of performance (Konge et al., 2012; Konge et al., 2013; Madsen et al., 2014).

Traditional examinee-based methods generally need to be modified to support the "well prepared to succeed" inferences of a mastery setting. The marginally acceptable performance of peers identified by the traditional borderline group method is not an appropriate final goal for mastery learners; on the other hand, benchmarking the performance of experts may result in standards that are inappropriately high and result in effort expended to little purpose. The "proficient group" approach (Gallagher et al., 2005; Gallagher, 2012) uses the performance scores observed from a developmentally appropriate benchmark group to guide standard setting. The proficient group performs a task such as knot tying in an instrumented environment (e.g., a virtual-reality simulator). Their performance data can then be used to guide standard setting; for instance, judges may deem it appropriate to set the average "time to secure knot" of the proficient group (second-year residents) as the mastery standard for first-year residents. A highly proficient or even expert benchmark group may be appropriate for learners transitioning to independent practice. However, experts may perform the task using procedural variants that would be inappropriate and unsafe for early trainees with limited clinical judgment and skills. Experts also may demonstrate behaviors that are not essential for safe practice at earlier stages of training, such as very rapid task performance. Measures of experience alone, such as years of practice, do not well predict acceptable performance (Choudhry, Fletcher, & Soumerai, 2005). Suitably proficient individuals are best identified based on a combination of clinical experience and scores on an objective measure of performance. The proficient group method has been applied repeatedly in procedural simulation in the simulation lab, operating room, and procedural suite (Rosenthal et al., 2010; Stefanidis et al., 2005; Seymour et al., 2002; Scott et al., 2008).

Comparison groups for contrasting groups methods used in mastery settings must be chosen with care. Several studies (e.g., Konge et al., 2012, 2013; Fraser et al., 2003) have compared medical students' performance of basic surgical skills on a simulator to that of practicing surgeons, and derived a cut score that maximally discriminated between the two groups. However, in mastery learning we rarely need assessments that can tell novices from experts; instead, we need assessments that discriminate between novices who are sufficiently competent to move on versus novices who are not, or that distinguish trainees who are not quite ready for unsupervised practice from those who can graduate and practice safely. This requires careful choice of comparison and benchmark groups depending on the stage of training and the specific inferences desired.

Performance data of expert or proficient groups should not form the basis for a mechanistic generation of a standard (e.g., arbitrarily choosing "expert score minus 1.5 standard deviations" or "the point of intersection between experts' and novices' score distributions"); rather, such data should serve as a point of departure for thoughtful deliberations among standard-setting judges about the importance of each metric for clinical and educational outcomes and the level of performance expected at different transition points. These deliberations are key to setting defensible, effective, and achievable mastery standards (Livingston & Zieky, 1982).

Test-Based or Compromise Procedures: Not Appropriate for Standards in a Mastery Context

The test-based *Hofstee method* (Hofstee, 1983), also called the whole test or compromise method (see Chapter 6), uses a combination of normative and criterion-based standards to ensure that the number of failed learners will be acceptable and the standards therefore implementable. The Hofstee method is arguably inappropriate for setting standards in a mastery context, in which practically all learners are expected to eventually achieve the specified standard and advance to the next phase of training. A curriculum in which required standards are lowered in order to meet constraints of acceptable fail rates would, by definition, be antithetical to a mastery learning approach. While one could pre-set minimum and maximum acceptable fail rates at 0% and 100% for mastery settings, eliminating fail-rate judgments would remove the essential characteristic of the Hofstee procedure.

Patient-Safety-Based Procedures for Mastery Standards

A key goal of milestones and EPAs is to ensure that learners are well prepared to transition safely and successfully to the next level of clinical training or practice. Mastery testing, often simulation-based, can support this goal by ensuring that students and residents acquire a suitable level of proficiency in skills prior to performing invasive procedures on live patients. When patient safety considerations are paramount, a conjunctive method such as the patient safety approach (Yudkowsky et al., 2014; Chapter 6) may be most appropriate. Traditional standard-setting procedures are compensatory across items: as long as examinees achieve the cut score, it does not matter which individual items are missed and which are accomplished. In clinical settings, however, the omission or incorrect performance of individual items may have a significant impact on patient safety and outcomes. The patient safety approach to setting mastery standards for basic procedural skills has judges rate each item as to its impact on dimensions such as patient safety, patient comfort, or procedure outcome, relying on evidence-based data when available; an item whose performance or non-performance impacts one of these dimensions can be considered "critical" or "essential." A similar approach can be taken for SP and mannequin scenario checklists that include many actions that contribute to good outcomes but only a few truly critical actions. Standards can be set separately for critical and non-critical checklist items such that performance of non-critical items does not compensate for omission or incorrect performance of critical items. Setting a conjunctive standard for critical items is also important when assessing maintenance of skills from initial testing to a delayed retest, to avoid having retention of non-critical items mask the decay of critical skills. While conjunctive standards increase the risk of incorrectly classifying a capable student as failing, one may choose to tolerate the higher error rate and require another round of testing in order to avoid the false positive of passing a student who is clinically unsafe.

Standards must be appropriate to the specific transition under consideration. For example, when setting standards for performing a lumbar puncture on a part-task trainer, we may be interested in whether the trainee is ready to perform the task on a live patient under close supervision later that week, or whether she is able to perform the procedure independently, in a variety of clinical settings, well into the future. These are very different inferences, and the metrics and standards we use to support these inferences need to be different as well.

Box 18.2 provides a summary of key considerations when setting standards in a healthcare mastery setting; Table 18.1 shows how these might apply to different types of tests.

Other Validity Evidence Regarding Consequences

In addition to information about standard-setting procedures and their outcomes, consequences evidence includes consideration of the impact of the assessment on curricula, learners, patients, and systems (Downing, 2003; Cook & Lineberry, 2016; Chapter 2).

Mastery testing has potentially widespread influence on curricula and training programs. Mastery standards mandate sufficient curricular time and resources for repeated practice, remediation, and retesting, thus reinforcing a competency-based approach to education (Frank et al., 2010). Poor initial performance and the need for repeated retests may highlight a gap between the experienced curriculum and faculty expectations, spurring curricular efforts to correct this gap. Conversely, mastery standards may disrupt scheduling within the curriculum and consume limited faculty and material resources for remediation and retesting. Additionally, instructors in a mastery learning context may identify common test errors and emphasize these points in subsequent sessions. While not inappropriate if these errors reflect key aspects of the task, such "teaching to the test" could undermine the validity of scores and inferences if it improves test performance without a concomitant improvement in true skill.

On an individual learner level, evidence can be sought of increased efficiency and effectiveness of study and practice strategies, increased attention to the critical elements of the assessed domain, more functional motivational orientations (Payne, Youngcourt, & Beaubien, 2007), and improved self-regulation of learning. The mastery approach—setting a high bar and practicing

---

Box 18.2 Considerations for Setting Mastery Standards

- Clarify the inferences and decisions that will be based on the mastery cut score. What is the "next step" of training or practice? When will it occur? What is the level of supervision at the next step?
- Identify essential content and, when appropriate, process variables such as speed or automaticity of response needed for a safe and successful transition to the next step.
- Use absolute or criterion-based standard-setting methods rather than normative methods.
- Consider conjunctive rather than compensatory standards for key knowledge and skill subdomains and for items that impact patient safety.
- Information about the performance of past examinees, especially first-time test-takers, is less helpful than performance of learners at the immediate next level of training or practice.
- Information about expert performance should be used with caution and as part of a thoughtful and deliberative standard-setting process.
- Information relating performance on the test to successful practice at the next stage of training is key to setting evidence-based mastery standards and should be a priority for mastery standards research.
- Traditional psychometric indices used to evaluate the quality of cut scores do not necessarily reflect measurement properties of mastery assessments and should be used with caution.

Table 18.1 Setting Standards for Different Types of Exams in Mastery Learning Settings

Type of Exam Data	Examples of Standard-Setting Considerations and Supporting Information in a Mastery Learning Setting[a]
Written exams such as multiple-choice questions Standardized patient checklists or rating scales	If using a modified Angoff method: • As supporting information, use benchmark performance data of students who were successful at later stages of curriculum. • Redefine borderline student from "minimally competent" to "well prepared for next stage." • Consider identifying critical items when patient safety issues are present.
Procedural skills checklists or rating scales Mannequin scenario checklists or rating scales	If passing the test will put live patients at risk: • As supporting information, identify subset of items critical to patient safety or procedure outcome (or other salient dimensions). • Note that item difficulty is less salient than item relevance and patient safety implications. • Set standards separately and conjunctively for critical and non-critical items.
Simulator-based performance metrics[b]	If using borderline group method: • As supporting information, identify appropriate benchmark group: solidly competent or proficient, rather than marginally or minimally competent. If using contrasting groups method: • As supporting information, identify appropriate "expert" or "passing" group: persons successful at the next stage of training or practice. Avoid contrasting novices with experts.

[a] Standard-setting methods shown are only examples; other standard-setting methods could be selected for the same type of exam data.

[b] Select relevant metrics with care; set mastery standards only for measures that have an impact on live performance.

until it is achieved—is consistent with a deliberate practice approach to attaining expertise (McGaghie, Issenberg, Cohen, Barsuk, & Wayne, 2011) and may encourage deliberate practice as a lifelong learning approach. However, mastery assessment systems that do not periodically reassess mastery may lead learners to focus on demonstrating mastery in the short term rather than maintaining mastery throughout their careers.

Mastery systems are meant to ensure that learners progress only when ready to do so, thus learner outcomes in subsequent educational experiences are a primary consequence of interest. However, drawing inferences about mastery assessments from learners' later progress can be challenging. If examinees' progress in later educational units is found to be subpar, it *may* be that one or more previous mastery standards were too lenient, but other factors could be at play. If their subsequent progress is satisfactory, the preceding mastery standards were arguably stringent enough, though more lenient standards might have yielded comparable results at less cost of learner time. The most powerful way to see if mastery assessment standards lead to desired outcomes would be to systematically experiment with the standards and observe how later outcomes are affected, though this can be logistically and sometimes ethically challenging.

Finally, evidence can be sought of an impact on outcomes for patients, the healthcare system, and society as a whole. For instance, Barsuk and colleagues found that a natural lapse in the provision of simulation-based mastery training of central line insertion corresponded with an increase in patient complications, providing evidence that adhering to the previous mastery standard had helped control complications (Barsuk et al., 2014).

SUMMARY AND CONCLUSIONS

Mastery learning systems have the potential to restructure health professions education towards the development of consistently high levels of achievement among learners, and as such fit well within current efforts to incorporate competency-based education in medical education. The assessment of learners' mastery and subsequent decision-making about learners' progress come with conceptual and methodological challenges, which are not necessarily more onerous than when conducting "traditional" assessments but do require different approaches. Box 18.1 provides a summary of the key considerations outlined here for validation and justification of mastery learning assessments.

ACKNOWLEDGEMENTS

This chapter is an updated and modified version of two papers that appeared in *Academic Medicine*, the journal of the Association of American Medical Colleges, in 2015:

Yudkowsky, R., Park, Y.S., Lineberry, M., Knox, A., Ritter, E.M. (2015). Setting Mastery Learning Standards. *Academic Medicine, 90*(11), 1495–1500.
Lineberry, M., Park, Y.S., Cook, D.A., Yudkowsky, R. (2015). Making the Case for Mastery Learning Assessments: Key Issues in Validation and Justification. *Academic Medicine, 90*(11), 1445–1450.

The authors are grateful to the publishers, Wolters Kluwer Health, for permission to reproduce here material from the papers. The original papers are available at the journal's website, https://journals.lww.com/academicmedicine.

Note: Additional material and resources may be available at the UIC AHPE website: https://go.uic.edu/AHPE

REFERENCES

American Educational Research Association, American Psychological Association, Joint Committee on Standards for Educational, Psychological Testing (US), & National Council on Measurement in Education. (1985). *Standards for educational and psychological testing.* Washington, DC: American Educational Research Association.
Angoff, W.H. (1971). Scales, norms, and equivalent scores. In R.L. Thorndike (Ed.), *Educational measurement.* Washington, DC: American Council on Education.
Arthur Jr., W., Bennett Jr., W., Stanush, P.L., & McNelly, T.L. (1998). Factors that influence skill decay and retention: A quantitative review and analysis. *Human Performance, 11*(1), 57–101.
Association of American Medical Colleges. (2014). *Core entrustable professional activities for entering residency: Curriculum developers' guide.* Washington, DC: Association of American Medical Colleges.
Barsuk, J.H., Cohen, E.R., Potts, S., Demo, H., Gupta, S., Feinglass, J., . . . Wayne, D.B. (2014). Dissemination of a simulation-based mastery learning intervention reduces central line-associated bloodstream infections. *BMJ Quality & Safety, 23*(9), 749–756.
Block, J.H. (Ed.). (1971). *Mastery learning: Theory and practice.* New York: Holt, Rinehart and Winston Inc.
Brent Stansfield, R., & Kreiter, C.D. (2007). Conditional reliability of admissions interview ratings: Extreme ratings are the most informative. *Medical Education, 41*(1), 32–38.
Choudhry, N.K., Fletcher, R.H., & Soumerai, S.B. (2005). Systematic review: The relationship between clinical experience and quality of health care. *Annals of Internal Medicine, 142*(4), 260–273.
Cizek, G.J. (1996). Standard-setting guidelines. *Educational Measurement: Issues and Practice, 15*(1), 13–21.
Cizek, G.J. (2012). Defining and distinguishing validity: Interpretations of score meaning and justifications of test use. *Psychological Methods, 17*(1), 31.
Cook, D.A., & Lineberry, M. (2016). Consequences validity evidence: Evaluating the impact of educational assessments. *Academic Medicine, 91*(6), 785–795.
Crocker, L., & Algina, J. (1986). Equating test scores from different tests. In: *Introduction to classical and modern test theory.* Belmont, CA: Wadsworth.
Downing, S.M. (2003). Validity: on the meaningful interpretation of assessment data. *Medical Education, 37*(9), 830–837.
Downing, S.M., Tekian, A., & Yudkowsky, R. (2006). Procedures for establishing defensible absolute passing scores on performance examinations in health professions education. *Teaching and Learning in Medicine, 18*(1), 50–57.
Embretson, S.E., & Reise, S.P. (2000). *Item response theory for psychologists.* Mahwah, NJ: Lawrence Erlbaum Associates.

Frank, J.R., Snell, L.S., Cate, O.T., Holmboe, E.S., Carraccio, C., Swing, S.R., . . . Dath, D. (2010). Competency-based medical education: theory to practice. *Medical Teacher, 32*(8), 638–645.

Fraser, S., Klassen, D., Feldman, L., Ghitulescu, G., Stanbridge, D., & Fried, G. (2003). Evaluating laparoscopic skills. *Surgical Endoscopy, 17*(6), 964–967.

Gallagher, A.G. (2012). Metric-based simulation training to proficiency in medical education: What it is and how to do it. *The Ulster Medical Journal, 81*(3), 107.

Gallagher, A.G., Ritter, E.M., Champion, H., Higgins, G., Fried, M.P., Moses, G., . . . Satava, R.M. (2005). Virtual reality simulation for the operating room: proficiency-based training as a paradigm shift in surgical skills training. *Annals of Surgery, 241*(2), 364.

Hambleton, R.K., & Slater, S.C. (1997). Reliability of credentialing examinations and the impact of scoring models and standard-setting policies. *Applied Measurement in Education, 10*(1), 19–28.

Hofstee, W.K. (1983). The case for compromise in educational selection and grading. *On Educational Testing,* 109–127.

Holmboe, E., Edgar, L., & Hamstra, S. (2016). *The milestones guidebook.* Chicago, IL: Accreditation Council for Graduate Medical Education.

Kane, M.T. (2013). Validating the interpretations and uses of test scores. *Journal of Educational Measurement, 50*(1), 1–73.

Konge, L., Annema, J., Clementsen, P., Minddal, V., Vilmann, P., & Ringsted, C. (2013). Using virtual-reality simulation to assess performance in endobronchial ultrasound. *Respiration, 86*(1), 59–65.

Konge, L., Clementsen, P., Larsen, K.R., Arendrup, H., Buchwald, C., & Ringsted, C. (2012). Establishing pass/fail criteria for bronchoscopy performance. *Respiration, 83*(2), 140–146.

Livingston, S.A., & Lewis, C. (1995). Estimating the consistency and accuracy of classifications based on test scores. *Journal of Educational Measurement, 32*(2), 179–197.

Livingston, S.A., & Zieky, M.J. (1982). *Passing scores: A manual for setting standards of performance on educational and occupational tests.* Princeton, NJ: Educational Testing Service.

Madsen, M.E., Konge, L., Nørgaard, L.N., Tabor, A., Ringsted, C., Klemmensen, Å., . . . Tolsgaard, M.G. (2014). Assessment of performance measures and learning curves for use of a virtual-reality ultrasound simulator in transvaginal ultrasound examination. *Ultrasound in Obstetrics & Gynecology, 44*(6), 693–699.

McGaghie, W.C. (1978). Competency-based curriculum development in medical education. An introduction. Public Health Papers No. 68.

McGaghie, W.C. (2015). Mastery learning: It is time for medical education to join the 21st century. *Academic Medicine, 90*(11), 1438–1441.

McGaghie, W.C., Issenberg, S.B., Cohen, M.E.R., Barsuk, J.H., & Wayne, D.B. (2011). Does simulation-based medical education with deliberate practice yield better results than traditional clinical education? A meta-analytic comparative review of the evidence. *Academic Medicine: Journal of the Association of American Medical Colleges, 86*(6), 706.

Mee, J., Clauser, B.E., & Margolis, M.J. (2013). The impact of process instructions on judges' use of examinee performance data in Angoff standard setting exercises. *Educational Measurement: Issues and Practice, 32*(3), 27–35.

Norcini, J.J., Stillman, P.L., Sutnick, A.I., Regan, M.B., Haley, H.L., Williams, R.G., & Friedman, M. (1993). Scoring and standard setting with standardized patients. *Evaluation & the Health Professions, 16*(3), 322–332.

Norman, G., Norcini, J., & Bordage, G. (2014). Competency-based education: Milestones or millstones? *Journal of Graduate Medical Education, 6*(1), 1–6.

O'Malley, K., Keng, L., & Miles, J. (2012). From Z to A: Using validity evidence to set performance standards. *Setting Performance Standards: Foundations, Methods, and Innovations,* 301–322.

Payne, S.C., Youngcourt, S.S., & Beaubien, J.M. (2007). A meta-analytic examination of the goal orientation nomological net. *Journal of Applied Psychology, 92*(1), 128.

Richland, L.E., Kornell, N., & Kao, L.S. (2009). The pretesting effect: Do unsuccessful retrieval attempts enhance learning? *Journal of Experimental Psychology: Applied, 15*(3), 243.

Rohrer, D., & Pashler, H. (2010). Recent research on human learning challenges conventional instructional strategies. *Educational Researcher, 39*(5), 406–412.

Rosenthal, M.E., Ritter, E.M., Goova, M.T., Castellvi, A.O., Tesfay, S.T., Pimentel, E.A., . . . Scott, D.J. (2010). Proficiency-based fundamentals of laparoscopic surgery skills training results in durable performance improvement and a uniform certification pass rate. *Surgical Endoscopy, 24*(10), 2453–2457.

Scott, D.J., Ritter, E.M., Tesfay, S.T., Pimentel, E.A., Nagji, A., & Fried, G.M. (2008). Certification pass rate of 100% for fundamentals of laparoscopic surgery skills after proficiency-based training. *Surgical Endoscopy, 22*(8), 1887–1893.

Seymour, N.E., Gallagher, A.G., Roman, S.A., O'brien, M.K., Bansal, V.K., Andersen, D.K., & Satava, R.M. (2002). Virtual reality training improves operating room performance: Results of a randomized, double-blinded study. *Annals of Surgery, 236*(4), 458.

Stefanidis, D., Korndorffer Jr,. J.R., Sierra, R., Touchard, C., Dunne, J.B., & Scott, D.J. (2005). Skill retention following proficiency-based laparoscopic simulator training. *Surgery*, *138*(2), 165–170.

Stefanidis, D., Scerbo, M.W., Montero, P.N., Acker, C.E., & Smith, W.D. (2012). Simulator training to automaticity leads to improved skill transfer compared with traditional proficiency-based training: a randomized controlled trial. *Annals of Surgery*, *255*(1), 30–37.

Subkoviak, M.J. (1988). A practitioner's guide to computation and interpretation of reliability indices for mastery tests. *Journal of Educational Measurement*, *25*(1), 47–55.

Webb, N.M., Shavelson, R.J., & Haertel, E.H. (2006). 4 reliability coefficients and generalizability theory. *Handbook of Statistics*, *26*, 81–124.

Yudkowsky, R., Tumuluru, S., Casey, P., Herlich, N., & Ledonne, C. (2014). A patient safety approach to setting pass/fail standards for basic procedural skills checklists. *Simulation in Healthcare*, *9*(5), 277–282.

Ziv, A., Wolpe, P.R., Small, S.D., & Glick, S. (2003). Simulation-based medical education: an ethical imperative. *Academic Medicine*, *78*(8), 783–788.

19

ITEM RESPONSE THEORY

Yoon Soo Park

INTRODUCTION

There are two dominant frameworks for scoring and analyzing assessments: (1) classical measurement theory (CMT; Lord & Novick, 1968) and (2) item response theory (IRT; Baker, 2001). Earlier chapters of this book focus on CMT—namely, classical test theory (CTT; Chapter 3) and generalizability theory (G theory; Chapter 4). CMT is perhaps the most widely used assessment framework in health professions education; CMT is simple to apply and implement in many assessment settings. The idea of CMT is straightforward—"observed scores" are a function of "true score" and "measurement error." On the other hand, inferences generated using CMT are sample specific, making comparisons of test statistics from different learner cohorts potentially confounded (Traub, 1997).

Item response theory refers to the theory and family of associated psychometric models that link learner performance to the probability of item responses on the assessment (Hambleton, Swaminathan, & Rogers, 1991). IRT conforms to a group of mathematical models that specifies the probability of learner success (i.e., that they will answer an item correctly) at the item level (Embretson & Reise, 2000). There are many IRT models available in the psychometric literature; different IRT models are used depending on the assessment context, item structure, and number of examinees (Park, Xing, & Lee, 2018). IRT resolves the circular dependency challenge posed by CMT approaches, and as such, it is used widely in national licensure and certification examinations (Ames & Penfield, 2015). The multiple-choice question components of the United States Medical Licensing Examination (USMLE), Medical Council of Canada Qualifying Examination (MCCQE), and the Medical College Admission Test (MCAT) are scored and analyzed using IRT.

In this chapter, we present an overview of IRT and its comparison to CMT. IRT-based item analysis and examples of IRT-based applications are presented with the purpose of providing an introduction for health professions educators. We also describe extensions of IRT, including computer-adaptive testing and test equating. This chapter is intended to provide an introduction to IRT. Interested health professions education researchers should pursue more advanced treatment and understanding of IRT concepts through additional resources beyond this chapter.

CLASSICAL MEASUREMENT THEORY: CHALLENGES IN SAMPLE-DEPENDENT INFERENCE

Consider a scenario. You are a biochemistry course director in a medical school. You administer a 100-item summative end-of-course assessment. Following test administration, you decide to compare the performance of your current students to students from last year. You find that this year's students performed significantly lower than last year's students. What happened? Did this year's students truly perform poorly? Was it due to new items administered this year? Were items more difficult? Consider a second scenario. You work for a national testing organization that administers certification assessments routinely, perhaps as often as four times a year. This requires different items in each test form, while measuring the same construct (e.g., assessment of clinical knowledge). Knowing that the item difficulty associated with test forms varies, how do you assemble items to form comparable assessments? How might you equate scores from one test form to another?

Challenges posed in these scenarios are common dilemmas faced by health professionals (Downing, 2003). Most assessments in health professions education are scored and analyzed using CMT. While CMT is relatively easy to use and apply in many situations (Chapters 3 and 5), inference drawn from CMT are *sample dependent*—that is, test scores (learner performance) and test characteristics (item difficulty and item discrimination) have a circular relationship. For example, if you administer easy items to poor-performing learners, your item statistics may indicate high difficulty (i.e., low p values); likewise, if you administer difficult items to high-performing learners, your results may indicate that items are easy (i.e., high p values).

Circular dependence limits meaningful comparison between learners and item characteristics—the "true" difficulty of items is confounded with learner's ability or proficiency level. These sample-dependent features in CMT place limits on item banking, on developing equated test forms, and on our ability to compare performance between assessments (Park, Lee, & Xing, 2016). In contrast, IRT was developed to resolve issues in sample dependence, by linking examinee performance and item characteristics to the same measurement scale (van der Linden, 1996).

CMT is used widely in local education programs because there are no limiting statistical requirements to perform CMT—or, more technically, CMT has weak theoretical assumptions. For example, if you have a multiple-choice question (MCQ) assessment, you can simply add the learner performance across items to obtain the total score. To conduct item analysis, you can calculate the proportion correct (difficulty) and point-biserial correlations (discrimination) to examine the quality of items. You can administer the assessment to a small group of learners and conduct these analyses without problems. This is the benefit of CMT. It is easy to apply in many situations without meeting rigorous statistical assumptions in the assessment data.

Comparison Between CMT and IRT

The overarching inference from CMT is at the test level. In IRT, the focus is on the item-level information. Table 19.1 shows a comparison of features between the CMT and IRT frameworks categorized by target inference, item statistics, assessment score, model assumptions, and sample size requirements. Besides the sample-dependent feature of CMT, other requirements for conducting analysis in the CMT framework are minimal. There are no theoretical assumptions, and sample size requirements are not as demanding when compared to IRT. The simplest IRT model (Rasch model) requires a strict minimum sample size of 100 examinees (Embretson & Reise, 2000; van der Linden, 1996). Perhaps the greatest benefit of conducting IRT-based analyses is the sample independence of results; that is, the circular dependence problem is resolved through the mathematical properties of the IRT models. This is known as the *invariance property* of IRT models (Lord & Novick, 1968). We review features of IRT in greater detail in the ensuing sections.

Table 19.1 Comparison Between Classical Measurement Theory and Item Response Theory

Feature	Classical Measurement Theory (CMT)	Item Response Theory (IRT)
Target Inference	Test-level information	Item-level information
Item Statistics	Sample dependent • Item difficulty: proportion correct • Item discrimination: item-total correlation (point-biserial correlation)	Sample independent • Item difficulty: IRT model intercept parameter (b) • Item discrimination: IRT model slope parameter (a)
Assessment Score (Person Statistic)	Sample dependent • Total score (sum total)	Sample independent • Common ability scale (θ)
Model Assumptions	None	Unidimensionality, local independence, and no item bias
Sample Size Requirements	None, but larger samples yield better results (e.g., over 30 learners)	Minimum of 100 for the most simple IRT model (500 or more for more complex IRT models)

ITEM RESPONSE THEORY: AN OVERVIEW

The development of IRT models date to the 1950s and into the 1960s through a convergence of research in mathematics, educational measurement, and quantitative psychology (Traub, 1997). In IRT, the focus is to create a model that links the probabilistic distribution of examinee success (getting an item correct) at the item level. Examinee ability (performance) and item characteristics are referenced to the same scale—this is an important innovation in measurement that overcomes the circular dependency. In CMT, the total score and item characteristics are not referenced to the same scale (Downing, 2003; de Champlain, 2010).

IRT Model: Logistic Parameter Model

IRT models have item-level parameters (difficulty and discrimination) and accompanying model equations for each item in the assessment. For example, if there are nine items in an assessment (see Table 19.2), there are nine mathematical equations that form the IRT model for an assessment. To date, there are three main IRT models that are widely used in educational measurement: the 1-, 2-, and 3-parameter logistic (PL) models (Ames & Penfield, 2015). The 1-PL model is also commonly referred to as the *Rasch model*, named by Benjamin Wright to honor the significant contributions by Georg Rasch. In this chapter, we present examples of the 2-PL model, as they are complementary to CMT models. The 2-PL model is also easily simplified to the Rasch model or extended to form the 3-PL model. The mathematical formula for the 2-PL model is shown below.

$$\Pr\left(Y_j = 1 \mid \theta\right) = 1 \, / \, [1 + \exp\left(-1.702 \, a_j \left(\theta - b_j\right)\right)] \tag{19.1}$$

In Equation (19.1), the probability of getting an item j correct, $\Pr\left(Y_j = 1\right)$, is modeled by an exponential function with two parameters: a_j (slope parameter: item discrimination) and b_j (intercept parameter: item difficulty). This probability is conditional on the ability of the examinee, modeled as a continuous latent ability score, known as theta (θ; examinee score).

Item Characteristic Curve

IRT models have the simple idea that learners with higher ability have a higher probability of answering an item correctly. Equation (19.1) may be best represented graphically through an item characteristic curve (ICC) presented in Figure 19.1.

In the 2-PL model, there are two item characteristics, modeled by discrimination (a) and difficulty (b) parameters. These parameters are item specific. In Figure 19.1, the X-axis is the

Table 19.2 Item Parameter Results: Classical Measurement Theory Versus Item Response Theory

Item	Classical Measurement Theory		Item Response Theory	
	Difficulty	Discrimination	Difficulty (SE)	Discrimination (SE)
1	.63	.37	−.47 (.07)	1.62 (.24)
2	.52	.22	−.15 (.12)	.66 (.12)
3	.80	.24	−1.71 (.24)	.92 (.16)
4	.44	.25	.33 (.11)	.82 (.13)
5	.23	.23	1.59 (.23)	.90 (.15)
6	.38	.28	.62 (.11)	.98 (.15)
7	.27	.11	2.84 (.87)	.36 (.11)
8	.86	.29	−1.71 (.19)	1.40 (.23)
9	.71	.18	−1.51 (.28)	.64 (.12)

Note: Values in parentheses are standard errors.

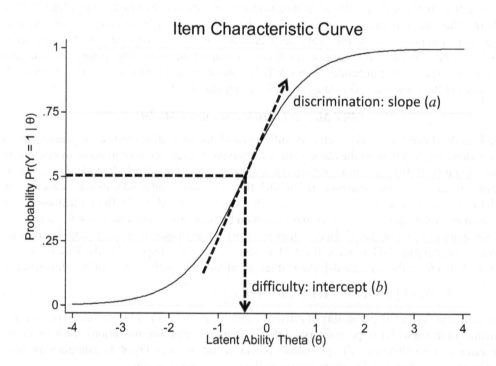

Figure 19.1 IRT item characteristic curve

latent ability scale, a standardized scale often specified with mean 0 and variance 1 (similar to a standardized z-scale). The Y-axis is the probability that an examinee gets the item correct; the higher the probability, the greater the likelihood of getting the item correct. As such, the IRT function links the relationship between the latent ability scale (X-axis) and the probability of correct answer (Y-axis) through a logistic curve characterized by the mathematical formula in Equation (19.1).

Item Difficulty

In IRT, the difficulty index (b) is the location on the ability scale where the probability of correct response is 50%. In Figure 19.1, the difficulty index (b) is −.50 (hypothetical value); that is, the latent ability score (θ; X-axis) corresponding to 50% probability of correct response is the difficulty index, which is $\theta = -.50$ in this example (half standard deviation below the mean). If the item characteristic curve shifts to the right, it signals a more difficult item, because the ability level corresponding to 50% probability of a correct response requires a higher ability level; in contrast, if the item characteristic curve shifts to the left, it signals an easier item, where the probability of 50% correct response can be reached by lower ability level.

Item Discrimination

The item discrimination index (a) is the slope of the item characteristic curve. If the slope is higher, it indicates a better discrimination of ability level given the probability of correct response. Imagine a flat horizontal line with slope = 0; in this case, the item is unable to discriminate the probability of correct response based on different levels of ability. As such, a higher slope indicates better discrimination. In Figure 19.1, the slope is $a = 1.00$.

Features of IRT

An important feature of IRT is the sample independence of item statistics (item difficulty and item discrimination). The ability level is also independent of the particular set of items administered. Since IRT model parameters are sample independent, we refer to them as *invariant*, prompting better understanding of assessment characteristics. The invariance property of IRT indicates stability of inference (examinee score distribution and item characteristics), regardless of examinee population or measurement conditions. A direct application of the item invariance characteristic of IRT is the ability to produce useful item banks. Item difficulty and discrimination indices are assumed to be stable over different test forms and difference examinees, allowing item properties to be easily used in creating new test forms and equating (Park et al., 2016).

Assumptions for Conducting IRT

There are three main assumptions required for conducting IRT analysis (Lord & Novick, 1968; Baker, 2001):

1. Unidimensionality: Assessment measures a single construct (single construct accounts for substantial portion of the overall assessment score variance).
2. Local independence: An item in the assessment is independent of another item (once you know a person's ability level, the learner's response to items are independent of one another).
3. No item bias: Items do not function differently across subgroups of learners (no differential item functioning [DIF]).

There are statistical tests in IRT that can be done to confirm these assumptions are met (Embretson & Reise, 2000; Park et al., 2016).

Rasch Model

In the Rasch model, the item discrimination parameter in Equation (19.1) is constrained to a fixed value, either to a value of "1" or a single value estimated by the software. Equation (19.2) shows the accompanying Rasch model:

$$\Pr(Y_j = 1 \mid \theta) = 1 / [1 + \exp(-1.702\,a_j\,(\theta - b_j))]$$
$$\rightarrow \{a_j = 1\} \text{ or } \{a_j = k\}, \text{ fix } a_j \text{ to a single value for all items} \qquad (19.2)$$

As such, the consequence to using a Rasch model is the assumption that all items discriminate learners at the same level. There are debates in the measurement literature on the pros and cons of the Rasch model assumption that all items have equal discrimination levels. For this reason, the 2-PL model is preferred as it allows differences in item discrimination to be modeled. However, the 2-PL model requires larger sample sizes, up to a minimum of 500 examinees, whereas the Rasch model has the convenience of stable estimation with as little as 100 examinees.

Application of IRT: An Example

This section demonstrates an example of IRT analysis. Consider the nine-item multiple-choice question quiz administered to medical students in Table 19.2 showing item characteristics based on CMT and IRT. For CMT, the difficulty and discrimination are measured using proportion correct and point-biserial correlation, respectively. Higher proportion correct indicates an easier item; higher point-biserial correlation indicates better ability for the item to discriminate between low- and high-performing learners.

In the right two columns, the corresponding IRT item characteristics are presented. The difficulty is the intercept parameter b_j in Equation (19.1); the discrimination is the slope parameter a_j in Equation (19.1). Compare the difficulty and discrimination indices between the two models. The results are highly correlated ($r > .90$). Both approaches identify difficult items and more discriminating items in a similar manner. For example, item 1 which has the highest CMT point-biserial correlation of .37 also has the highest IRT slope parameter discriminating of 1.62. Likewise, item 8 which is the easiest item with CMT proportion correct of .86 also has the lowest IRT intercept parameter of −1.71.

IRT creates separate mathematical functions for each item, generating nine distinct item characteristic curves. Figure 19.2a shows ICCs for all nine items and Figure 19.2b shows ICCs for selected two items.

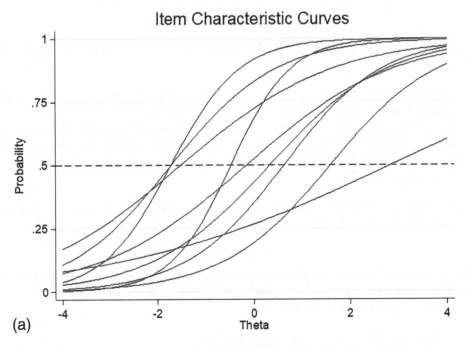

Figure 19.2 Item characteristic curves: all items (Figure 19.2a) and two selected items (Figure 19.2b)

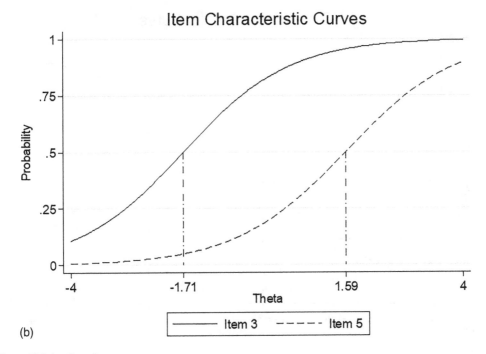

Item Characteristic Curves

(b)

Figure 19.2 (continued)

In Figure 19.2a, a range of curves are illustrated, showing varying items of difficulty and discrimination. To illustrate this difference in greater detail, the ICCs for items 3 and 5 were selected (Figure 19.2b). The ICC for item 3 is to the left, where the 50% probability of correct response relates to an ability level of −1.71 (i.e., 1.71 standard deviation units below the mean); on the other hand, the difficulty level for item 5 is to the right, where the 50% probability of correct response relates to an ability level of 1.59. These values correspond to the difficulty indices (b_j) for items 3 and 5, respectively. The two curves have similar discrimination (a_j) of .92 and .90, respectively.

To translate the ability level to the actual raw score, a test characteristic curve (TCC) can be created in IRT analysis. Figure 19.3a shows the TCC for this nine-item quiz. As illustrated in the figure, the relationship between ability level (θ, X-axis) and raw score (expected score, Y-axis) is curvilinear. For example, the ability level −.587 corresponds to a raw total score of 4. This is a distinction between CMT and the 2-PL model, where classical models assume equal weighting of items; the IRT model weights each item based on their difficulty and discrimination to derive the total score.

Another distinct feature of IRT models is the derivation of a test information function, which shows the ability level corresponding to the greatest score precision. In Figure 19.3b, test information is maximized at −.59 (hypothetical). In other words, a raw cut score of 4 points (translating to ability score of −.59) would yield the most precise information for this particular quiz.

OTHER APPLICATIONS OF IRT

Computer-Adaptive Testing

The item invariance property of IRT allows a specialized form of assessment known as computer-adaptive testing (CAT). This differs from computer-based testing (CBT), which is simply a

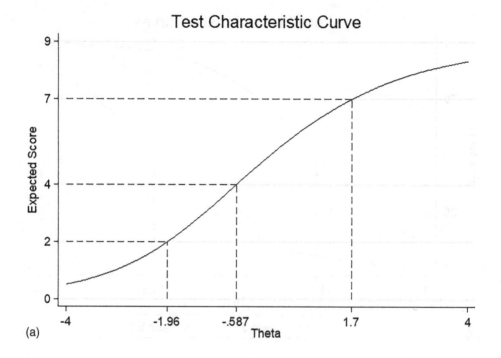

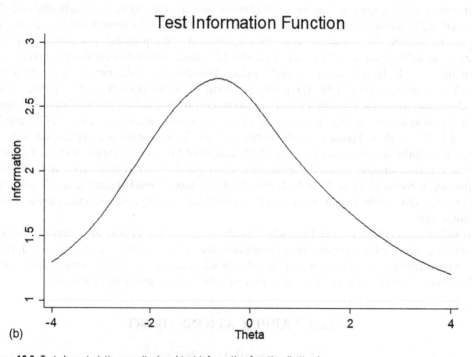

Figure 19.3 Test characteristic curve (top) and test information function (bottom)

computerized version of a paper-pencil assessment. In CAT, the items are adaptive to the response pattern of the examinee. For example, if the examinee gets a particular item correct, an item specific to that ability level is given (e.g., more difficult item) until the computer program converges to arrive at a precise estimate of the learner's performance level. Unlike CBT, which is based on linear-testing format (everyone receives the same items in a linear process), CAT has shown to yield more precise scores (lower measurement error) with a variable number of items needed to estimate the learner's ability level. CAT can only be achieved when item statistics are sample independent; and as such, IRT is needed to conduct CAT.

Test Equating

Test equating refers to a group of techniques that allow assessments with different items measuring the same construct to be placed on the same scale. For example, consider two test forms with 21 items in Form X and 24 items in Form Y administered to different examinees; further, assume that both forms share 12 common items (anchor items). This design, known as a nonequivalent group with anchor test (NEAT), is a widely used assessment format for equating scores (Kolen & Brennan, 2014). This is illustrated in Figure 19.4a. Using IRT, test characteristic curves can be derived by calibrating items. Using the ability scale as the common metric, scores from Form X can be linked to scores on Form Y as illustrated in Figure 19.4b. For example, for score 8 in Form X, this translates to an ability scale score (θ) of .007914321; this ability scale score of .007914321, in turn, translates to Form Y score of 10.90723. In this manner, scores from two assessment forms with varying items can be placed on the same measurement scale to equate test scores. This is the basic principle behind test equating. For further materials, readers should reference Kolen and Brennan (2014).

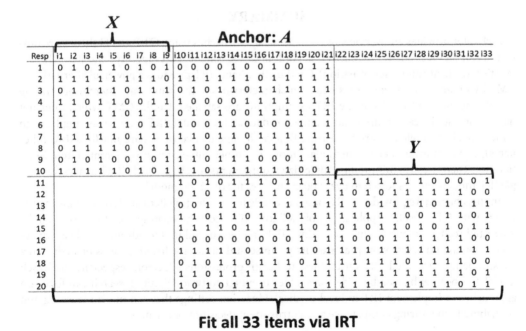

Fit all 33 items via IRT

Figure 19.4a Test equating using IRT: non-equivalent groups with anchor test

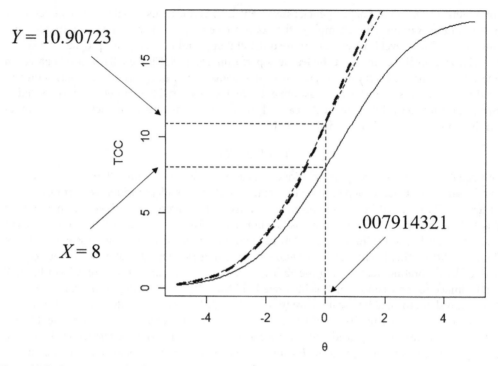

$Y = 10.90723$

$X = 8$

.007914321

Figure 19.4b Test equating using IRT: concurrent calibration—an example

SUMMARY

This chapter provides an overview of IRT. Classical approaches using CTT and G theory are limited in sample-dependent inferences that confound assessment scores (ability) and item characteristics (difficulty and discrimination). On the other hand, IRT provides a powerful alternative to CMT by linking assessment scores and item characteristics to the same scale, thereby generating sample independent results, if the IRT assumptions are satisfied. Unlike CMT, which does not have strong statistical requirements (sample or data assumptions), IRT requires assumptions in dimensionality (single construct measured), local independence (items are not linked to other items), and item invariance (no item bias among examinee subgroups; no differential item functioning). There are also minimum sample size requirements that begin with 100 learners for simple IRT models such as Rasch to over 500 examinees for the 2-PL model.

In this chapter, we provide an IRT-based example for conducting item analysis, comparing the results with CTT results. Applications of IRT for CAT and test equating are also described for interested readers to pursue further reading. IRT can be a useful tool to advance medical education research and assessment practices. Its promise and utility for health professions educators are still being uncovered. IRT's usefulness to health professions educators, especially the Rasch model, has been enhanced by widely available computer software. Future research can focus on approaches to implement IRT in local medical education settings that can inform learning and contribute to measuring competence and entrustment decisions of learners.

Note: Additional material and resources may be available at the UIC AHPE website: https://go.uic.edu/AHPE

REFERENCES

Ames, A.J., & Penfield, R.D. (2015). An NCME instructional module on item-fit statistics for item response theory models. *Educational Measurement: Issues and Practice, 34*(3), 39–48.

Baker, F.B. (2001). *The basics of item response theory* (2nd ed.). Washington, DC: Office of Educational Research and Improvement.

de Champlain, A.F. (2010). A primer on classical test theory and item response theory for assessments in medical education. *Medical Education, 44,* 109–117.

Downing, S.M. (2003). Item response theory: Applications of modern test theory in medical education. *Medical Education, 37,* 739–745.

Embretson, S.E., & Reise, S.P. (2000). *Item response theory for psychologists.* Mahwah, NJ: Lawrence Erlbaum Associates.

Hambleton, R.K., Swaminathan, H., & Rogers, H.J. (1991). *Fundamentals of item response theory.* Newbury Park: Sage.

Kolen, M.J., & Brennan, R.L. (2014). *Test equating, scaling, and linking.* New York: Springer.

Lord, F.M., & Novick, M.R. (1968). *Statistical theories of mental test scores.* Reading, MA: Addison-Wesley.

Park, Y.S., Lee, Y.S., Xing, K. (2016). Investigating the impact of item parameter drift for item response theory models with mixture distributions. *Frontiers in Psychology, 7,* 255.

Park, Y.S., Xing, K., & Lee, Y.-S. (2018). Explanatory cognitive diagnostic models: Incorporating latent and observed predictors. *Applied Psychological Measurement, 42*(5), 376–392.

Traub, R.E. (1997). Classical test theory in historical perspective. *Educational Measurement: Issues and Practice, 16*(4), 8–14.

van der Linden, W.J. (1996). *Handbook of modern item response theory.* New York: Springer.

20

ENGAGING WITH YOUR STATISTICIAN

Alan Schwartz and Yoon Soo Park

INTRODUCTION

Many assessment projects involve the use of quantitative methods and data analyses. Not all health professions education researchers conduct their own analyses; many prefer to engage the services of professional data analysts, statisticians, or psychometricians, as collaborators, co-investigators, or consultants. This chapter offers suggestions for how to facilitate these collaborations, which constitutes an important aspect of successfully conducting assessment projects and assessment research.

Throughout this chapter, we use "statistician" informally to refer to anyone with expertise in the design and analysis of research yielding quantitative data. We include in this category not only those with bona fide graduate degrees in statistics, but others with training or experience in statistical analysis. That is, we treat the statistician as a role played by a member of the research team. Moreover, guidelines offered in this chapter extend beyond assessment-related research to health professions education research more broadly where quantitative data analyses are used.

PLANNING FOR DATA ANALYSIS

Finding the Appropriate Statistician

Analysis of educational data is an entrustable professional activity (Chapter 1 and ten Cate, 2005). You will entrust your statistician to conduct the analysis and should find a statistician who is both competent and trustworthy. Analytic competence includes not only experience with appropriate methods for the research question and data, but also strong oral and written communication skills to facilitate both the statistician's understanding of the researcher's needs and the analyst's ability to explain the methods and results in a way that will facilitate interpretation. The components of trustworthiness—truthfulness, discernment, and conscientiousness—are equally important (Kennedy, Regehr, Baker, & Lingard, 2008). Prefer a statistician who understands his or her limits, has a strong sense of research integrity, and can collaborate reliably.

Methods used in quantitative analyses in assessment research can differ substantively from those used in biomedical sciences, public health, and other social sciences more broadly. For example, estimating reliability of an objective structured clinical examination (OSCE) would be straightforward for a psychometrician working in medical education, but statisticians working in other disciplines may not be familiar with statistics of testing (Chapter 5) or generalizability theory (Chapter 4) and the technical details accompanying this approach. Standards for reporting results also differ among disciplines. As such, identifying a statistician who is familiar with conceptual frameworks, vocabulary, and applications in assessment approaches within health professions education further facilitates collaboration.

When and What to Present to Your Statistician

Research data analysis is a process of asking questions and using data to propose answers: telling an intriguing story about how something takes place and how we learn about it. Clear research questions make for satisfying narratives (Bordage & Dawson, 2003) and help the statistician understand what kinds of approaches will be fruitful rather than trivial. The research question should always precede and inform decisions about variables, instrumentation, and analytic methods.

A too-common scenario sees a researcher presenting a collected data set to a statistician at first meeting and asking him or her to "run the numbers." Involving the statistician at a far earlier stage—during the design of the study—is more productive for both statistician and researcher. A good statistician will compare and propose potential analytic methods at the outset, ensure that the data collection plan, sample size, and instruments will yield usable data, and assist in performing a power calculation or drafting an analytic plan for a grant proposal, IRB protocol, or future publications. Depending on the study design, the types of quantitative methods available to the statistician can vary, possibly affecting the interpretation of results. The value of a sound data collection plan is also often overlooked, but will impact the variables collected and the time required for the statistician to clean and compile the data.

A particularly useful document is a table of constructs. A table of constructs is much like a codebook for a data set, but rather than describing the format and contents of data that *have been* collected, the table of variables describes the constructs included in the research question and how they *will be* measured in the data collection to come. Because a given construct can be operationalized and measured in several ways, a table of constructs helps the statistician develop analytics plans that are appropriate to the research question and the nature of the measures. Such tables are also valuable in grant proposals.

The nature of the question and study design should dictate the columns in the table, including the role (outcome or predictor) and measurement level (continuous or categorical) of the constructs. For example, a longitudinal study might include columns relating to measurement time points. The statistician can help define useful columns—and can question why a researcher is gathering a particular variable if it seems to have no role in a research question. Table 20.1 is an example of a table of constructs for a study designed to address a stylized research question, "How do the spacing and amount of simulated practice affect the mastery of surgical knot-tying in two different task trainer models?" Notice that it also helps reveal a data-handling question related to measuring frequency: if skills are practiced for two, four, or eight weeks, should we treat practice time as a categorical, ordinal, or interval variable?

Another very helpful kind of table is the "mock table." Imagine that you've collected your data and are preparing a manuscript or a slide presentation. What do you expect to see in Table 20.1? Participant demographics? Draw an empty Table 20.1 with rows and columns labeled to indicate the demographics you expect to report and among which groups (if you're comparing an intervention group and a control group, add a column for each and a column to report the p-values of the comparisons too). Will Table 20.2 present the results of testing the primary study hypothesis?

Table 20.1 An Example of a Table of Constructs for a Study of Learning Knot-Tying

Construct	Variable Name	Role	Instrumentation	Measurement Level
Surgical knot-tying skill	Errors	Outcome	Observation of performance at end of practice	Counted (likely to be many zeros)
Surgical knot-tying skill	Speed	Outcome	Observation of performance at end of practice	Continuous (likely to be normally distributed)
Task trainer model	TrainingModel	Predictor	Each learner completes an attempt on each of the two models	Categorical, 2 levels (model 1, model 2)—within-subject (learners do both levels)
Practice	SpacingCondition	Predictor	Assignment to one of two spacing conditions during weeks of practice	Categorical, 2 levels (spaced, bunched)—between-subject
Practice	PracticeWeeks	Predictor	Number of weeks of practice (2, 4, or 8)	To be determined: could be treated as categorical, ordinal, or continuous, depending on hypothesized relationship and study context—between-subject

Table 20.2 An Example of a Properly Formatted Data Spreadsheet for the Study of Learning Knot-Tying

ID	SpacingCondition	PracticeWeeks	TrainingModel	Errors	Speed
101	B	2	1	3	1.3
101	B	2	2	1	1.0
102	S	2	1	0	1.0
102	S	2	2	1	0.9
103	S	8	1		
103	S	8	2	0	0.5

Note: Learner 103 has missing data for task trainer model 1 (e.g., because the model was being repaired the day learner 3 was tested).

Draw an empty Table 20.2 with labels that explain what you plan to present. Sharing these mock tables with your statistician will allow him or her to quickly see what's important to you and what kinds of results you'll need to fill them in. You can do the same with mock figures as well—drawing stylized versions freehand is usually sufficient.

In many studies (especially field studies in medical education assessment), complete data without missing records is so unusual as to be cause for celebration. More often, participants will leave items blank, fall sick during testing sessions, or drop out of the study altogether. Sometimes a study will have missing data by design ("structural missing data"), such as when branching logic is used in an adaptive test to ask certain questions only of certain respondents. Analytic methods differ in how robust they are to missing data of various sorts, and handling missing data requires both understanding of the processes that cause the data to be missing and considerable judgment on the part of the statistician and researcher. Anticipate missing data and discuss the likely nature of missing data with the statistician. These early discussions will also inform the presentation of descriptive statistics that reveal the degree of missing data or participant attrition.

COLLABORATING DURING ANALYSES

Talking Through the Analysis Plan

Even if you have delegated conducting the analyses and writing up the methods and results to your trustworthy statistician, you are ultimately responsible for understanding the nature of your data and defending the interpretation of the results. Moreover, when researchers present their findings orally (at a podium or in front of a poster), they are expected to discuss all aspects of the study; the statisticians are seldom immediately available. A valuable exercise is for you to "teach back" the analysis plan to the statistician by reviewing the proposed methods and what each is expected to demonstrate in your own words. The teach-back confirms a shared mental model of the research among the research team (including the statistician), provides an opportunity for the statistician to correct misunderstandings (or to revise the analysis plan), and lets the researcher practice for eventual presentation. A teach-back might (eventually) sound like this:

> We're going to compare the mean knot-tying speed among the six study groups (spaced or bunched practice for either 2, 4, or 8 weeks) using an analysis of variance. That will tell us the effect of spacing, on average, the effect of the amount of practice, on average, and whether the effect of spacing differs depending on the amount of practice. We'll treat amount of practice as three categories for this analysis, which doesn't require us to assume each additional week of practice has the same effect, or to assume that more practice is necessarily better at all (but may be a less powerful or sensitive test than if we were willing to make those assumptions).

Creating Data Files

Very few research data analyses are conducted in spreadsheet software: the set of functions and formulas is generally too limited, and the cell-based approach is too difficult to debug and replicate. Expect your statistician to want to read your data into statistical software (e.g., R, Stata, SPSS). At the same time, your statistician should not expect you to provide data in the native format of their software (to which you may not have access). Spreadsheet or spreadsheet-like text files (e.g., Microsoft Excel or comma-separated value files) are the de facto lingua franca for translating data from collection to analysis.

The most versatile arrangement for study data in spreadsheets is for each row of data (after the header row) to represent an individual participant at a single measurement period or condition. In a cross-sectional study, this means each participant will be represented as a single data row. In a longitudinal study, each participant will be represented by several data rows ("long format"), each containing the participant's ID in one column and a value representing the measurement period in another column. When there are a small number of repeated measures (e.g., a single pre-test score and a single post-test score), some analysts may prefer each participant to be on a single row (with a pre-test score column and a post-test score column) and others may prefer each participant to be represented by two rows (with a participant ID column, a time column for pre or post, and a score column for the participant's score at the given time). Accompany the data with a reasonably detailed codebook that describes the variables in the data. It is generally better to have all data in a single spreadsheet rather than multiple files that may require further data cleaning and compilation by the analyst (for example, each file will need to be individually checked to ensure the data are represented consistently, the variables have the same names, and any obvious data entry errors have been corrected).

When using spreadsheet files for data, avoid anything that won't translate into the statistician's software. Generally, that means avoid anything in cells except numbers and text. Specifically, avoid at all costs:

- Spreadsheet formulas
- Colors or highlighting that have any meaning or analytic import

- Blank rows or blank columns
- "Total" rows (rows at the end of the data that represent the total or average or other summaries of variables)
- Relying on the order of the rows or row numbers themselves to mean anything

For example, some researchers would like to use blank rows or colors to separate groups of participants in the data file. This violates several of the above taboos (color, blank rows, relying on row order). Instead, add a column and use values in the column to identify groups. For example, the "SpacingCondition" column in our data file could contain values "S" (spaced) or "B" (bunched) for each participant's rows, to indicate to which group they were assigned.

When a participant is represented by multiple rows in a data file (e.g., because they participated in multiple sessions over time), each row should be complete on its own. Don't fill out the participant ID on the first session's row and then leave it blank in the subsequent sessions' rows. Although that's more readable to human beings, it violates the principle of row order being meaningless, and statistical software will happily treat those subsequent rows as not being associated with any participant.

The representation of missing data will depend on how it is to be handled in the analysis. For many studies, it can be appropriate to leave missing cells empty, which will cause most statistical software to appropriately consider the data missing. In other situations, it may be necessary to use explicit numeric values—those that could not be mistaken for an actual response—to denote missing data (e.g., -99, -98, etc.). Using numeric values has the advantage of producing a data file that has entries in every cell, so you can easily distinguish a row that is incomplete (for example, because you haven't yet entered the data) from a row that is complete but contains missing values. Explicit missing values are also useful when there are multiple ways a data point can be missing, and it is important to distinguish between them (for example, data could be missing due to a refusal to respond vs. a failure to present an item). When explicit missing values are used, however, it is critical that the statistician be informed so their statistical software can be informed to treat those values as missing—including a couple of -99 values in calculating a mean will invalidate the results.

With categorical variables, the researcher is often faced with the choice between recording them in text (e.g., "S" or "B" for "spaced" or "bunched," respectively) or as numbers (e.g., 1 or 2 for "spaced" or "bunched," respectively). Text has the advantage of being easier for humans to read and less prone to misinterpretation ("did 1 mean spaced or bunched?"). On the other hand, most statistical software is case-sensitive and will consider "B" and "b" to be different text values, so it is critical that researchers and statisticians check text cells to be sure they contain only the desired values. Blank spaces present a similar difficulty. It is easy for a column that is supposed to contain A or B to end up with a small number of values that are "A " (an A followed by a space), which are indistinguishable from "A" to the human eye. Researchers who wish to use text values should do a "search and replace" in text columns to remove spaces.

Alternatively, using numerical codes (1, 2, 3, etc.) avoids this danger but requires that the values of the codes be clearly conveyed to the statistician. Never mix numerical and text values in the same variable.

Yes/No responses are a very common special case. They should be coded as either Y/N, y/n, or 1/0 (which has a natural interpretation as present vs. absent). Given a choice, 1/0 is least likely to result in confusion by the statistician, as it offers no chance of confusion due to case sensitivity or extra blanks. Variables coded as 1/0 are known as "indicator variables." For example, in an experimental study, learners may be randomized to "control" or "intervention" groups; this can be represented using an indicator "intervention" variable with values 0 for control and 1 for intervention groups, respectively. Consult your statistician on strategies for appropriately coding complex categorical data.

Table 20.2 illustrates a well-formatted data file corresponding to the table of constructs for the knot-tying study.

Exploratory Work Before Planned Analyses

It is critical that both you and your statistician have a good understanding of the nature of the data set and its constituent variables. Exploratory data analysis methods focus on helping you visualize relationships in data by means of tables and charts, and also serve an important purpose in checking data quality (Tukey, 1977). For example, the scatterplot in Figure 20.1 not only suggests that both Speed and Age are distributed roughly normally, but that they have a positive association, and that some kind of data entry error was likely made for the Age variable. Asking your statistician to produce histograms showing the distribution of each variable is helpful.

Exploratory Work After Planned Analyses

Often, the results of planned analyses suggest new ideas or questions that might be explored in the data. The danger, however, is that these new questions are based not on a theoretical rationale or expectation, but on the data as they actually turned out. It is easy to devise a test that "discovers" an effect with the benefit of hindsight and poor science to report such a discovery as if it were made without foreknowledge.

Your statistician wants to help you understand your data, describe it clearly, and test your study hypotheses convincingly. His or her responsibility is not only to you but also to the field of medical education. Although atheoretical data mining, or "fishing," is widely condemned (Picho & Artino, 2016), we suspect it is nevertheless widely practiced. If you ask your statistician to go on a fishing expedition, he or she is likely to oblige you, but express concern by (appropriately) hedging the findings as "post hoc," "exploratory," "secondary analysis," "unplanned comparisons," or similar expressions. Understand this for what it is: discomfort with the possibility of indiscriminately testing an unplanned hypothesis to find a significant effect (sometimes referred to as "p-hacking")

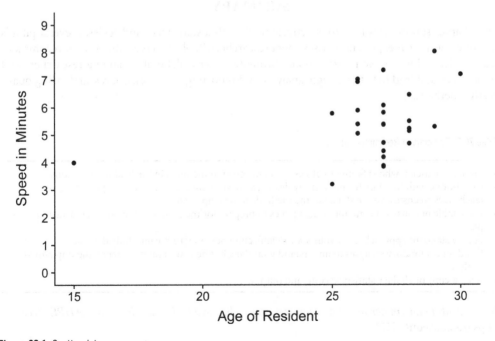

Figure 20.1 Scatterplot

(Simmons, Nelson, & Simonsohn, 2011). This discomfort is a sign of a good statistician. Carefully consider whether and how you disseminate such results.

WRITING THE MANUSCRIPT AND BEYOND

You should expect your statistician to stand by the results of his or her analysis, but only if your paper or presentation correctly reflects the analysis. Your statistician should provide a suitable description of the analysis plan for any paper that presents his or her work, and you should ask your statistician to review and revise your presentation of the findings and your discussion of inferences based on those findings to be sure they properly convey the results and do not overgeneralize the conclusions. If, as this chapter suggests, your statistician contributed to the study design or analysis, revised the manuscript, approved the final version, and agrees to be accountable for the work, he or she qualifies as an author according the ICMJE criteria (International Committee of Medical Journal Editors, 2018), and should be an author on the paper. If for some reason your statistician is unable to contribute to revising and approving the manuscript, an acknowledgement (but not authorship) is appropriate.

Although we often think of publication as the end of the research process, secondary analyses of existing data, including meta-analyses of multiple studies' data, have an important place in medical education research (Schwartz, Pappas, & Sandlow, 2010). Accordingly, you should ensure that your statistician shares with you a copy of the complete statistical code necessary to reproduce your results when applied to your original data file (and, if a substantial amount of manual data cleaning was necessary, a copy of the cleaned data file); you will also want a copy of the output generated by running the code on your data, in case a future version of the statistical software should make the code inoperable. Store the data files, codebooks, analysis code, and analysis output together; label the files with a date or version stamp when possible. Requesting your statistician to annotate certain areas of the syntax code is often helpful. Make a backup.

SUMMARY

This chapter summarizes how to effectively work with a statistician and reviews several pitfalls that often ensnare inexperienced assessment researchers. Table 20.3 recapitulates our recommendations. The principles we present should promote better collaboration among researchers and statisticians and lead to better design, analysis, and reporting of assessment research using quantitative methods.

Table 20.3 Summary of Recommendations

- Find a statistician who is familiar with assessment research methods in the health professions.
- Collaborate with the statistician on study design, analysis planning, and manuscript writing; use a teach-back to ensure you understand the methods to be employed.
- Use a table of constructs and mock data tables to prepare for the nature of the expected data and clarify plans.
- Follow standard approaches (or your statistician's guidance) in structuring study data files.
- Conduct exploratory analyses to understand your data, but be conservative in reporting unplanned analyses.
- Keep a copy of all data, statistical code, and output.

Note: Additional material and resources may be available at the UIC AHPE website: https://go.uic.edu/AHPE

REFERENCES

Bordage, G., & Dawson, B. (2003). Experimental study design and grant writing in eight steps and 28 questions. *Medical Education, 37*(4), 376–385.

International Committee of Medical Journal Editors. (2018). Defining the roles of authors and contributors. Retrieved from www.icmje.org/recommendations/browse/roles-and-responsibilities/defining-the-role-of-authors-and-contributors.html. Accessed April 25, 2018.

Kennedy, T.J., Regehr, G., Baker, G.R., & Lingard, L. (2008). Point-of-care assessment of medical trainee competence for independent clinical work. *Academic Medicine, 83*(10), S89-S92.

Picho, K., & Artino Jr., A.R. (2016). 7 Deadly sins in educational research. *Journal of Graduate Medical Education, 8*(4), 483–487.

Schwartz, A., Pappas, C., & Sandlow, L.J. (2010). Data repositories for medical education research. *Academic Medicine, 85*(5), 837–843.

Simmons, J.P., Nelson, L.D., & Simonsohn, U. (2011). False-positive psychology undisclosed flexibility in data collection and analysis allows presenting anything as significant. *Psychological Science, 22*(11), 1359–1366.

ten Cate, O. (2005). Entrustability of professional activities and competency-based training. *Medical Education, 39*(12), 1176–1177.

Tukey, J.W. (1977). *Exploratory data analysis,* Vol 2. Reading, MA: Addison-Wesley.

CONTRIBUTORS

Mark D. Adler, MD

Mark D. Adler is Professor of Pediatrics and Medical Education at Northwestern University Fein-berg School of Medicine. He is the Director and Founder of Kidstar Medical Education program, and an attending physician in Pediatric Emergency Medicine at the Ann and Robert H Lurie Chil-dren's Hospital of Chicago. His research interests include curriculum development and assess-ment of learners at the graduate medical education level. He has served on multiple international simulation-based educational organizations.

Georges Bordage, MD, MSc, PhD

Georges Bordage is Professor Emeritus in the Department of Medical Education in the College of Medicine at the University of Illinois at Chicago. He is the recipient of four honorary doctoral degrees (Sherbrooke, Moncton, Louvain, Laval) and is a visiting professor at the universities of Bern (Switzerland) and Tokyo (Japan). He taught courses in Scholarship and Current Issues in Health Professions Education, Research Design and Grant Writing, and Scientific Writing. His research includes the study of clinical reasoning, the written and oral assessment of clinical decisions, the "key features" approach (first developed for the Medical Council of Canada in the early 1990s and now used worldwide), the hypothesis-driven approach to teaching and assessing the physical exam, and scientific writing. Dr. Bordage is the recipient of multiple awards, including the Abraham Flex-ner Award of the American Association of Medical Colleges for extraordinary contributions to the medical education community, the John P. Hubbard Award from the National Board of Medical Examiners for significant contributions to the pursuit of excellence in the field of evaluation in medicine, the American Education Research Association Distinguished Career Award, and the Dr. Louis Levasseur Distinguished Service Award for Outstanding Contributions to the Vision and Mission of the Medical Council of Canada. He consults worldwide on educational matters.

David Cook, MD, MHPE

David Cook is Professor of Medicine and Medical Education in the Mayo Clinic College of Med-icine; Director of Education Science in the Mayo Office of Applied Scholarship and Education

Science; Director of the Data, Analytics, and Quality Section in the Mayo Clinic School of Continuous Professional Development; Research Chair for the Mayo Multidisciplinary Simulation Center; and a practicing physician specializing in the diagnosis and treatment of complex medicine problems. He is currently a Deputy Editor for the journal *Medical Education*, and an editorial board member for the journal *Simulation in Healthcare*. Dr. Cook's research interests include the theory and design of online learning and other educational technologies, the quality of medical education research methods and reporting, clinical reasoning, and assessment of clinical performance. Dr. Cook is the Scoutmaster for his younger sons' Boy Scout troop, and serves as a youth leader in the Church of Jesus Christ of Latter-Day Saints. He and his wife Jennifer are the parents of five incredibly wonderful children.

Luke A. Devine, MD

Luke A. Devine is Assistant Professor of Medicine, Director Undergraduate Medical Education at the University of Toronto, and the Site Lead for the Division of General Internal Medicine at Mount Sinai Hospital, Toronto. He is the Simulation Lead for the HoPingKong Centre for Excellence in Education and Practice (CEEP) at the University Health Network. His main interests are the curricular integration of simulation into undergraduate and postgraduate internal medicine education and the use of simulation in the assessment of learners at all stages of training.

Steven M. Downing, PhD

Steven M. Downing has worked with high-stakes testing programs in medicine and the professions throughout his career. Dr. Downing joined the faculty of the University of Illinois at Chicago, Department of Medical Education, in 2001, where he taught courses in testing and assessment for the Master of Health Professions Education (MHPE) program. Formerly, he was Director of Health Programs at the American College Testing Program (ACT), Director of Client Programs and Deputy Vice President at the National Board of Medical Examiners (NBME), Senior Psychometrician at the American Board of Internal Medicine (ABIM), and Director of Psychometrics and Senior Program Manager for the Institute for Clinical Evaluation (ICE) at the American Board of Internal Medicine. Dr. Downing consults with various national and international testing programs in all areas of test development and psychometrics, with particular interests in selected-response formats, test validity issues, testing program evaluation, and computer-based testing. Dr. Downing was the senior editor for a comprehensive book on test development, *Handbook of Test Development*, published by Lawrence Erlbaum in January 2006.

Nancy Dudek, MD, MEd

Nancy Dudek is Professor in the Faculty of Medicine at the University of Ottawa. She has a diverse clinical practice and works at the Ottawa Hospital Rehabilitation Centre, the Ottawa Children's Treatment Centre, and the Children's Hospital of Eastern Ontario. Dr. Dudek's academic interests are in medical education. Her focus is the assessment of medical students and residents with a particular interest in work-based assessment, and she holds several grants related to research in this area. Dr. Dudek has served as the University of Ottawa's undergraduate coordinator for musculoskeletal medicine and as the Director for the Physical Medicine & Rehabilitation Residency Program. She is the recipient of several national awards for her work in medical education. She currently works as a Clinician Educator for the Royal College of Physicians and Surgeons of Canada.

Sylvia Heeneman, PhD, MHPE

Sylvia Heeneman is Professor of Health Profession Education at the Faculty of Health, Medicine and Life Sciences (FHML), School of Health Profession Education (SHE), Maastricht University.

Her current research interests in the health professions education field are (programmatic) assessment in undergraduate and post-graduate medical education, professional performance, portfolio, and mentoring. Within the FHML, she was the program coordinator of the Physician-Clinical Investigator program (2011–2017); programmatic assessment was implemented in this program in 2011 and was a stepping-stone for implementation in other FHML programs. Currently, she is the program coordinator of the Bachelor International Track of Medicine and the Chair of the Board of Examiners of the Biomedical Sciences program. In addition, she is involved in teacher professionalization and education in postgraduate medical education and gives workshops worldwide to educate professionals in the use of (programmatic) assessment and mentoring in their courses and programs.

Barry Issenberg, MD

Barry Issenberg is Professor of Medicine and Medical Education, Senior Associate Dean for Research in Medical Education, and Senior Associate Dean for Continuing Medical Education at the University of Miami Miller School of Medicine. Dr. Issenberg's career focus has been in the research, development, implementation, and evaluation of simulation and e-learning systems, outcome measures to assess student and physician competencies, and implementation of faculty development programs for teaching and research.

Dorthea Juul, PhD

Dorthea Juul joined the American Board of Psychiatry and Neurology (ABPN) in June 1990, after working at the University of Illinois College of Medicine's Department of Medical Education for many years. In addition to supervising examination scoring and reporting, Dr. Juul is vice president for research and development activities of the ABPN. She teaches test development and assessment courses in UIC's Department of Medical Education.

Aaron Knox, MD, MHPE

Aaron Knox is a plastic and reconstructive surgeon in Calgary, Alberta, Canada, with special interest in competency-based medical education and assessment in surgical education. He completed a medical education fellowship at the Wilson Centre in Toronto and graduated from the University of Illinois at Chicago with a Master in Health Professions Education. Clinical interests include hand, wrist, and peripheral nerve surgery.

Clarence D. Kreiter, PhD

Clarence D. Kreiter is a professor specializing in medical education at the University of Iowa Carver College of Medicine. His research interests include generalizability theory, medical education, admission and selection, Bayesian reasoning, validity theory, psychological measurement, assessing clinical reasoning, simulation-based assessment, and classical test theory. He teaches two graduate-level courses on educational measurement and test design.

Matthew Lineberry, PhD

Matthew Lineberry is Director of Simulation Research, Assessment, and Outcomes for the Zamierowksi Institute for Experiential Learning (ZIEL), a partnership of the University of Kansas Medical Center and University of Kansas Health System. Previously, he served as a Research Psychologist for the US Navy's training systems command, and then as Assistant Professor of Medical Education at the University of Illinois at Chicago. Dr. Lineberry's research is focused on (1) designing and investigating the validity and consequences of assessments, (2) self-regulated learning, (3) computer-adaptive training, and (4) healthcare simulation instructional design.

Mary E. McBride, MD, MEd

Mary E. McBride is an attending physician in the cardiac intensive care unit at Ann & Robert H. Lurie Children's Hospital of Chicago and Associate Professor of Pediatrics & Medical Education in the Divisions of Cardiology and Critical Care Medicine at Northwestern University Feinberg School of Medicine in Chicago. She is the Director of Critical Care Education within the Kid-STAR simulation laboratory at Lurie Children's. Dr. McBride's research interests include medical education, resuscitation, and simulation.

William C. McGaghie, PhD

William C. McGaghie is Professor of Medical Education and Professor of Preventive Medicine at the Northwestern University Feinberg School of Medicine in Chicago. He previously held faculty appointments at the University of Illinois College of Medicine, the University of North Carolina School of Medicine, and the Loyola University Chicago Stritch School of Medicine. Dr. McGaghie has been a medical education scholar for over four decades, writing about topics including personnel and program evaluation, research methodology, medical simulation, and medical education translational science. He serves on the editorial boards of five scholarly journals and consults with a variety of professional boards, agencies, institutes, and medical schools worldwide.

Gordon Page, EdD

Gordon Page is Emeritus Professor, Department of Medicine, University of British Columbia. Dr. Page is a professional educator, and for 30 years was Director of the Health Sciences Division of Educational Support and Development at UBC. Throughout his career, he has worked locally, nationally, and internationally with academic and professional groups concerned with the quality of health professions education, and with assessing the competence of health professionals in training and in practice. He has been a visiting professor at numerous universities and colleges in Canada, Australia, New Zealand, Europe, the USA, China, Japan, the United Arab Emirates, and Southeast Asia. Dr. Page's major research and development interests are directed toward the assessment of medical trainees and practitioners. In recognition of his contributions, he has been the recipient of multiple awards, including the following: (1) The Royal College of Physicians and Surgeons of Canada, Duncan Graham Award, in recognition of outstanding lifelong contribution to medical education, (2) The Medical Council of Canada, "Dr. Louis Levasseur Distinguished Service Award," (3) The Association of Faculties of Medicine of Canada, "AFMC-AstraZeneca Award for Exemplary Contribution to Faculty Development in Canada," (4) The Medical Council of Canada, "Outstanding Achievement Award for Contributions to the Assessment of Clinical Competence," and (5) The Canadian Association for Medical Education Ian Hart Award for Distinguished Contribution to Medical Education.

Miguel Paniagua, MD

Miguel Paniagua served as the internal medicine residency program director at Saint Louis University School of Medicine for five years prior to joining the staff of the National Board of Medical Examiners®. In addition to multiple teaching awards while a faculty member, Dr. Paniagua is a forum member representative to the Institute of Medicine (IOM) Global Forum on Innovations in Health Professions Education, a member of the ACGME's National Collaborative to Improve the Clinical Learning Environment (NCICLE), and a member of the Alpha Omega Alpha medical honor society. He is a fellow of the American College of Physicians, the American Academy of Hospice and Palliative Medicine, and the College of Physicians of Philadelphia. Dr. Paniagua currently serves as Medical Advisor for Test Development Services at the National Board of Medical Examiners (NBME). His work at NBME includes research on wellness and burnout, and on how race, ethnicity, and patient characteristics impact exams. Dr. Paniagua is working towards development of assessments of competencies such as communication skills and interprofessional teamwork, as well as other innovations across various NBME examinations. He has served on multiple item writing and reviewing committees at the NBME over the last decade, and has served as a representative member of the National Board of Medical Examiners governance from 2011 to 2014 and on the Executive Board of the NBME from 2013 to 2014. He is the co-editor of the fifth edition of the "Essential Practices of Palliative Medicine (UNIPAC)" book series and the fourth edition of the NBME publication "Constructing Written Test Questions for the Basic and Clinical Sciences."

Yoon Soo Park, PhD

Yoon Soo Park is Associate Professor and Associate Head of the Department of Medical Education at the College of Medicine at the University of Illinois at Chicago. He is also Director of Research, Office of Educational Affairs at the University of Illinois College of Medicine. Dr. Park's research agendas have focused on statistical modeling of educational and psychological processes that span wide applications in assessment, learning, and behavioral sciences. His experiences include both academic and industry settings, across multiple disciplines in psychometrics, education, biostatistics, and medicine. Dr. Park serves on editorial boards of leading education, measurement, and statistics/applied mathematics journals. He is Vice President and Council Member for the American Educational Research Association (AERA), serving Division I: Education in the Professions.

Harold I. Reiter, MD

Harold I. Reiter is Professor in Oncology at McMaster University. Aside from his radiation oncology clinical practice, he was Chair of Admissions at the Michael G. DeGroote School of Medicine at McMaster University for nine years and Assistant Dean, Director of the Program for Educational Research and Development at McMaster for four years. He is a co-creator of the multiple mini-interview as well as CASPer and continues as an active academic in the research and development of tools measuring personal and professional characteristics.

E. Matthew Ritter, MD, FACS

E. Matthew Ritter is Professor of Surgery and Vice Chairman for Education in the Department of Surgery at the Uniformed Services University & Walter Reed National Military Medical Center, and the Program Director of the General Surgery residency program and the ACS-AEI Accredited Surgical Education Fellowship. Dr. Ritter has deployed multiple times in direct support of Operations Iraqi and Enduring Freedom; his stateside clinical practice focuses on advanced laparoscopic, gastrointestinal, and hernia surgery. His research focuses on applying simulation solutions to surgical education. He is an active member of the Association of Program Directors in Surgery (APDS), the Association for Surgical Education (ASE), the American College of Surgeons (ACS), and the Society of American Gastrointestinal and Endoscopic Surgeons (SAGES), where he is a member and leader of multiple education-based committees.

Christopher Roberts, MBBS, MBChB, PhD

Christopher Roberts is Associate Professor in Medical Education, based at the Northern Clinical School and the Office of Education at Sydney Medical School. Previously he worked as Associate Director (Education) in the Charles Perkins Centre, Head of the Office of Medical Education, and then the Office of Postgraduate Medical Education in Sydney. He is a past Chair of the Medical and Dental Admission Committee. He undertakes consultancy in medical education, particularly around selection-focused assessment.

Daniel J. Schumacher, MD, MEd

Daniel J. Schumacher's career in medical education began in graduate medical education administration at the Boston Combined Residency Program in Pediatrics and has since transitioned to research at Cincinnati Children's Hospital Medical Center. He has presented and published widely in the area of competency-based assessment, has led multi-site national research studies, and has participated in efforts in this arena with several national and international organizations. Highlights of this work include serving as one of eight members of the Pediatrics Milestone Project Working Group that authored the pediatrics milestones now being used for resident and fellow assessment in all pediatric residency and fellowship programs accredited by the Accreditation Council for Graduate Medical Education.

Suzanne Schut, MSc

Suzanne Schut is a staff member of the School of Health Professions Education (SHE) at Maastricht University. She is an educational advisor within the Assessment Taskforce and responsible for the assessment and quality assurance of assessment within the Faculty of Health, Medicine and Life Sciences. She is chair of the review committee for knowledge testing. She is experienced in educational development and design, teaching, and faculty development, focusing on educational design and innovation and on item and scenario writing, assessment, and feedback within the workplace. In her research, she aims to unravel and validate the concepts underlying the theoretical model of programmatic assessment. Topics of interest are assessment for learning, self-regulated learning, and student-teacher relationships within the assessment environment.

Alan Schwartz, PhD

Alan Schwartz is the Michael Reese Endowed Professor of Medical Education, the Interim Head of the Department of Medical Education, and Research Professor in the Department of Pediatrics at the University of Illinois at Chicago. His research interests include the psychology of decision-making in both patients and physicians, and research infrastructure and competency-based assessment in medical education. He serves as Editor-in-Chief of the journals *Medical Decision Making* and *Medical Decision Making Policy & Practice* and as Director of the Association of Pediatric Program Directors Longitudinal Educational Assessment Research Network (APPD LEARN).

Kimberly A. Swygert, PhD, FCPP

Kimberly A. Swygert has 20 years of experience as a psychometrician and is the Director of Research and Development in Test Development Services at the National Board of Medical Examiners® (NBME®). She is responsible for designing and implementing NBME's test development research, as well as managing multiple cross-functional test development units including test construction, multimedia, and test materials. She has been a key player in research and operations related to item creation, scoring, and score reporting for multiple NBME examinations, including Step 2 CS and Step 3. Her chapter on performance assessments in credentialing examinations appeared in the updated *Handbook of Test Development* in 2015. She is the coeditor and coauthor of the most recent edition of the item writing guidebook *Constructing Written Test Questions for the Basic and Clinical Sciences*, published in early 2017. In addition, she has taught graduate courses in biostatistics and psychometrics for Drexel University and the Uniformed Services University of the Health Sciences (USUHS). She currently serves on advisory boards and technical advisory panels for organizations such as USUHS and the Federation of State Boards of Physical Therapy, and was recently elected to the Board of Directors for the Association of Test Publishers (ATP). She was inducted in November 2018 as a Fellow of the College of Physicians of Philadelphia due to her contributions to the medical education literature.

Ara Tekian, PhD, MHPE

Ara Tekian is Professor and Director of International Affairs at the Department of Medical Education (DME), and the Associate Dean for the Office of International Education at the College of Medicine, the University of Illinois at Chicago (UIC). He joined DME in 1992, where he teaches courses offered in the Master of Health Professions Education (MHPE) program and advises graduate students. He is the senior author of the book *Innovative Simulations for Assessing Professional Competence: From Paper-and-Pencil to Virtual Reality*, published in 1999. His consultations and workshops have focused on curriculum development, assessment, program evaluation, simulations, and international medical education. He has received numerous honors and awards including the 2012 ASME (Association for the Study of Medical Education) Gold Medal Award, as well as the Ellis Island Medal of Honor in 2017. His scholarship in health professions education is reflection in numerous publications in the premiere medical education journals.

Cees van der Vleuten, PhD

Cees van der Vleuten has been at the University of Maastricht since 1982. In 1996, he was appointed Professor of Education and chair (until 2014) of the Department of Educational Development and Research in the Faculty of Health, Medicine and Life Sciences. Since 2005, he has been the Scientific Director of the School of Health Professions Education. He is also the Director of the European Board of Medical Assessors (EBMA). A full CV can be found at www.ceesvandervleuten.com.

Rachel Yudkowsky, MD, MHPE

Rachel Yudkowsky is Professor and Director of Graduate Studies in the Department of Medical Education at the University of Illinois at Chicago College of Medicine. She co-edited with Steven M. Downing the first edition of this book, published in 2009. She served as Director of the Dr. Allan L. and Mary L. Graham Clinical Performance Center from 2000 to 2018, where she developed standardized patient and simulation-based programs for the instruction and assessment of students, residents, and staff. She also served as Director of the University of Illinois Health Sciences Simulation Consortium from 2009 to 2018. She was the founding Co-President of the Chicago Simulation Consortium (CSC) in 2013. She served on the Editorial Board of the journal *Simulation in Healthcare* from 2008 to 2017, and as an Associate Editor from 2015 to 2017. She received the Outstanding Educator Award from the Association of Standardized Patient Educators in 2009, and the Society for Simulation in Healthcare SP SIG Award in 2016. Areas of research interest include performance assessment using standardized patients and other simulations, and setting passing standards for performance tests.

Nikki L. Zaidi, PhD

Nikki L. Zaidi is the Evaluation and Assessment Director for Michigan Medicine's Research. Innovation. Scholarship. Education (RISE) program. Prior to this role, Dr. Zaidi served as Associate Director of Advancing Scholarship at the University of Michigan Medical School where she helped develop and disseminate the school's education research and promote an infrastructure to produce high-quality scholarship. She has contributed to undergraduate medical education in other capacities, holding positions in both admissions and student affairs. She earned a PhD in quantitative research methods with a focus in generalizability theory and repeated measurement designs.

INDEX

Note: Page numbers in *italics* indicate figures and in page numbers in **bold** indicate tables on the corresponding pages.

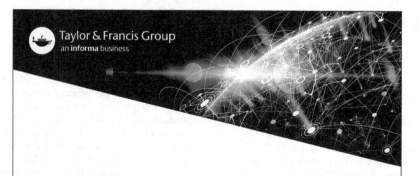